# Review in
# Medical Physiology

## for Undergraduate Students

### Third Edition

# Review in
# Medical Physiology

## for Undergraduate Students

### Third Edition

**Mohini Khullar** MD
Professor and Head
Department of Physiology
Manav Rachna Dental College
Faridabad, Haryana

**Shilpa Khullar** MD
Assistant Professor
Department of Physiology
ESIC Dental College and Hospital
Rohini, Delhi

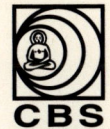

**CBS Publishers & Distributors** Pvt Ltd

New Delhi • Bengaluru • Chennai • Kochi • Pune
• Hyderabad • Kolkata • Mumbai • Nagpur • Patna

**Review in**
**Medical Physiology**
for Undergraduate Students
Third Edition

ISBN: 978-81-239-2339-0

**Third Edition: 2013**
First Edition: 1998
Second Edition: 2000

Published by Satish Kumar Jain for
**CBS Publishers & Distributors** Pvt Ltd
4819/XI Prahlad Street, 24 Ansari Road, Daryaganj, New Delhi 110 002, India.
Ph: 23289259, 23266861, 23266867      Website: www.cbspd.com
Fax: 011-23243014                     e-mail: delhi@cbspd.com; cbspubs@airtelmail.in.
*Corporate Office:* 204 FIE, Industrial Area, Patparganj, Delhi 110 092
Ph: 4934 4934       Fax: 4934 4935       e-mail: publishing@cbspd.com; publicity@cbspd.com

*Branches*

- **Bengaluru:** Seema House 2975, 17th Cross, K.R. Road, Banasankari 2nd Stage, Bengaluru 560 070, Karnataka
  Ph: +91-80-26771678/79       Fax: +91-80-26771680       e-mail: bangalore@cbspd.com
- **Chennai:** 20, West Park Road, Shenoy Nagar, Chennai 600 030, Tamil Nadu
  Ph: +91-44-26260666, 26208620       Fax: +91-44-42032115       e-mail: chennai@cbspd.com
- **Kochi:** 36/14 Kalluvilakam, Lissie Hospital Road, Kochi 682 018, Kerala
  Ph: +91-484-4059061-65       Fax: +91-484-4059065       e-mail: kochi@cbspd.com
- **Pune:** Bhuruk Prestige, Sr. No. 52/12/2+1+3/2 Narhe, Haveli (Near Katraj-Dehu Road Bypass), Pune 411 041, Maharashtra
  Ph: +91-20-64704058, 64704059, 32342277 Fax: +91-20-24300160       e-mail: pune@cbspd.com

*Representatives*

- **Hyderabad**   0-9885175004
- **Mumbai**   0-9833017933
- **Patna**   0-9334159340
- **Kolkata**   0-9831437309, 0-9051152362
- **Nagpur**   0-9021734563

*Printed at Shree Maitrey Printech Pvt. Ltd., Noida*

# Preface to the Third Edition

The third edition of *Review in Medical Physiology for Undergraduate Students* has been rendered necessary by the changing trends in the examination pattern in recent years.

The primary aim of this book is to help undergraduate students of MBBS, BDS and all allied courses in doing a 'quick revision' before their final examinations. It will help them get trained in writing answers in the examination, which in itself is an art.

The *salient features* of this book are:

- The text has been divided into 11 chapters and each chapter is further divided into sub-sections according to the topics covered.

- The questions on 'Blood' and 'General Physiology' have been divided into two separate sections which had been merged in the earlier edition to make reading easier.

- Question papers (primarily of Delhi University) from the year 2000 onwards have been included in this edition.

- The text material has been edited, modified and updated wherever considered necessary.

- Questions on 'normal values' and 'definitions' have been deleted keeping the current trend of question papers in mind.

- To enhance the lucidity of the text, flowcharts, tables and diagrams have been modified and new ones added.

- This edition is produced in full colour to render vividness to graphics and improve readability.

We are greatly indebted to our family, friends, teachers, students and well-wishers for their constant support and encouragement in completing this arduous task.

We express our deepest gratitude to the staff of CBS Publishers & Distributors, especially Mr YN Arjuna, Senior Director—

Publishing, Editorial and Publicity, for their immense cooperation in completing this edition successfully.

It is not possible for any book to be entirely free from human errors, some inaccuracies, ambiguities and typographical mistakes. We would, therefore, welcome feedback and suggestions from students and teachers alike for further improvement of this book.

**Mohini Khullar**
**Shilpa Khullar**
Email:drshilpakhullar@gmail.com

# Preface to the First Edition

Answering questions correctly is a natural concern of every student. To this end, through this book, an attempt has been made to guide the students on answering questions in the examinations.

Examples of all types of questions, i.e. long, short and very short, have been included. In addition, it will enable the students to revise the subject matter in a short time. All the chapters have been written with the intention of making the book comprehensive and relevant. The book, however, is not intended to be a textbook, but only a useful accompaniment.

**Mohini Khullar**

## List of Books Referred

1. *Ganong's Review of Medical Physiology,* 24th edition
   BARRETT, KIM E et al
   Tata McGraw-Hill
2. *Textbook of Medical Physiology,* 11th edition,
   GUYTON and HALL
   Elsevier
3. *Samson Wright's Applied Physiology,* 13th edition
   KEELE, NEIL and JOELS
   Oxford University Press
4. *Medical Physiology,* 3rd edition
   MARYA, RK
   CBS Publishers & Distributors
5. *Textbook of Physiology,* 3rd edition
   AHUJA
   CBS Publishers & Distributors
6. *Textbook of Physiology,* 4th edition
   JAIN, AK
   Avichal Publishing Company
7. *Essentials of Medical Physiology*
   KHURANA, INDU
   Elsevier
8. *Understanding Medical Physiology,* 4th edition
   BIJLANI, RL and MANJUNATHA, S
   Jaypee Brothers
9. *Hutchison's Clinical Methods,* 23rd edition
   GLYNN AND DRAKE
   Saunders Ltd.
10. *Renal Physiology,* 4th edition
    ARTHUR VENDOR
    McGraw-Hill
11. *Best and Taylor's Physiological Basis of Medical Practice,* 10th edition
    Ed. BROBECK, JOHN R
12. Various internet sources

# Contents

---

*Note for the Readers*

Along with the topics/headings in the text of the book, marks in red colour and year of examination/question paper in parentheses are given for the readers' information. For example:

**ENDOPLASMIC RETICULUM**                          **2.5 (1993)**

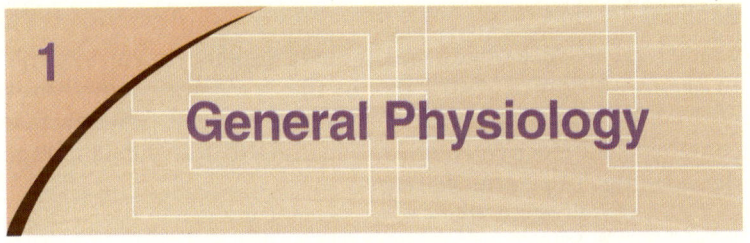

# General Physiology

### ENDOPLASMIC RETICULUM        2.5 (1993)

Endoplasmic reticulum is an important cellular organelle. It is constituted by an extensive interlacing network of membrane lined tubules. Endoplasmic reticulum (ER) is of 2 types:

1. **Granular or rough ER:** Having ribosomes attached on the cytoplasmic side of the membrane. Ribosomes contain RNA and proteins and are the site of protein synthesis, e.g. secretions and enzymes.

2. **Agranular or smooth ER:** They have no ribosomes attached to them. Their function is synthesis of lipids, e.g. steroid hormones. It is also the site of detoxification of drugs in the liver. In the muscles ER provides $Ca^{++}$ for the process of contraction.

### LYSOSOMES        2 (2000)

These are large irregular structures surrounded by unit membrane and are found in the cytoplasm. A typical cell contains several hundred lysosomes. It is filled with large number of small granules which contain variety of enzymes called lysozymes.

### Functions

1. Acts as a form of digestive system for the cell, because enzymes present in it can digest essentially all the macromolecules.
2. Engulf worn out components of the cells in which they are located.
3. Engulf exogenous substances, e.g. bacteria and degrade them.
4. When a cell dies lysosomal enzymes cause autolysis of the remnants, therefore, they are called suicidal bags.

## Applied

Congenital absence of any one of the lysosomal enzymes results in accumulation of substrates in the lysosomes which they normally degrade. This finally disrupts the cell function that contains the defective lysosomes leading to lysosomal storage diseases, e.g. *Tay-Sachs disease*.

## TYPES OF PROTEINS PRESENT IN CELL MEMBRANE       2 (2004)

1. **Structural proteins**
2. **Transport proteins**
   a. *Channels:*
      i.   Continuously open, e.g. water channel
      ii.  Gated
         • Voltage-gated, e.g. $Na^+$
         • Ligand-gated
           External, e.g. hormones
           Internal, e.g. $Ca^{++}$, cAMP
         • Mechanical: In hair cells of organ of Corti
   b. *Carriers:*
      i.   Uniport, e.g. glucose transporter
      ii.  Symport, e.g. absorption of $Na^+$ and glucose in intestines and kidney tubules
      iii. Antiport, e.g. $Na^+$ and $Ca^{++}$ exchange in cardiac muscle.
3. **Pumps:** Enzymes with ATPase activity which actively transport ions across cell membrane: $Na^+ - K^+$ pump
4. **Receptors:** Bind to specific ligands (hormones and neuro-transmitters)
5. **Enzymes:** Catalyse chemical reactions
6. **Glycoproteins:** For antibody processing and self-recognition from non-self
7. **Cell adhesion molecules:** Anchor cells to each other and basal lamina.

## INTERCELLULAR JUNCTIONS

## COMPARE GAP JUNCTIONS AND TIGHT JUNCTIONS
2.5 (2004, 2007)

Cells are structurally and functionally connected to each other through intercellular junctions.

**Following types of junctions are present**

1. **Tight junctions:** Formed by ridges between the cells which are formed by the fusion of the cell membranes of adjacent cells, thus forming a belt between them. Such junctions prevent transport of substances between cells. Such type of junctions are located in epithelium lining intestinal mucosa, walls of renal tubules and choroid plexus. These prevent passage of substance from the lumen to epithelial cells.

2. **Desmosomes:** Button like junctions are there between cells through thickened spots on both cells and their membranes do not come in contact at desmosomes.

   At the site of desmosome towards the cytoplasmic side are filamentous structures radiating from the thickened membrane.

   Desmosomes hold cells together and also attach them to the basement membrane providing strength and stability to the tissues.

3. **Gap junctions:** At gap junctions a 2–3 nm gap exists between adjacent cells. The gap is traversed by hollow cylindrical channels formed by regular arrangements of protein units **(connexons)**. The channel allows the passage of ions and other small molecule with molecular weight up to 1000. Gap junctions thus allow the rapid propagation of electrical activity from one cell to another and are present in smooth muscles and cardiac muscles. The diametre of these channels is regulated by intracellular $Ca^{++}$, pH and voltage.

## MEMBRANE POTENTIALS

### RESTING MEMBRANE POTENTIAL      2.5 (1989)

In many body cells specially excitable tissues, i.e. nerve and muscles, a potential difference is present across the cell membrane, when the tissue is at rest called the resting membrane potential (RMP). Inside of the cell RMP is negative in relation to the outside. Magnitude of RMP varies between –10 and –100 mV. Minus sign signifies, it is negative inside. In nerve RMP is –70 mV and in skeletal muscle –90 mV. RMP is generated due to the following factors:

   i. Selective permeability of cell membrane. It is permeable to $K^+$ and impermeable to protein anions.

ii. Activity of $Na^+$-$K^+$-ATPase pump present in the cell membrane. It pumps out $3Na^+$ and $2K^+$ enters the cell.

As a result of the above-mentioned factors an excess of negative ions is present inside the cells as compared to the exterior and RMP is generated.

## EQUILIBRIUM POTENTIAL

Equilibrium potential is the potential difference across the membrane at which there is no net movement of an ion, i.e. influx and efflux are equal.

Movement of ions across the cell membrane is guided by two factors:

i. **Concentration gradient:** Due to the difference in intracellular and extracellular concentration.

ii. **Electrical gradient:** Inside of the membrane is negatively charged and favors entry of anions towards inside and opposes that of cations.

For example, there are 3 important ions of physiologic importance:

a. $K^+$: Concentration gradient favors efflux, whereas electric gradient favors influx.

b. $Na^+$: Concentration gradient directed towards inside and electrical gradient is also in the same direction.

c. $Cl^-$: Concentration gradient favors influx, whereas electrical gradient favors efflux.

Magnitude of equilibrium potential (EP) can be calculated from the **Nernst equation**.

$$EP = \frac{RT}{FZ} \frac{[C_o]}{[C_i]} = 61 \log \frac{[C_o]}{[C_i]}$$

R—Gas constant

T—Absolute temperature

F—Faraday constant

Z—Valence of the ion.

Substituting values for monovalent ions at 37°

for example, $K^+$

$$= 61 \log \frac{[K_o^+]}{[K_i^+]} = -61 \log \frac{155}{4} = -97 \text{ mV}$$

Similarly, EP for $Na^+$ = + 60 mV

EP for $Cl^-$ = − 70 mV

## GENESIS OF RMP                                2 (2007)

Following factors generate resting membrane potential:

1. Difference in concentration of $K^+$ in extra and intracellular fluid.
2. Impermeability of membrane to protein anions (at normal body pH (7.4) protein ionize as anions).
3. Membrane is poorly permeable to $Na^+$.
4. Activity of $Na^+$–$K^+$-ATPase pump in membrane.

### MAGNITUDE OF RMP CAN BE CALCULATED USING GOLDMAN CONSTANT FIELD EQUATION

$$V = \frac{RT}{F} \ln \left( \frac{P_{K^+}[K_o^+] + P_{Na^+}[Na_o^+] + P_{Cl^-}[Cl_i^-]}{P_{K^+}[K_i^+] + P_{Na^+}[Na_i^+] + P_{Cl^-}[Cl_o^-]} \right)$$

$V$—Membrane potential

$R$—Gas constant

$T$—Absolute temperature

$F$—Faraday constant

$P_{K^+}, P_{Na^+}$ and $PCl^-$—Permeability to $K^+$, $Na^+$ and $Cl^-$ respectively

[o]—Concentration outside

[i]—Concentration inside

Extracellular $K^+$ concentration is major component influencing V as the membrane permeability to $Na^+$ is negligible at rest.

## TRANSPORT ACROSS CELL MEMBRANES

### MECHANISM OF TRANSPORT OF SUBSTANCES ACROSS THE CELL MEMBRANE                  2.5 (1991)

### SECONDARY ACTIVE TRANSPORT                  2.5 (2010)

Transport of substances across the cell membrane occurs:

i. Through the lipid layer of membrane

ii. Across special ionic channels in the membrane.

Various mechanisms of transport across cell membranes are:
1. **Diffusion:** A physical process and occurs along the concentration and electric gradient.
2. **Solvent drag:** Bulk flow of solvent drags solute molecules along with it.
3. **Osmosis:** Movement of water across a semipermeable membrane.
4. **Carrier mediated:** With the help of a **carrier molecule.** Speed of transport is increased manifold with the help of a carrier. It is of two types:
   a. **Facilitated diffusion:** Occurs along with the gradient
   b. **Active transport:** Occurs against the concentration gradient and requires energy in the form of ATP
      **It is of two types:**
      i. Primary active transport
      ii. Secondary active transport
5. **Filtration:** Fluid under pressure is forced through membrane, e.g. glomerular filtration.
6. **Endocytosis**
7. **Exocytosis,** e.g. of secretory granules

## CO-TRANSPORT ACROSS CELL MEMBRANE (Fig. 1.1) 2.5 (1992)

Co-transport across cell membrane is a type of coupled transport mechanism. In this mode of transport, two substances are simultaneously transported across the membrane. It requires a carrier to which both the substances must be bound for the transport. It requires energy in the form of ATP. In this system one of the substances is transferred with the gradient and the other against the concentration gradient. One example is mechanism of absorption of glucose or amino acids across the intestines along with $Na^+$.

Na$^+$ and glucose are both bound to carrier proteins present on the membrane. $Na^+$ moves into the cell with the concentration gradient and also takes glucose along with it. Inside the cell glucose and sodium are released. $Na^+$ is reabsorbed into lateral intercellular space by active process and glucose diffuses into the interstitium and then into the blood. Hence, glucose is co-transported with $Na^+$ (Fig. 1.1). This mode of transport is also called **secondary active transport.**

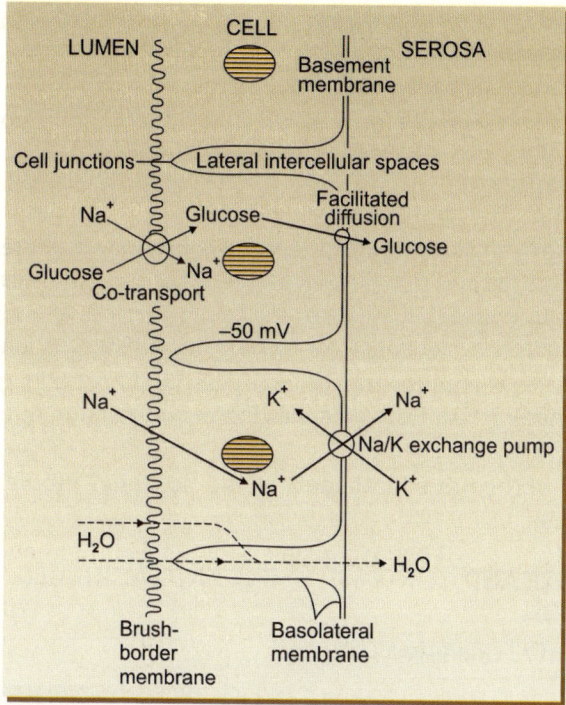

**Fig. 1.1:** Glucose, sodium, and water transport across the intestinal epithelium

## COMPARE AND CONTRAST PRIMARY AND SECONDARY ACTIVE TRANSPORT          2 (2003)-IPU, 2 (2004)

Active transport refers to the mechanism of transport of substances against the chemical and/or electrical gradient. It involves the expenditure of energy which is liberated by breakdown of high energy compounds like ATP.

The active transport is of two types:
- Primary active transport
- Secondary active transport

**Primary active transport:** The energy is derived directly from the breakdown of ATP or some other high-energy phosphate compounds. Some of the examples are:
- $Na^+ - K^+$ pump
- $Ca^{2+}$ pump
- $K^+ - H^+$ pump

**Secondary active transport:** The energy is derived secondarily from the energy, which has been stored in the form of ionic concentration difference between the two sides of the membrane, created in the first place by primary active transport. At many areas in the body transport of some other substances is coupled with active transport of $Na^+$. This may occur in the form of sodium co-transport or sodium counter-transport.

- **Sodium co-transport of glucose:** Absorption of glucose from the intestine and renal tubules
- **Sodium counter-transport:** Antiport carriers are used, i.e. sodium ion is exchanged for some other substances, e.g.
  - $Na^+$–$Ca^{2+}$ counter-transport occurs in almost all cell membranes with sodium ions moving in and calcium outside the cell
  - $Na^+$–$H^+$ counter-transport in the proximal tubules of the kidney.

## COMPARE AND CONTRAST: SIMPLE AND FACILITATED DIFFUSION 2 (2003)-IPU

### Short Note Facilitated Diffusion

Diffusion is a passive process by which molecules move from area of high concentration to area of lower concentration (**concentration gradient**) or cations move to negatively charged areas, whereas anions move to positively charged areas (**electrical gradient**). It is of two types—simple diffusion and facilitated diffusion. In facilitated diffusion carrier proteins are involved.

There are **three main** differences between simple and facilitated diffusion:

- **Specificity:** The carrier proteins in facilitated diffusion are highly specific for different molecules.
- **Saturation:** In simple diffusion the rate of diffusion increases proportionately with the increase in the concentration of the substance and there is no limit to it. However, in facilitated diffusion the rate of diffusion increases with increase in concentration gradient to reach a limit beyond which a further increase in rate of diffusion does not occur. This is called saturation point and here all the binding sites on the carrier proteins are occupied and the system functions at the maximum of its capacity.

- **Competition:** When two molecules are carried by the same protein, there occurs a competition between the two molecules for transport. An increase in concentration of one will decrease the transport of the other and *vice versa*. No such competition occurs in simple diffusion.

## COMPARE FACILITATED DIFFUSION AND ACTIVE TRANSPORT                                    2 (2003)

**Facilitated transport:** This is a form of passive transport that does not need energy. It is a carrier-mediated process that enables molecules that are too large to flow through membrane channels by simple diffusion to cross the membrane.

- It is much faster than simple diffusion.
- Transport is along their electrochemical gradient
- Examples:
  - Glucose transport by the glucose transporters (GLUT) across the intestinal epithelium
  - Transport of glucose into RBCs, muscles and adipose tissue in the presence of insulin.

**Active transport:** This involves the expenditure of energy which is liberated by the breakdown of high energy compounds like ATP.

- Transport is against the electrochemical gradient
- Examples: It is of two types:
  - Primary active transport: $Na^+ - K^+$ pump, $Ca^{2+}$ pump and $K^+ - H^+$ pump
  - Secondary active transport: $Na^+$ co-transport and counter-transport.

  **(Refer previous question for details)**

## BODY WATER AND BODY FLUIDS

## DESCRIBE THE MECHANISMS BY WHICH THE BLOOD VOLUME IS MAINTAINED IN THE BODY                           10 (1990)

## DESCRIBE THE HORMONAL REGULATION OF BLOOD VOLUME                                              5 (1991)

**Blood volume:** In a normal adult blood volume is 8% of body weight. In an adult weighing 70 kg, it is approximately 5.6 liters. Blood volume is controlled with a great degree of precision in spite of changes in water and electrolyte intake. In the body there exists a basic feedback mechanism for the control of:

- ECF volume
- Blood volume
- Cardiac output
- Arterial blood pressure

These are all inter-related, i.e. ECF determines blood volume, which determines the cardiac output. It in turn determines the arterial BP. Arterial BP regulates ECF by influencing urinary output.

↑Blood volume →↑CO→↑ BP→↑Urine output →↓Blood volume.

**Control of ECF:** It involves the control of two factors:
   i.  ECF volume
   ii.  Tonicity of ECF

### Control of ECF Volume

Primarily controlled by the amount of osmotically active $Na^+$ as it is the most abundant ion in the ECF.

**$Na^+$ balance in the body is controlled by:**

a. **Kidney:** $Na^+$ ion is filtered in the kidney at the glomerulus and a constant fraction is reabsorbed in the proximal tubule known as glomerulotubular balance.

b. **Aldosterone:** Influences the reabsorption of $Na^+$ at distal convoluted tubules. Aldosterone secretion is controlled by renin-angiotensin system, whose secretion is in turn controlled by the level of $K^+$ and $Na^+$ in the ECF.

c. **Atrial natriuretic peptide (ANP):** It is secreted from the atrial muscles and promotes the excretion of $Na^+$ through kidney when ECF volume increases.

### Role of ADH

For control of blood volume it acts through low pressure atrial receptors which reflexly control ADH secretion, e.g.

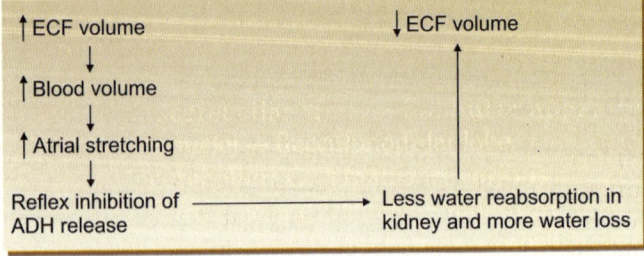

Role of ADH in ECF control

## Angiotensin II

Angiotensin II secretion is related to renin secretion which in turn is controlled by level of $Na^+$ and $Cl^-$ reaching the **macula densa** in the DCT.

When $Na^+$ and $Cl^-$ levels increase in blood, its amount increases in the filtrate and more is presented to macula densa and renin secretion is stimulated as a consequence.

– If $Na^+$ decreases →↓ Renin →↓ Angiotensin II

**Angiotensin II has the following actions:**

1. ↑Aldosterone →↑ $Na^+$ reabsorption →↑ ECF volume.

2. ADH →↑ reabsorption of water by kidney →↑ ECF volume.

3. Stimulates thirst →↑ ECF volume.

## CONTROL OF TONICITY OF ECF

Basically determined by the amount of $Na^+$ in the ECF and it is responsible for exerting 90% of osmotic pressure of ECF.

Change in tonicity occurs when there is a disproportionate loss or gain of water or electrolytes in the body.

### Regulatory Mechanisms

  i. Hypothalamic osmoreceptors
 ii. Thirst mechanism

  i. **Osmoreceptors:** Act by controlling the ADH secretion. These are neurons (in hypothalamus) sensitive to changes in the osmolarity or tonicity of interstitial fluid around them.

    If osmolarity is lowered → osmoreceptors swell →↓rate of impulses to ADH secreting neurons →↓ ADH → more water loss → osmolarity is restored.

 ii. **Thirst mechanism:** The 'thirst centre' is located in the lateral hypothalamus which when stimulated, there is conscious desire to drink water. Neurons are stimulated when osmolarity of the interstitium increases. Hence, neurons function the same way as osmoreceptors. Once the ECF volume is regulated, plasma volume is regulated and parallel changes in number of blood cells takes place, hence the blood volume is maintained.

## HORMONAL REGULATION OF BLOOD VOLUME 5

Discuss the role of:

- ADH
- Aldosterone
- Angiotensin II
- ANP

  **(Refer to previous questions)**

## MISCELLANEOUS

### APOPTOSIS                                    2.5 (2003)

This is a process of programmed cell death in which body cells die and get absorbed under genetic control. It can be called **cell-suicide** in the sense that the cell's own genes play an active role in its demise. It should be distinguished from necrosis (cell murder) in which healthy cells are destroyed by external processes such as inflammation.

**Mechanism:** Apoptosis may be initiated by:

- Internal stimuli
- Fas, a transmembrane protein produced by natural killer cells and T-lymphocytes
- Tumour necrosis factor (TNF).

  The activated apoptotic genes cause the cell to undergo DNA fragmentation, condensation of cytoplasm and chromatin. Finally, the cells break up and remnants are removed by phagocytes.

**Physiological significance:** It plays an important role during embryonal development and also in adulthood. For example:

- Responsible for regression of the duct system during sex differentiation in the foetus.
- Degeneration and regeneration of neurons within the CNS and during the formation of synapse.
- Removal of inappropriate clones of immune cells and lytic effects of glucocorticoids on lymphocytes.
- Cyclical shedding of the endometrium during menstruation.
- Cell shedding from the tip of the villi in small intestine.

Abnormal apoptosis occurs in autoimmune diseases, degenerative diseases and cancer.

## NERVE GROWTH FACTOR  2 (2003), 2.5 (2003)–IPU

A number of proteins necessary for growth and survival of neurons are called neurotrophins. These are produced in the muscles and other structures that the neurons innervate. In CNS these are produced by astrocytes. They bind to receptors at the endings of neurons. They are carried by retrograde transport to the neuronal cell body, where they foster the production of proteins associated with neuronal development, growth and survival.

- **Nerve growth factor (NGF)** was the first neurotrophin to be characterised, necessary for the growth and maintenance of sympathetic neurons and some sensory neurons.
- It is made up of $2\alpha$, $2\beta$ and $2\gamma$ subunits with the $\beta$ subunit having similar structure to that of insulin.
- **Function:** It is necessary for the growth and maintenance of sympathetic neurons, sensory neurons and cholinergic neurons in the basal forebrain and striatum.

## STARLING FORCES  2.5 (1990), 2.5 (2010)

Capillary osmotic pressure across the capillary wall helps to maintain fluid exchange at tissue level. The rate of filtration and absorption at any point along the capillary depends upon a balance of forces which are called **Starling forces** (Fig. 1.2). These include the following factors:

1. Hydrostatic pressure across the capillary wall
2. Capillary osmotic pressure across capillary wall
3. Hydrostatic pressure in interstitial fluid
4. Interstitial fluid osmotic pressure

Factors 3 and 4 tend to cancel each other, hence forces which determine fluid exchange at the tissue level depend on factors 1 and 2 mainly.

Hydrostatic pressure at the arteriolar end is 37 mm Hg, therefore, some fluid is forced out of the capillary bed, whereas hydrostatic pressure at the venous end is 15 mm Hg by which some fluid is pulled back by osmotic forces.

## Applied Aspect

1. **Hypoprotienemia:** Decrease in plasma protein level causes decrease in colloidal osmotic pressure because of which increased filtration occurs at the arterial end and decrease in absorption of fluid occurs at the venous end. This results in abnormal collection of fluid in the interstitial fluid (oedema).

2. When capillary permeability is increased all the proteins escape much more readily from the capillary into the interstitial spaces producing oedema.

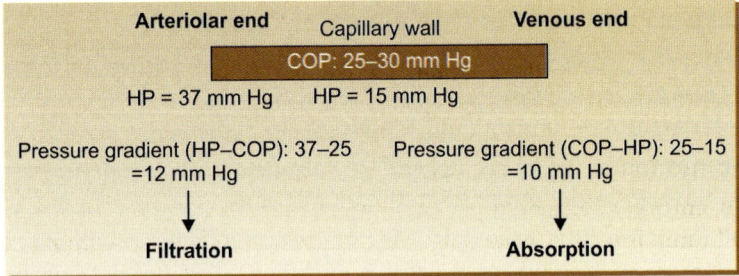

**Fig. 1.2:** Starling forces—pressure gradient across most capillary walls (COP Colloidal osmotic pressure, HP Hydrostatic pressure)

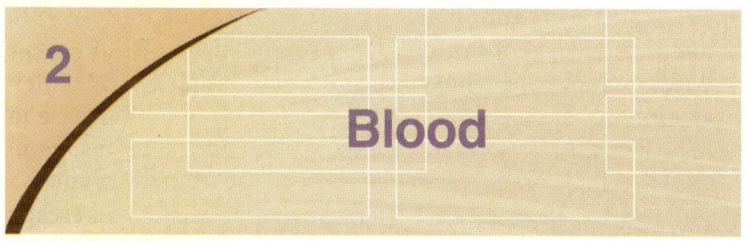

**2**

# Blood

**FUNCTIONS OF PLASMA PROTEINS**    **5 (1986, 1992), 2 (2006)**

**FORMATION AND FUNCTIONS OF PLASMA PROTEINS**    **2.5 (2004)**

### Formation of Plasma Proteins

**In embryo:** Mesenchymal cells form plasma proteins. First the albumin is synthesised and rest of plasma proteins are synthesised later.

**In adults:**

   i. Albumin is formed from the liver

  ii. Fibrinogen is also formed in the liver

 iii. Globulin is synthesised from:

- Tissue macrophages: Liver (particularly $\alpha$ and $\beta$ globulin), spleen and bone marrow
- Plasma cells
- Lymphocytes synthesise $\gamma$ globulin.

Plasma proteins have the following functions:

1. **Osmotic pressure:** Plasma proteins are responsible for exerting osmotic pressure of plasma which influences the exchange of fluid between blood and interstitial fluid. It is of the magnitude of 25 mm Hg. Albumin contributes the major portion towards osmotic pressure.

2. **Viscosity:** Plasma proteins along with blood cells provide viscosity to blood, which maintains the peripheral resistance and hence arterial blood pressure. Fibrinogen because of its shape contributes as much as albumin though it is present in smaller amount.

3. **Transport function:** Plasma proteins combine loosely with many chemicals, transport them, release them slowly, act as their reservoir, and prevent their excretion, e.g.
   - Albumin: transports
     - Calcium
     - Bilirubin
   - α globulins
     - Cortisol
     - Thyroxine
   - β globulins
     - Cholesterol
     - Iron
     - Insulin
   - γ globulins
     - Histamine

4. **Buffering effects:** In alkaline medium plasma proteins partially ionize as acid and donate $H^+$. They can also accept hydrogen ions if plasma becomes acidic. So they act as blood buffers and account for 1/6th of the buffering power of blood.

5. **Antibodies:** γ-globulins or immunoglobulins. These are formed by B-lymphocytes in response to specific antigens and destroys them by antigen–antibody reactions, protecting the body from their harmful effects.

6. **Carrier for lipids:** Lipoproteins in globulin fraction act as carrier of cholesterol, phospholipids and free fatty acids and transport them in blood.

7. **Blood coagulation:** Fibrinogen and prothrombin are essential for blood clotting and hence haemostasis.

## HAEMOGLOBIN

### WHAT WILL HAPPEN AND WHY TO Hb WHEN IT IS FREE IN THE CIRCULATION                    1 (2002)

If Hb was found free in the plasma, it would lead to:
- Increase in the viscosity of plasma, causing a rise in the blood pressure.
- Increase in the osmotic pressure of plasma.

Both these factors will interfere with fluid exchange across the capillaries.

- Loss of Hb through the kidneys **(haemoglobinuria)** may lead to kidney damage.
- Free Hb may be taken up rapidly by the tissue macrophage system and destroyed.

## COMPARE MYOGLOBIN AND HAEMOGLOBIN     2 (2006)

| Myoglobin | Haemoglobin |
|---|---|
| • This is an iron-containing pigment found in skeletal muscles. It binds 1 mol of oxygen | • It is an iron-containing pigment found in RBCs which binds 4 mol of oxygen |
| • It contains only 1 atom of iron per molecule, therefore, its MW is 1/4th compared to Hb | • It contains 4 atoms of iron per molecule, therefore, the molecular weight is four times higher compared to myoglobin |
| • Its curve is to the left of oxygen–Hb dissociation curve and is a rectangular hyperbola | • The oxygen–Hb dissociation curve is sigmoid in shape |
| • It takes up oxygen at lower pressures compared to Hb Therefore, it is found in muscles specialised for sustained contracttion where the $pO_2$ is close to zero | • It takes up oxygen at higher partial pressures compared to myoglobin transporting oxygen from the lungs to the tissues |

## EXPLAIN WHY REDUCED Hb IS A BETTER BUFFER THAN OXY-Hb     1 (2004)

The buffering action of Hb is mainly due to imidazole group of histidine residues. This imidazole group of deoxyhaemoglobin, i.e. reduced Hb dissociate less than that of oxyhaemoglobin, therefore, reduced Hb produces less $H^+$ than oxyhaemoglobin at a given pH making it a weaker acid and a more effective buffer compared to oxyhaemoglobin.

## RED BLOOD CELLS

**ERYTHROPOIESIS**      **2.5 (1991)**

**DEFINE ERYTHROPOIESIS. DESCRIBE THE VARIOUS STAGES OF ERYTHROPOIESIS. DESCRIBE THE FACTORS REGULATING IT**      **1 + 4 + 3 = 8 (2012)**

**STAGES OF ERYTHROPOIESIS**      **2 (2008), 2.5 (2011)**

Erythropoiesis is the process of formation of RBCs. In an adult it takes place in the red bone marrow of flat bones and ends of long bones.

RBCs originate from pluripotent stem cells and passes through the successive stages to mature cells as follows:

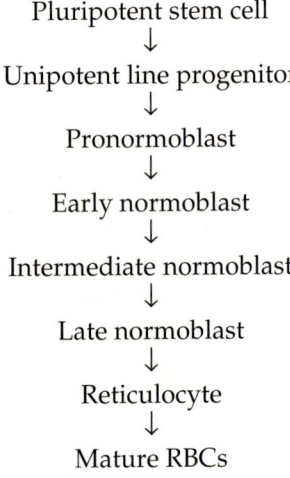

Pluripotent stem cell
↓
Unipotent line progenitor
↓
Pronormoblast
↓
Early normoblast
↓
Intermediate normoblast
↓
Late normoblast
↓
Reticulocyte
↓
Mature RBCs

In general, it undergoes the following changes:

- Decreases in size
- Cytoplasm increases in amount and the nucleus decreases in size
- Nucleoli disappear
- Chromatin becomes progressively coarser
- Nucleus is gradually lost
- Staining reaction of cytoplasm changes from deep basophilic to polychromatophilic to acidophilic due to gradual reduction in the amount of RNA.

Development from pronormoblast to reticulocytes takes 3 days and reticulocytes mature in 4 days, hence in 7 days complete formation of mature RBCs occurs.

## REGULATION OF ERYTHROPOIESIS            2.5 (1992)

## ERYTHROPOIETIN                           2 (2004)

Normally, erythropoiesis is so regulated that number of RBCs and haemoglobin is maintained within a narrow range. There exist a feedback mechanism between RBC count and formation of fresh RBCs.

**Factors regulating erythropoiesis:** This is classified into two categories:

I. **General factors:** Hypoxia

II. **Special maturation factors:**

   i.  Dietary factors

   ii. Castle's intrinsic factor

   iii. Extrinsic factors

**I. General factors: Hypoxia** This is the most potent stimulus for the formation of RBCs. It causes the stimulation of bone marrow increasing RBC production. This effect is mediated by erythropoietin.

### Erythropoietin

This is also called erythrocyte stimulating factor or erythropoiesis stimulating hormone.

### Source and Metabolism

1. 85% is secreted by the kidneys probably by the interstitial cells of the peritubular capillaries.

2. 15% is produced by extrarenal sources: Liver parenchymal cells and tissue macrophage system.

Hypoxia of the kidneys causes release of REF or erythrogenin that acts on the plasma substrate, eryhtropoietinogen, an $\alpha$-globulin to form erythropoietin.

## Mode of Action

1. Causes early differentiation of erythropoietin sensitive stem cells in the bone marrow into proerythroblasts and hence mature RBCs.
2. Increases release of reticulocytes from the bone marrow.
3. Increases synthesis of RNA, DNA, globin and ferritin which increase haem synthesis, thus increasing haemoglobin synthesis in the already existing normoblasts.

### Factors that affect erythropoietin production

1. Increase
   - Hypoxia
   - Vasoconstrictor agents
   - Nucleotides
   - Products of RBC destruction
   - Hormones (thyroxine, anterior pituitary hormones and androgens)
2. Decrease
   - Estrogen
   - Chronic renal diseases
   - Protein deficiency
   - Cirrhosis of liver
   - Chronic inflammatory diseases

## II. Special Maturation Factors

### Dietary factors

i. Globin helps in protein formation.
ii. Iron, manganese, copper, cobalt, iron and nickel help in haem formation.
iii. Calcium increases iron absorption from GIT.
iv. Vitamin C, $B_{12}$ and folic acid help in synthesis of nucleic acid.

## Castle's Intrinsic Factor

This is a glycoprotein secreted by the parietal (oxyntic) cells of the stomach which helps in the absorption of vitamin $B_{12}$ from the stomach. One molecule of intrinsic factor (IF) combines with one molecule of vitamin $B_{12}$ that binds to specific receptors in the ileal mucosa. IF splits from the complex and vitamin $B_{12}$ is released into the portal blood. This process does not require energy but is calcium dependant occurring optimally at a pH of 7.0.

## Extrinsic Factors

These are present in certain foods and are essentially folic acid and vitamin $B_{12}$.

Intrinsic factor along with extrinsic factor forms the haematinic principle which helps in the maturation of RBCs. Therefore, deficiency of any of the two leads to maturation failure and hence megaloblastic anaemia.

## FATE OF RBCS                                    2.5 (1986)

Lifespan of mature RBCs is 120 days. RBCs cannot survive longer as they do not contain nucleus, mitochondria and contain cytoplasmic enzymes capable only of metabolising glucose by glycolytic processes and thus generating a few ATPs. However, this metabolic system becomes progressively weak with time. As a result following changes take place:

  i. Flexibility of membrane decreases.
 ii. Transport across membrane and hence ionic composition in the cell cannot be maintained.
iii. Keeping the iron of haemoglobin in ferrous state becomes difficult.
 iv. Inhibition of oxidation of proteins in RBCs cannot be maintained.

Cells progressively become more fragile and break down as they pass through narrow capillaries specially in the spleen. As cells are broken, their Hb is phagocytosed by the reticuloendothelial cells. Iron and globin are removed and rest through successive stages is converted into bilirubin which is carried to the liver where it is conjugated with glucuronic acid and secreted in the bile into the duodenum.

In intestine it is partially reabsorbed and partially converted into urobilinogen and stercobilinogen by bacterial action and lost from the urine and stool respectively. Iron and globin are reused for synthesis of fresh Hb. Rest of the bilirubin is reabsorbed and transported to the liver via enterohepatic circulation.

## WHY RBC DIE AFTER AVERAGE LIFESPAN OF 120 DAYS    2, 3

Energy in the form of ATP is generated in RBCs by anaerobic metabolism by cytoplasmic enzymes capable of metabolising glucose. ATP serves to maintain stability and pliability of cell membrane and also transport of ions across the membrane.

However, this metabolic (anaerobic) metabolism becomes progressively less and less active with time and RBCs become more fragile as the membrane becomes fragile, the cells rupture during their passage through minute capillaries specially when passing through the red pulp of spleen and die off.

## LAB-CLASSIFICATION OF ANAEMIA    5 (1989)

Lab-classification of anaemia is based on calculation of certain blood indices from the values of the following:

i. Hb content of patient's blood
ii. RBC count
iii. Haematocrit or packed cell volume (PCV)

From these values 3 indices are calculated:

i. **MCV:** Mean corpuscular volume, i.e. average volume of RBCs.

$$MCV = \frac{PCV/Liter}{RBC \ count \ in \ million/cu \ mm} \ in \ \mu^3$$

For example, PCV = 40%
RBC count = 5 million/cu mm

$$MCV = \frac{40 \times 10}{5} = 80 \ \mu^3$$

**Normal range** = 78 – 94 $\mu^3$

When MCV is less than normal cells, it is known as microcytes and anaemia is called microcytic, e.g. iron deficiency anaemia.

If MCV is more than normal, it is macrocytic anaemic, e.g. folic acid deficiency and $B_{12}$ deficiency anaemia.

ii. **MCH:** Mean corpuscular haemoglobin, i.e. average amount of Hb in RBCs.

Formula for calculating MCH

$$MCH = \frac{Hb/Liter}{RBC \ in \ million/cu \ mm} \ in \ picograms \ (pg)$$

For example, Hb = 15 gm/dL, RBC = 5 million/cu mm

$$MCH = \frac{15}{5} \times 10 = 30 \text{ pg}$$

**Normal range** = 29.5 ± 2.5 pg

MCH may vary with variation in RBC size.

iii. **MCHC:** Mean corpuscular haemoglobin concentration, i.e. degree of saturation of RBCs with Hb. As size of the RBCs is also taken into consideration unlike for calculating MCH, it is a more informative index.

$$MCHC = \frac{Hb \text{ in gm/dL}}{PCV} \times 100$$

For example, Hb = 15 gm/dL

PCV = 45%

$$MCHC = \frac{15}{45} \times 100 = 33.3\%$$

**Normal range** = 32 ± 3%

MCHC in normal range – normochromic cells.

Less than normal – hypochromic cells.

MCHC cannot be more than normal as Hb saturation of RBCs cannot be beyond a certain limit.

Based on these indices, anaemia can be classified as:

1. **Microcytic hypochromic**–iron deficiency anaemia, thalassemia.
2. **Macrocytic normochromic**–folic acid and $B_{12}$ deficiency.
3. **Normocytic normochromic**–after acute haemorrhage, aplastic anaemia and all haemolytic anaemias except iron deficiency anaemia.

## HEMOLYTIC ANAEMIAS                                    (2001)

This is a type of anaemia which is produced due to the destruction of RBCs. It is further divided into intracorpuscular defects and extracorpuscular defects.

**Intracorpuscular** defects are hereditary in nature:

- Hereditary spherocytosis
- Haemoglobinopathies like sickle cell anaemia and thalassemia

- Erythroblastosis foetalis
- G6PD deficiency.

**Extracorpuscular** defects are acquired in nature:

- Antigen–antibody reactions
- Infections like malaria
- Drugs/Poisons like quinine, aspirin, burns, snake venom, etc.
- Hypersplenism which causes overactivity of normal destructive mechanisms.

## WHAT WILL HAPPEN AND WHY IF A PATIENT OF PERNICIOUS ANAEMIA IS GIVEN FOLIC ACID (1991)

## COMPARE FOLIC ACID AND VITAMIN $B_{12}$ DEFICIENCY ANAEMIA (2001)

Both the vitamins are required for maturation of RBCs during erythropoiesis. Their deficiency leads to macrocytic or megaloblastic anaemia. In addition, vitamin $B_{12}$ is essential for nutrition of nerves, hence its deficiency leads to neurological symptoms due to involvement of sensory and motor columns of spinal cord called subacute combined degeneration of the cord.

Under these circumstances folic acid is not an effective substitute and may worsen the neurological symptoms.

## EXPLAIN WHY ANAEMIA OCCURS IN KIDNEY DISEASES
1 (2004)

Around 85% of the circulating erythropoietin is secreted by the kidneys probably by the interstitial cells (or cells in the endothelium) of the peritubular capillaries. This stimulates the process of erythropoiesis, increasing the number of circulating RBCs. Hence, anaemia occurs in kidney disorders due to deficiency of erythropoietin.

## EXPLAIN WHY MACROCYTIC ANAEMIA OCCURS IN VITAMIN $B_{12}$ DEFICIENCY
1 (2004)

Vitamin $B_{12}$ is required for the synthesis of DNA and maturation of nucleus in developing red cells. Therefore, in the deficiency of this vitamin cells remain large (called megaloblasts) due to reduction in cell division.

## WHAT WILL HAPPEN AND WHY IF A PERSON WITH SICKLE CELL ANAEMIA IS EXPOSED TO HYPOXIA  1 (2010)

When a person with sickle cell anaemia is exposed to hypoxia, HbS present in the RBCs becomes much less soluble and precipitates into crystals within the RBCs. These crystals elongate producing change in the shape of the cells from biconcave to sickle shape. These cells are less flexible compared to RBCs leading to blockage of the microcirculation. As they are more fragile and hence liable to haemolysis, they produce sickle cell anaemia.

## JAUNDICE

## EXPLAIN WHY IN OBSTRUCTIVE JAUNDICE PATIENTS AFTER SOMETIME IF OBSTRUCTION IS NOT RELIEVED SUFFER FROM BLEEDING DISORDERS  1 (2003)-IPU

Liver plays an important role in the coagulation mechanism:

- **Synthesis of procoagulants:** It is the site of synthesis of factors V, VII, IX and X, prothrombin and fibrinogen.
- **Removal of activated procoagulants:** Liver removes the activated coagulants from the blood.
- **Synthesis of anti-coagulants:** Liver also synthesises anti-coagulants like heparin, antithrombin III and protein C.

Hence, patients with obstructive jaundice suffer from bleeding disorders, if their obstruction is not relieved due to liver failure that leads to hypocoagulability of blood.

## EXPLAIN WHY THERE IS AN INCREASE IN FAECAL FAT IN OBSTRUCTIVE JAUNDICE  1 (2007)

Faecal fat increases by 40–50% in obstructive jaundice because of deficiency of bile in the intestine because of which emulsification and absorption of fat is inadequate. This produces bulky, pale, greasy and foul smelling stools. This condition is called steatorrhoea.

## EXPLAIN WHY PHOTOTHERAPY IS GIVEN IN CASES OF PHYSIOLOGICAL JAUNDICE OF THE NEWBORN  1 (2008)

Exposure of skin to white light converts bilirubin to lumirubin which has a shorter half-life than bilirubin. It acts by photo-isomerisation of bilirubin to soluble forms which are easily excreted. Therefore, phototherapy is of value in treating infants in jaundice irrespective of the cause.

## WHITE BLOOD CELLS

### PHAGOCYTOSIS                                              3 (2004)-IPU

Neutrophils are the major cells that carry out phagocytosis. They play an important role in bacterial inflammation, thus called the **first line of defence** against bacterial infections. The process of phagocytosis involves the following steps:

- **Diapedesis:** Neutrophils migrate from the bloodstream into tissues by passing through the junction between the endothelial cells lining the blood vessels called **diapedesis**.

- **Chemotaxis:** Bacterial products interact with plasma proteins to produce chemotactic agents that attract neutrophils to the site of injury or inflammation called **chemotaxis**. As a result, neutrophils adhere to each other and become immobile. The chemotactic agents include:
  - Components of complement system $C_{5a}$
  - leukotrienes
  - polypeptides from lymphocytes, basophils and mast cells.

- **Opsonisation:** Opsonins coat the bacteria and make them tasty to the phagocytes, a process called opsonisation. The opsonins are naturally acting factors and include IgG and opsin fragments of complement proteins.

- **Phagocytosis:** The coated bacteria bind to receptors on the neutrophil cell membrane which increases the motor activity of the cell. The increased motor activity leads to prompt ingestion of the bacteria by endocytosis which is called phagocytosis.

- **Degranulation:** After phagocytosing the bacteria, bacteriocidal substances called defensins such as lysozymes and peroxidises are released from the lysosomal granules into the digestive pouch (degranulation) where they kill and digest the bacteria. There is a sharp increase in oxygen uptake and metabolism in the neutrophils which is called the respiratory burst that results in generation of superoxide radical ($O_2^-$) and hydrogen peroxide ($H_2O_2$).

- **Inflammatory response:** Release of lysosomal enzymes, histamine and 5-HT into the ECF produces the inflammatory response.

- **Limiting inflammation:** Fusion of phagocytic vacuole with lysosomes causes release of thromboxanes (that produce vasoconstriction and platelet aggregation) and prostaglandins that have an anti-inflammatory effect. Both these factors limit inflammation.

## PLATELETS

### FUNCTIONS OF PLATELETS                              2.5 (2004)

Platelets contain various granules which are released when platelets are activated and perform a number of important functions.

a. **Dense granules** contain ADP and serotonin
b. **α-granules** contain clotting proteins and platelet derived growth factors (PDGF).

### FUNCTIONS

i. Plays a role in **haemostasis** by:
   a. Forming a platelet plug at the site of injury which helps to arrest bleeding.
   b. Secrete serotonin—a potent vasoconstrictor that helps in arrest of bleeding in the earliest stage.
   c. Plays a role in coagulation by producing platelet factor 3 which helps in conversion of prothrombin to thrombin by factors V and X.
ii. **Clot retraction:** Platelets contain contractile proteins which contract and cause shortening of fibrin fibres attached to them.
iii. **Phagocytosis:** Platelets phagocytose immune complexes, carbon particles and viruses.
iv. **Storage and transport functions:** Platelets contain histamine and 5-HT which are released as platelets disintegrate. They can actively take up 5-HT.

### WHAT WILL HAPPEN AND WHY WHEN THE PLATELET COUNT IS DECREASED                                              1 (2006)

Platelets form an important part of the clotting mechanism. When the platelet count is decreased, clot retraction is deficient and there is poor constriction of ruptured blood vessels. The resulting clinical syndrome is called **thrombocytopenic purpura** and is characterised by easy bruisability and multiple subcutaneous haemorrhages.

## BLOOD GROUPS

### EXPLAIN LANDSTEINER'S LAW                          2.5 (1988)

Landsteiner's law is related to blood groups. It states that if an agglutinogen is present on the red cells, the corresponding agglutinin must be absent in the plasma, e.g. if blood group agglutinogen A is present on RBCs, anti-A will be absent in plasma. It further states if agglutinogen is absent, the corresponding agglutinin must be present, i.e. if A-agglutinogen is absent on RBCs, then anti-A must be present in plasma. Both the parts of the law are applicable in ABO system of blood grouping as shown in Table 2.1.

| Table 2.1 | | |
|---|---|---|
| **Blood groups** | **Antigen on RBC** | **Agglutinins in plasma** |
| A | A | Anti-B |
| B | B | Anti-A |
| AB | A and B | None |
| O | None | Anti-A and anti-B |

The law does not hold good in Rh type of blood grouping. In Rh +ve person antigen-D is present on RBCs, and anti-D is absent in the plasma. But in Rh –ve individual though D-agglutinogen is absent on RBCs, anti-D antibodies are naturally not present in plasma.

### INCOMPATIBLE BLOOD TRANSFUSION                     (1991)
### DANGERS OF BLOOD TRANSFUSION            2 (2002), 2.5 (2003),
###                                                3 (2004)-IPU

Incompatible transfusion or mismatched transfusion means that the cells of the donor and agglutinins of recipient are not matching and as a result RBCs in transfused blood are agglutinated by the agglutinins in the recipient plasma. This can occur due to ABO incompatibility or Rh incompatibility.

Agglutinated RBCs are entrapped and block the peripheral blood vessels causing acute pain. Over a period of hours the entrapped cells are haemolysed and phagocytosed by macrophages and their Hb is liberated into circulation. Hb is ultimately converted into bilirubin, thereby increasing blood levels of bilirubin and may produce jaundice.

Occasionally, antibodies are sufficiently potent and cause immediate haemolysis of donor cells and release the Hb, thus increasing bilirubin levels of blood producing jaundice.

If the liver function is normal, jaundice does not occur unless a large volume of (300–500 ml) mismatched blood is transfused.

Effects of incompatible blood transfusion:

1. **Inapparent haemolysis:** Injected RBCs are destroyed rapidly, the recipient's blood returning within a week or less to the pre-transfusion state.

2. **Post-transfusion jaundice:** Heamolysed RBCs cause increased release of haemoglobin which gets metabolised to bilirubin producing haemolytic jaundice.

3. **Severe reactions with haemoglobinuria and renal failure:** After a few ml of blood has been transfused patient complains of violent pain in the back and tightness in the chest because agglutinated RBCs form clumps that can block the capillaries.

   This may also lead to oliguria. Later anuria sets in due to vascular disturbances involving the glomeruli. Still later it may lead to lethargy, coma and death within 8–10 days.

4. **Mechanical overloading** leads to hypervolaemia.

5. **Chemical risks:**
   - As stored blood looses potassium ions to the external plasma, therefore, following excessive transfusion death may occur due to hyperkalaemia
   - With massive transfusion of citrated blood, normal conversion of citrate to bicarbonate may be delayed. Patient may suffer from lack of ionised calcium producing tetany and alkalosis may develop in patients with defective kidney functions.

6. **Pyogenic reactions** like fever with chills and rigors.

7. **Allergic reactions:** Rash, anaphylactic shock, angioneurotic oedema, urticaria, etc.

8. Transmission of **diseases** like malaria, syphilis, AIDS and jaundice.

## Rh FACTOR                                    5 (1986), 2.5 (1993)
## Rh INCOMPATIBILITY                                      2 (2007)
## WHAT WILL HAPPEN AND WHY IF Rh +VE BLOOD IS
## TRANSFUSED TO A Rh–VE PERSON              1 (2004)

Rh factor or Rhesus factor is a blood group antigen present in about 85% of the population known as Rh +ve people and absent in the remaining 15% known as Rh –ve. It was initially discovered in Rhesus monkey and hence the name Rhesus factor. There are several varieties of Rh-antigen and the commonest is 'antigen-D'. Rh +ve people have antigen-D on the RBCs like the antigen of ABO groups. At the same time antibodies against anti-D is not naturally present in the plasma of a Rh –ve person. Anti-D formation can only be induced in a Rh –ve subject to Rh +ve cells are injected in him.

### Clinical importance of Rh factor

1. When blood transfusion is to be given Rh factor must be considered. A Rh –ve person should not be transfused with Rh +ve blood lest anti-D formation should occur and cause agglutination of donors cells.

2. Rh factor is especially important in females. During pregnancy if the mother is Rh –ve, father Rh +ve and the child may be Rh +ve or –ve. If the child is Rh +ve and if Rh +ve cells happen to cross the placental barrier, it will cause the production of anti-D in maternal blood, anti-D can cross and reach the foetal blood and destroy the RBCs. This can cause complications of varying severity in the foetus.

    Normally, Rh +ve cells of the child do not cross in sufficient numbers during pregnancy and no harm is done in the first pregnancy. Rh +ve cells cross in substantial amount after separation of the placenta and after delivery large amount of anti-D is formed in the maternal blood which could be harmful in a subsequent pregnancy.

    Hence, nowadays as a precautionary measure anti-D is injected after delivery in Rh –ve mother, if the child is Rh +ve. This prevents the formation of anti-D in the mother later on as all cells containing antigen-D which have reached maternal blood are destroyed and further children to be born are protected.

## WHAT WILL HAPPEN AND WHY WHEN A Rh –VE MOTHER IS CARRYING A Rh +VE FOETUS DURING HER FIRST, SECOND AND THIRD PREGNANCY                                  2.5 (1989)

## WHAT WILL HAPPEN AND WHY IF Rh –VE WOMAN IS TRANSFUSED WITH Rh +VE BLOOD                                1 (2011)

When a Rh –ve mother is carrying a Rh +ve foetus, harm to the baby can occur when RBCs containing D-antigen from the foetus cross the placental barrier and reach maternal circulation.

In maternal blood they stimulate the formation of anti-D antibodies, which can gain access to foetal circulation and destroy foetal red blood cells. Damage will depend on:

1. Degree of maternal anti-D response

2. Amount of antibodies that can cross the placental barrier.

- Under normal circumstances during the first pregnancy placental barrier is not broken during pregnancy and usually no harm is done and condition may pass unnoticed.

- During the second pregnancy foetus may be harmed to variable extent because Rh +ve foetal cells crossover after the delivery when maternal blood sinuses get exposed during the first pregnancy. Anti-D antibodies are already present in the maternal blood which if they cross, the placenta will harm the Rh +ve foetus. Haemolytic disease due to destruction of foetal RBCs can occur, but it may not be a severe reaction except for neonatal jaundice.

- In the third pregnancy chances of greater damage to the foetus in the form of **hydrops foetalis**, death or a still birth can occur.

## ERYTHROBLASTOSIS FOETALIS AND ITS TREATMENT  5 (2004)-IPU

In case of Rh incompatibility there may be no anaemia at birth but may develop in a few days because at birth excessive destruction of RBCs is compensated by an intense normoblastic response of the marrow associated with high reticulocyte count and many nucleated RBCs in the circulation. This is called **erythroblastosis foetalis**. Free anti-D derived from the mother is present in the infant's blood for at least one week after birth and continues to destroy the infant's cells though at diminished rates.

## Treatment

Exchange blood transfusion soon afterbirth, i.e. after removing small quantities of infant's blood successively from inferior vena cava and replacing an equal volume of compatible Rh –ve blood. Thus infant's Rh +ve RBCs prone to destruction are removed from the circulation.

## CLOTTING MECHANISMS

### COMPARE HAEMOSTASIS AND HOMEOSTASIS      2 (2002)

**Haemostasis** is a collective term used for various body mechanisms which arrest bleeding and hence prevent the blood loss, via spasm of local vessels (vasoconstriction), platelet plug formation and blood coagulation.

**Homeostasis** maintenance of constancy of internal environment of body, i.e. constancy of volume, temperature, electrolytes and pH. All the body systems contribute towards homeostasis.

### HAEMOSTASIS      2, 3

Haemostasis is the spontaneous arrest or prevention of bleeding by physiological processes:

1. Spasm or constriction of injured blood vessels due to:
   a. Mechanical stimulation
   b. Release of 5-HT from tissues which is a potent vasoconstrictor.
2. Collection and aggregation of platelets at the site of injury forming a temporary haemostatic plug that is a prompt response.
3. Conversion of temporary haemostatic plug to definitive haemostatic plug.

### MECHANISMS THAT KEEP BLOOD FLUID      2, 3

Blood is kept in the fluid state as a result of a balance between clotting and anticlotting mechanism. The mechanisms which prevent clotting are:

1. Smooth vascular endothelium lining the vessel prevents activation of factor XII needed for clotting of blood.
2. Anticlotting mechanisms:
   a. **Antithrombin III**—inhibits active forms of factors IX, X, XI and XII.

b. **Thrombomodulin**—a thrombin binding protein produced by all endothelial cells except that in the cerebral circulation.

c. **Plasmin**—previously known as fibrinolysin is an enzyme that causes the lysis of fibrin and fibrinogen forming fibrin degradation products (FDP) that inhibit thrombin.

d. **Heparin**—naturally, present in the blood and facilitates the action of antithrombin III.

## ANTIHAEMOPHILIC GLOBULIN 2.5 (1993)

Antihaemophilic globulin (AHG) is a protein normally present in the blood. It is also known as antihaemophilic factor or blood clotting factor VIII.

It is essential for the formation of prothrombin activator by the intrinsic pathway. It is consumed during the process of blood coagulation. Deficiency or absence of this factor leads to prolongation of clotting time. **Haemophilia** is a clinical condition in which clotting time is prolonged due to congenital absence of AHG. The condition arises out of abnormality of a gene on X-chromosome. It is inherited by males as X-linked recessive character from females, who do not suffer themselves. Factor VIII is destroyed when blood is stored at 4°C. Hence, haemophiliacs are transfused with fresh blood. Plasma can be frozen and factor VIII separated and given to them as well.

## EXPLAIN WHY VITAMIN K IS GIVEN IN PREMATURE BABIES 1 (2008)

Premature babies are likely to develop vitamin K deficiency and thus haemorrhagic disorders because bacterial gut flora which synthesise vitamin K is not developed satisfactorily in early infancy. Hence, vitamin K is given to premature babies.

## INTRINSIC PATHWAY OF CLOTTING 2.5 (1992)
## COMPARE INTRINSIC AND EXTRINSIC COAGULATION MECHANISMS (Fig. 2.1) 2 (2005)

• Intrinsic pathway of clotting involves the formation of prothrombin activator by the activation of mechanisms present in the blood.

- It includes a cascade of reactions in which inactive enzymes which are clotting factors are activated which in turn activate other enzymes in series and lead to the formation of prothrombin activator which in turn converts prothrombin to thrombin.

- *In vivo*, it is activated when blood clotting factors come in contact with collagen of the damaged vessel wall and change in the blood constituents.

- *In vitro*, it is activated when blood comes in contact with wettable surface like glass.

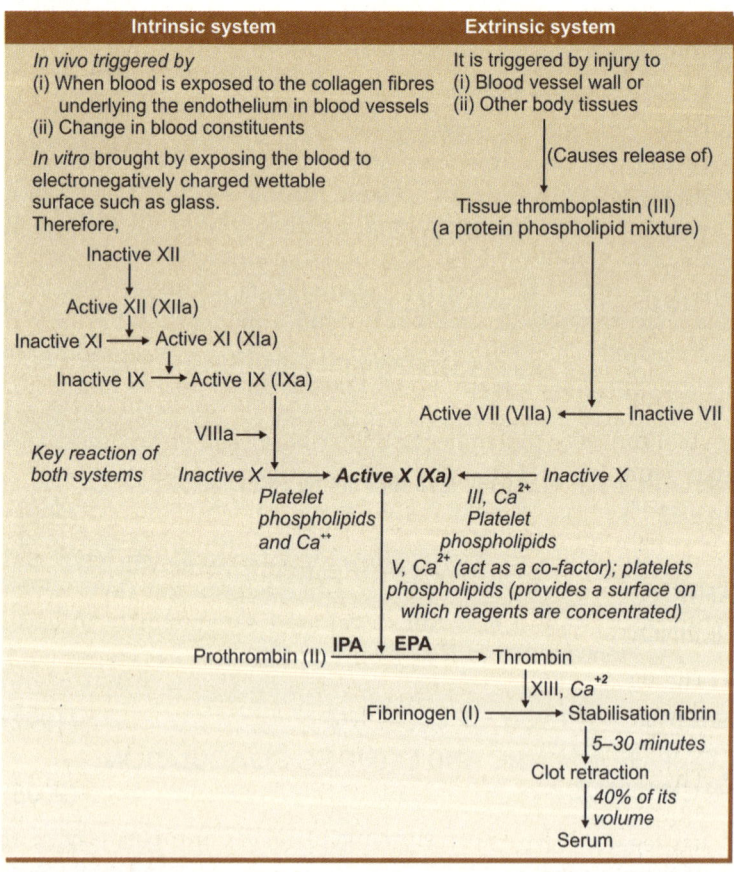

**Fig. 2.1:** Schematic diagram of clotting mechanism

## Extrinsic Pathway of Clotting

This is triggered by injury to the blood vessel wall and other body tissues causing releasing of tissue thromboplastin III that leads to activation of factor VII.

In both these pathways key reaction is activation of factor X to its active form which in turn interacts with factor V, $Ca^{2+}$, platelet, phospholipids to form prothrombin activator. In this stage factor V acts as a cofactor and phsopholipids provide a surface on which the reagents are concentrated.

## ROLE OF VITAMIN K IN BLOOD COAGULATION     2.5

Vitamin K is required for the synthesis of a number of clotting factors in the liver. These are:

- Factor II—Prothrombin
- Factor VII—Proconvertin
- Factor IX—Christmas factor
- Factor X—Stuart-Prower factor

If vitamin K is deficient, clotting time is prolonged and bleeding tendency can occur. In addition, vitamin K is required for synthesis of:

a. **Protein C:** It is a circulating inhibitor of intravascular clotting. It functions by inactivating active factors V and VIII.

b. **Protein S:** It activates protein C. Vitamin K plays a role in conversion of a number of glutamic acid residues to carboxyglutamic acid before the abovementioned clotting factors and compounds are released into the circulation.

## ANTICLOTTING MECHANISMS     3 (2004)-IPU
## FIBRINOLYTIC SYSTEM     2.5 (2002), 2 (2008), 2 (2010)

- The tendency of blood to clot *in vivo* is balanced by reactions that prevent formation of blood clots inside blood vessels, break down any clot that do form or both mechanisms.
- These reactions include the interaction between platelet aggregating effects of **thromboxane $A_2$** and the anti-aggregating effects of **prostacyclin**, which causes clots to form at the site where a blood vessel is injured but keeps the vessel lumen free of clots.

- **Antithrombin III** is a protease inhibitor that blocks the activity of clotting factors IX, X, XI and XII. This binding is facilitated by heparin, a naturally occurring anticoagulant first isolated in the liver. It is secreted by the granules of the mast cells and circulating basophils.

- The endothelium of blood vessels also plays an active role in the extension of the clot. All endothelial cells except those in the cerebral microcirculation produce **thrombomodulin**, a thrombin-binding protein on their surface. This thrombin-thrombomodulin complex activates **protein C**. Activated protein C (APC) along with its cofactor **protein S**, inactivates factors V and VIII and inactivates an inhibitor of tissue plasminogen activator, increasing the formation of plasmin (Fig. 2.2).

- **Plasmin (fibrinolysin)** is the active component of **plasminogen (fibrinolytic)** system. This enzyme lyses fibrin and fibrinogen with the production of fibrin degradation products that inhibit thrombin. Plasmin is formed from its inactive precursor

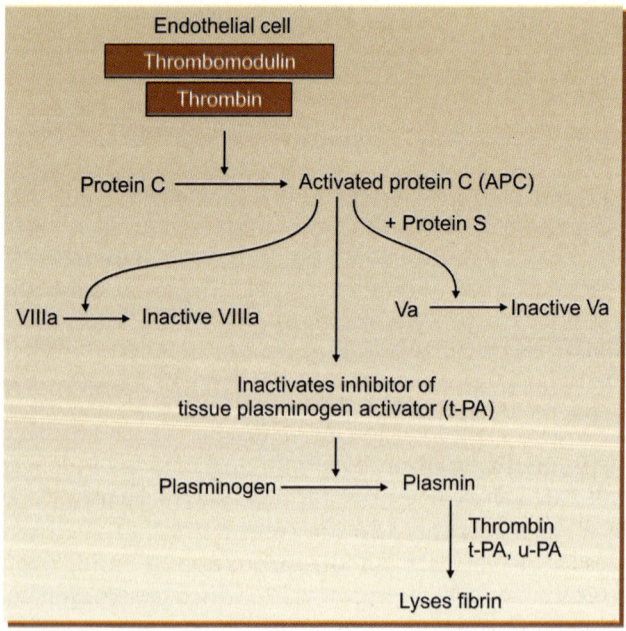

**Fig 2.2:** Fibrinolytic system and its regulation by protein C

plasminogen by action of thrombin and tissue type plasminogen activator **(t-PA)** as well as urokinase type plasminogen
activator **(u-PA)**.

* Plasminogen receptors are located on the surface of many types
of cells and are plentiful on endothelial cells. When plasminogen binds to its receptors it becomes activated, so intact
blood vessels are provided with a mechanism that discourages
clot formation.

## ANTICOAGULANTS                                    2.5 (2003)

Anticoagulants are chemicals that inhibit the process of blood
coagulation by acting at different steps. Some anticoagulants are
naturally present in circulation and prevent intravascular clotting
and are called *in vivo* anticoagulants. These are:

   i. Heparin—acts as antithrombin

  ii. Protein C—inactivates active factors V and VIII

 iii. Fibrinolytic system—active component is plasmin which
causes the lysis of fibrin and fibrinogen.

   Certain chemicals prevent coagulation of blood outside the body
and are used in laboratory for blood collection and are called
*in vitro* anticoagulants, e.g.

1. Oxalates of $K^+$ and ammonium
2. Na citrate—chelates $Ca^{2+}$
3. EDTA—chelates $Ca^{2+}$
4. Heparin—it has antithrombin action

**Therapeutically used anticoagulants:** To prevent intravascular
clotting (thrombosis) in patients, e.g. vitamin K antagonists like
dicoumarol and warfarin.

## BLOOD PRODUCTS FOR TRANSFUSION                          3

In some patients instead of whole blood, only a component is
sufficient and supplying only that component is advantageous.
This has the following advantages:

   i. Lowers the risk of transmitting infections
  ii. Avoids other complications due to mismatched transfusions
 iii. Prevents circulatory overload
  iv. Other components may be used for some other patients.

Various components that can be used are:

a. **Packed RBCs:** Prepared by separating RBCs by centrifugation of blood and removal of plasma. Useful in patients suffering from severe anaemia.

b. **Platelet concentrates:** Prepared by centrifugation of platelet rich plasma and given in platelet deficient cases.

c. **WBC concentrates:** Given in severe deficiency of WBCs.

d. **Fresh plasma:** In cases with severe fluid loss (e.g. burns) or in deficiency of a clotting factor (e.g. haemophilia).

e. **Freeze dried plasma:** Reconstituted with sterile water and given to replace fluid loss.

## IMMUNITY

### EXPLAIN WHY AIDS CAUSE EVENTUAL LOSS OF IMMUNE FUNCTION                                           1 (2003)-IPU

AIDS is caused by HIV (human immunodeficiency virus) which binds to $CD_4$ causing a decrease or loss of helper T cells. As a result of this, there is failure of proliferation of $T_8$ cells (suppressor and cytotoxic T cells) and B-lymphocytes, resulting in loss of immune functions and death from infections and cancer.

### COMPARE CELL-MEDIATED AND HUMORAL IMMUNE RESPONSE                                    2 (2003)-IPU, (2011)
### SHORT NOTE ON CELLULAR IMMUNITY                    2 (2007)

| Cell-mediated response | Humoral response |
|---|---|
| 1. This involves the T-lymphocytes that are further divided into four types: Cytotoxic, helper, suppressor and memory T-lymphocytes | 1. This involves the B-lymphocytes that are further divided into plasma and memory B cells |
| 2. This does not involve the production of antibodies | 2. Antibody production is involved |
| 3. It is responsible for delayed allergic reaction, rejection of transplanted foreign tissue and lysis of tumour cells | 3. It is a major defence against bacterial infections |
| 4. Effect of stimulation: | 4. Effect of stimulation: |

*Contd.*

*Contd.*

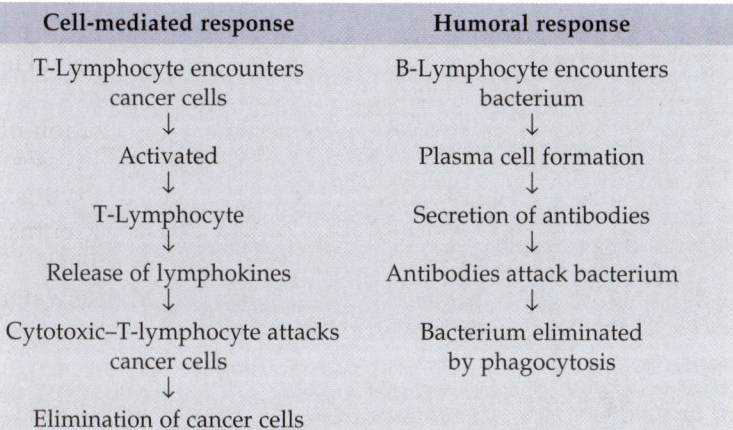

| Cell-mediated response | Humoral response |
|---|---|
| T-Lymphocyte encounters cancer cells<br>↓<br>Activated<br>↓<br>T-Lymphocyte<br>↓<br>Release of lymphokines<br>↓<br>Cytotoxic–T-lymphocyte attacks cancer cells<br>↓<br>Elimination of cancer cells | B-Lymphocyte encounters bacterium<br>↓<br>Plasma cell formation<br>↓<br>Secretion of antibodies<br>↓<br>Antibodies attack bacterium<br>↓<br>Bacterium eliminated by phagocytosis |

## COMPARE T- AND B-LYMPHOCYTES    2 (2004)-IPU

| T-Lymphocytes | B-Lymphocytes |
|---|---|
| 1. They are responsible for cell-mediated immune response | 1. They are responsible for humoral immunity |
| 2. They are divided into four types: Cytotoxic T cells, helper T cells, suppressor T cells and memory cells | 2. These are divided into two types: Plasma cells and memory cells |
| 3. Development of T cells takes place in the thymus gland | 3. Development takes place in the liver, spleen and bone marrow |
| 4. It is responsible for delayed allergic reaction, rejection of transplanted foreign tissue and lysis of tumour cells | 4. It is a major defence against bacterial infections |

## COMPARE ACTIVE AND PASSIVE IMMUNITY    2000, DU

| Active immunity | Passive immunity |
|---|---|
| 1. Antibodies are produced by the body's own immune system in response to antigens introduced naturally or artificially in the body | 1. It is produced by administration of readymade antibodies to the host |

*Contd.*

*Contd.*

| Active immunity | Passive immunity |
|---|---|
| 2. Active immunity develops after a latent period of 4 days to 4 weeks which is required for generation of antibodies and immunocompetent cells | 2. There is no latent period as passive immunity is effective immediately |
| 3. Due to immunological, memory the secondary response is more enhanced | 3. There is no immunological memory because subsequent administration of antibodies is less effective due to immune elimination |
| 4. This is long lasting | 4. This is short lasting |
| 5. This is more effective and confers better protection | 5. This is less effective and provides inferior immunity |
| 6. Active immunity is not applicable in immunodeficient individuals | 6. This is applicable in immunodeficient individuals |

## COMPARE INNATE AND ACQUIRED IMMUNITY    2 (2010)

**Innate immunity:** This is due to the genetic and constitutional make-up of an individual. Prior contact with micro-organisms and their products is not essential. It may be specific against a particular organism or non-specific. It is further divided into species, racial or individual immunity:

- **Species:** It is relative or total resistance to a pathogen shown by all the members of a species, e.g. all humans are resistant to plant pathogens or to some animal pathogens.
- **Racial:** Within a species there may be marked racial differences in resistance to infections, e.g. negroes are more susceptible to tuberculosis compared to whites.
- **Individual:** Different individuals in a race differ in their resistance to microbial infections, e.g. if one homozygous twin develops tuberculosis, there is a 75% chance that the other twin will also develop tuberculosis.

**Acquired immunity:** Most potential pathogens are checked by innate immunity before they establish an overt infection. If these defences are breached, the acquired immune system come into play. The resistance that an individual acquires during his lifetime is called acquired immunity. It is antigen specific and may be antibody-mediated or cell-mediated. It is further divided into active and passive immunity.

**(Refer to question on difference between active and passive immunity).**

## NATURAL KILLER CELLS                    2 (2005), 2 (2008)

They are large lymphocytes that make-up 10–15% of the circulating granulocytes. They are special type of cytotoxic lymphocytes also called **non-T, non-B-lymphocytes**. There are certain characteristic features of their action:

- They kill antigens without any prior sensitisation and without the involvement of major histocompatibility gene.
- They destroy cancerous cells, thus helping in prevention of cancerous conditions.
- They attack viruses killing antibody-coated viruses.
- Their activity is increased by interleukin-2 (IL-2).

They represent a primitive immune system from which the T and B cell system evolved. They represent an important first line of defence against viral infections combating the spread of diseases while more specific T and B cell responses are activated.

## IMMUNOGLOBULINS                         2.5 (2006)

The B-lymphocytes that are responsible for humoral immunity are divided into plasma cells and memory cells. The plasma cells secrete large quantities of antibodies that circulate in the γ-globulin fraction of plasma and are called immunoglobulins.

The immunoglobulins contain 4 polypeptide chains linked by disulphide bonds. There are two identical light chains and two identical heavy chains (Fig. 2.3).

Both the heavy and light chains are divided into a constant and variable regions. The amino acid sequence in the constant region being very similar in different types of immunoglobulins and are involved in the effector function of antibodies. The amino acid sequence of the variable region is distinct for each antibody and allows for vast number of unique antibodies each of which bind with different antigens with specific affinities.

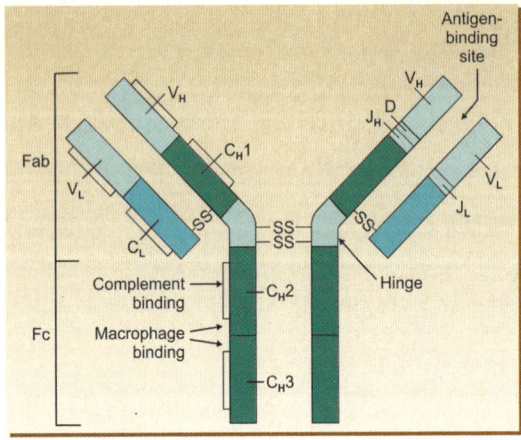

**Fig. 2.3:** Structure of immunoglobulin

Immunoglobulins are divided into **five types** based on the differences in the constant regions of their heavy chains. There are five types of heavy chains:

- γ (gamma): IgG
- α (alpha): IgA
- μ (mu): IgM
- δ (delta): IgD
- ε (epsilon): IgE

There are **two types of light chains κ (kappa) and λ (lambda)**. Both light chains in any antibody are either of kappa or lambda type:

- The major **functions** of each type of immunoglobulins are as follows:
  - **IgG:** These are involved in the secondary immune response against major antiviral, antibacterial and antifungal activity in the serum. They may also serve as opsonins and promote chemotactic activity of WBCs.
  - **IgA:** They occur in the plasma and are also secreted in the tears, saliva, intestinal juices, respiratory secretions and colostrum where they provide localised immunity.
  - **IgM:** They are mainly involved in the primary immune response, e.g. α and β antibodies of the ABO blood group system. In addition, they activate the complement system,

promoting phagocytosis and causing cell lysis by digesting holes in the cell membrane at the site of antibody attachment.
- **IgD:** They are present on the surface of B-lymphocytes with IgM, therefore, involved in antigen recognition
- **IgE:** They play an important role in allergies, skin infestations, parasitic infections and anaphylactic type of immediate hypersensitivity disorders.

## T-LYMPHOCYTES                                    2.5 (1993)

T-Lymphocytes are a type of lymphocytes which are processed in thymus gland to gain maturity for providing immunity against diseases. T-Lymphocytes are responsible for providing cellular immunity.

It provides defence against
1. Infections such as:
   - Viruses
   - Fungi
   - Some bacteria like tubercular bacteria
2. Responsible for delayed allergic reaction.
3. Rejection of foreign tissue transplant.
4. Defence against tumour cells.

There are **four** different types of T-lymphocytes:
1. **Helper or inducer T cells** regulate antibody production by B-lymphocytes.
2. **Suppressor T cells** regulate antibody production by B-lymphocytes.
3. **Cytotoxic or killer cells** destroy foreign cells.
4. **Memory T cells** converted to cytotoxic cells on subsequent encounter with foreign cells.

## HUMORAL IMMUNITY                                   4 (1985)

Humoral immunity is a defence against foreign antigens by elaborating antibodies against them in the circulation. Antigen may be bacteria, viruses or any other foreign protein.

Antibodies are produced by the B-lymphocytes, which are processed in gut related lymphoid tissues. Antibodies are γ-globulins and a specific type of antibody is produced in response to a specific foreign antigen.

## Steps Involved in Production of Antibodies

1. Antigen is ingested by the macrophages.
2. Macrophages expose antigen and protein of major histo-compatibility (MHC) on their surface.
3. Macrophages then contact and activate helper-T cells, i.e. $T_4$ cells.
4. $T_4$ cells in turn stimulate B-lymphocytes.
5. B-Lymphocytes are activated and they proliferate producing:
   a. Memory B cells
   b. Plasma cells
6. Plasma cells then secrete large amount of antibodies which are γ-globulins and are also known as immunoglobulins. B-Lymphocytes can recognise a large number of antigens and this property is innate. Accordingly, stem cells destined to form B-lymphocytes differentiate into a very large number of lymphocytes and each can recognize a different antigen and accordingly a specific antibody is produced by them.
7. Memory B cells respond quickly when body is exposed to the same antigen in future.

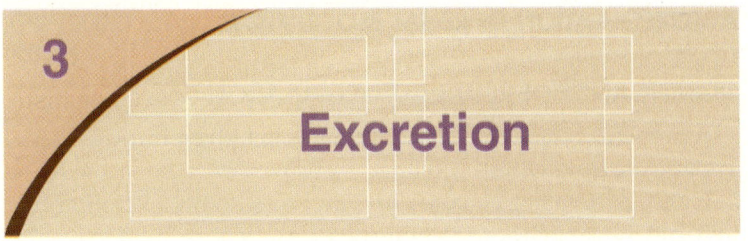

# Excretion

**3**

## NON-EXCRETORY FUNCTIONS OF THE KIDNEY   2 (2010)

The non-excretory functions of the kidney are:

1. *Homeostatic function*: Kidneys maintain constancy of the internal environment of the body by regulating the volume and composition of the ECF via the conservation or excretion of water and solutes. The major homeostatic mechanisms operate through the kidneys and the lungs to maintain the tonicity, volume and ionic composition particularly the $H^+$ ion concentration of ECF.

2. *Endocrine functions*: Kidneys have the following endocrine functions:

   - *Renin*: This is the major component of the renin-angiotensin-aldosterone mechanism that helps to regulate blood pressure.

   - *Renal erythropoietin:* Hypoxia causes release of erythropoietin from the kidney which promotes erythropoiesis.

   - **1, 25 DHCC (dihydrocholecalciferol)**

     Dietary vitamin $D_3$

     $\downarrow$

     25 HOCC (hydroxycholecalciferol)

     $\downarrow$ 1-$\alpha$ hydroxylase in the kidney PCT

     1,25 DHCC (biologically most active form of vitamin D)

3. *Gluconeogenic functions:* The kidneys acquire the important ability to synthesis and secrete glucose produced from non-carbohydrate sources in abnormal situations like prolonged starvation.

## AUTOREGULATION OF RENAL BLOOD FLOW   3 (2002)-IPU, 2.5 (2002)

### SIGNIFICANCE OF RENAL AUTOREGULATION

1. It prevents major blood flow changes in kidney during arterial pressure fluctuation.
2. It prevents major changes in water and solute excretion that could occur if there is a significant change in glomerular filtration rate. Autoregulation is not perfect and smaller changes occur with changes in arterial pressure but a major change is prevented. Autoregulation is not effective below 70 and above 180 mm Hg mean pressures. It is influenced by the activity of sympathetic nervous system and renin angiotensin system even within the autoregulatory range.

### EXPLAIN WHY THERE IS ALBUMINURIA IN NEPHRITIS   1 (2006)

The presence of significant amount of albumin in urine is called albuminuria. The normal amount of protein in urine is generally less than 100 mg/day and most of this is not filtered but comes from shed tubular cells. In nephritis, the glomerular membrane is damaged and negative charges in the glomerular wall are dissipated. Hence, albuminuria can occur for this reason without an increase in size of pores of the membrane.

### EXPLAIN WHY FILTRATION OF ANIONIC SUBSTANCE 4 nm IN DIAMETRE THROUGH THE GLOMERULAR CAPILLARIES IS LESS THAN HALF OF NEUTRAL SUBSTANCE OF THE SAME SIZE   1 (2003)-IPU

Neutral substances with effective molecular diametre of less than 4 nm are freely filtered and the filtration of neutral substances with diametres of more than 8 nm approaches zero. Sialoproteins in the glomerular capillary wall are negatively charged and studies with negatively and positively charged dextrans indicate that negative charges repel negatively charged substances in blood, with the result that filtration of anionic substances 4 nm in diametre is less than half of neutral substances of the same size.

### RENIN-ANGIOTENSIN SYSTEM   5 (1985, 1990, 1991)

Renin-angiotensin system comprises a protease hormone renin produced by the kidneys and a circulating peptide angiotensin.

Renin is secreted from the cells of juxtaglomerular apparatus. It acts on a circulating glycoprotein in a globulin fraction of plasma protein known as angiotensinogen or renin substrate. Angiotensinogen is converted to angiotensin I which is physiologically inactive.

Angiotensin I is converted to angiotensin II by the action of angiotensin converting enzyme (ACE). This enzyme is located in endothelial cells in various tissues but most of the conversion occurs in the lungs. Angiotensin II is a physiologically active substance with the following actions:

1. It is a potent vasoconstrictor and brings about an increase in systolic as well as diastolic blood pressure.
2. It acts on the adrenal cortex and stimulates the release of aldosterone.
3. Facilitates the release of norepinephrine from postganglionic sympathetic ganglion.
4. Causes contraction of mesangial cells in the kidney and thereby decreases GFR.
5. Increases water intake, by acting on thirst centre in brain and regulate ECF volume.

## Regulation of Renin-angiotensin System

i. Intra-renal baroreceptor mechanism: When intra-arteriolar pressure at level of JG cells is decreased, renin secretion is increased and *vice versa*. Renin secreting cells themselves act as baroreceptor.

ii. Cells of macula densa sense the amount of $Na^+$ and $Cl^-$ ions in the filtrate reaching the distal tubule and amount of renin secreted is inversely proportional to $Na^+$ and $Cl^-$, i.e. decrease amount of $Na^+$ and $Cl^-$ reaching this part of nephron stimulates renin secretion.

iii. Amount of angiotensin II controls renin secretion by negative feedback mechanisms by direct action on JG cells.

iv. Vasopressin also inhibits renin secretion.

v. Renal sympathetic nerves:
    1. By constricting afferent arterioles decreases intra-arteriolar pressure. It stimulates intrarenal baroreceptors and controls renin secretion.

2. By direct stimulation via $\beta_1$ adrenergic receptors on renin secreting granular cells. Direct affect is more sensitive. Renin secretion is promoted by certain stimuli:
   a. Sodium depletion
   b. Hypotension
   c. Haemorrhage
   d. Dehydration
   e. Cardiac failure
   f. Liver cirrhosis
   g. Psychological stimuli

### Applied Physiology of Renin-angiotensin System

Inhibitor of angiotensin converting enzymes, e.g. captopril is used in treating hypertension. Saralasin acts as a competitive inhibitor of angiotensin II at its receptor level. It is also used in treating hypertension.

### JUXTAGLOMERULAR APPARATUS      2.5 (1986)

Juxtaglomerular apparatus is a complex, present in the kidney. Its various components can be seen in (Fig. 3.1):

1. **Juxtaglomerular cells or JG cells:** These are specialized epithelial cells present in the tunica media of afferent arteriole,

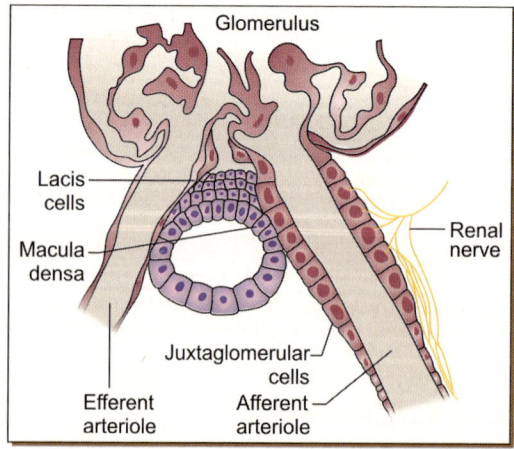

**Fig. 3.1:** Glomerulus, showing the juxtaglomerular apparatus

where it enters the glomerulus. They contain membrane lined renin granules.

2. **Macula densa:** A modified region of tubular epithelium of distal tubule, where it touches the arterioles of the glomerulus from which the tubule has originated. It is in close proximity to JG cells.

3. **Lacis cells:** Located in the triangular space bounded by afferent and efferent arterioles and macula densa. These cells are also known as **mesangial cells**. Juxtaglomerular complex secretes renin and plays an important role in regulation of BP.

## MECHANISM OF FORMATION OF URINE

### FILTRATION FRACTION                     2.5 (1986, 1989)

**Filtration fraction** is the ratio of glomerular filtration rate to renal plasma flow, e.g. if the normal GFR in an adult is 125 ml/min and renal plasma flow is 700 ml/min, therefore, the filtration fraction is 125/700 = 0.18

**Normal range:** 0.16 – 0.20

GFR varies less than RPF with changes in blood pressure.

If blood pressure falls, RPF decreases more than the decrease in GFR. This is because fall in blood pressure causes sympathetic stimulation with constriction of both afferent and efferent arterioles and consequent rise of GFR due to constriction of efferent arterioles. As GFR rises, filtration fraction is also increased.

### FACTORS AFFECTING GFR                     2.5 (2007)

The factors that affect the GFR include:

- **Changes in the renal blood flow:** GFR changes in linearity with changes in the RBF.
- **Changes in the hydrostatic pressure in the glomerular capillaries:**
  - **Changes in the blood pressure:** Changes in the hydrostatic pressure in the glomerular capillaries is directly proportional to BP below 60 mm Hg and above 220 mm Hg (as between 90 and 220 MBP the changes in hydrostatic pressure are subject to autoregulation)
  - **Afferent or efferent arteriolar constriction:** Constriction of the afferent arteriole reduces both the renal plasma flow

(RPF) and GFR, whereas efferent arteriole constriction reduces RPF but increases GFR. However, GFR tends to be maintained when efferent arteriolar constriction is greater than afferent arteriolar constriction.

- **Hydrostatic pressure in the Bowman's capsule:** Ureteral obstruction and oedema of kidneys in tight renal capsule increase the hydrostatic pressure inside Bowman's capsule which decreases the GFR as it opposes filtration.

- **Changes in the concentration of plasma proteins:** Hypoproteinemia decreases the colloidal osmotic pressure inside the glomerular capillaries which increases the GFR, whereas dehydration increases the colloidal osmotic pressure that decreases the GFR.

- **State of the glomerular membrane:** Glomerular membrane is absolutely impermeable to molecules more than 4 nm in diametre or molecular weight more than 70,000. Since sialoproteins present in the glomerular membrane are negatively charged hence filtration of cationic substances is slightly greater than that of neutral or anionic substance of the same size.

- **Size of the capillary bed:** Contraction of the mesangial cells decreases the surface area available for filtration. This decreases the $K_f$ (filtration coefficient) which then decreases the GFR.

- GFR decreases with advancing age due to decrease in renal plasma flow, cardiac output and renal tissue mass.

### WHAT IS GFR? WRITE A SHORT NOTE ON THE METHOD OF DETERMINATION OF GFR     2.5

GFR is the volume of glomerular filtrate formed each minute by all the nephrons in both the kidneys.

**Normal value:** 125 ml/min

It can be determined by finding out the renal clearance of a substance which satisfies the following criteria:

1. Freely filtered at glomerulus
2. Not reabsorbed in the tubules
3. Not secreted into the tubular lumen
4. Not metabolized in the kidney
5. Non-toxic

One such substance that meets all the above criteria is **inulin**.

Inulin clearance is calculated by infusing it at a steady rate and maintaining its concentration in blood. It is then determined by the following equation:

Clearance = **UV/P**

**U** – Urinary concentration of inulin in mg/ml

**V** – Urinary volume in ml/min

**P** – Plasma concentration of inulin in mg/ml

Value of inulin clearance normally is 125 ml/min.

## FACULTATIVE REABSORPTION IN KIDNEY            2.5 (1991)

Facultative reabsorption means varies reabsorption of a substance, e.g. reabsorption of water in collecting ducts of the kidney occurs under the influence of ADH secreted by the posterior pituitary. ADH facilitates water reabsorption by increasing permeability of tubular epithelial cells to water. Facultative reabsorption results in concentration of urine and hypertonic urine is excreted.

Facultative reabsorption of water varies according to body needs. If fluid intake is excessive, reabsorption is decreased and vice versa. This is achieved through regulation of ADH secretion.

## WHAT WILL HAPPEN AND WHY TO GLUCOSE REABSORPTION IN KIDNEYS IF BLOOD GLUCOSE LEVEL BECOMES 220 mg
### 2 (2012)

The renal threshold for glucose is the plasma level at which the glucose first appears in the urine in more than the normal minute amounts. The predicted value of this is 300 mg/dL but the actual renal threshold corresponds to 200 mg/dL of arterial plasma and 180 mg/dL of venous blood. The actual renal threshold is less than the predicted value for two reasons:

- The ideal curve shown in the diagram (Fig. 3.2) would be seen if the $Tm_G$ (transport maximum for glucose) in all the tubules was identical.

- If all the glucose were removed from each tubule when the amount filtered was less than the $Tm_G$.

This is not the case in humans, hence the actual curve is rounded and deviates considerably from the ideal curve which is called **splay** (Fig. 3.2). The magnitude of this splay is inversely

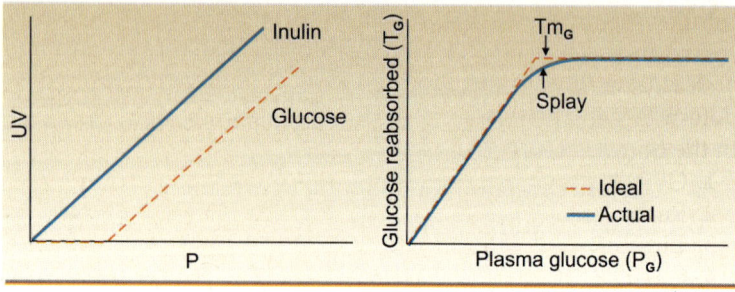

**Fig. 3.2:** Relation between plasma glucose level ($P_G$) and amount of glucose reabsorbed ($T_G$)

proportional to the avidity with which the transport mechanism binds the substance it transports.

Hence, at plasma glucose level of 220 mg/dL renal threshold for glucose is crossed and it appears in the urine.

## HANDLING OF GLUCOSE BY THE KIDNEY     3 (1992)

About 100 mg of glucose is filtered per minute at the glomerulus. Almost 100% of this is reabsorbed in the proximal convoluted tubules. Normally, glucose is not present in the urine. Reabsorption occurs by a process of secondary active transport along with sodium.

Up to a limit called the **Tubular maximum for glucose ($Tm_G$)** reabsorption is proportional to the amount filtered. $Tm_G$ is 375 mg/min and it corresponds to a plasma glucose level of 300 mg/dL, i.e. if plasma level of glucose is more than 300 mg/dL further reabsorption will not occur and some glucose will appear in the urine. The plasma level beyond which glucose appears in urine is called the renal threshold of glucose. The actual renal threshold of glucose is 200 mg/dL and not 300 mg/dL as predicted from $Tm_G$ value of 375 mg/min. The disparity between the two values is called 'splay' and is due to the following two facts:

  i. Not all the tubules are working at their maximum capacity at one time.

  ii. All the nephrons do not have $Tm_G$ of 375 mg/min.

## REGULATION OF SODIUM EXCRETION BY KIDNEY    2.5 (1986)

Amount of $Na^+$ excreted is regulated by the amount filtered at glomerulus, and reabsorbed as the filtrate passes through the tubules. The amount excreted is adjusted depending on the $Na^+$ intake and body needs.

$Na^+$ is the main ion present in the ECF which primarily determines ECF volume so a number of mechanisms are present in the body to regulate its excretion:

1. GFR is regulated by tubuloglomerular feedback.
2. Reabsorption is governed by glomerulotubular balance
3. Circulating levels of aldosterone
4. Circulating levels of atrial natriuretic peptide (ANP)
5. Renin-angiotensin mechanism
6. Rate of tubular secretion of $K^+$ and $H^+$.

## DESCRIBE BRIEFLY THE REGULATION OF GLOMERULAR FILTRATION. DESCRIBE ONE METHOD OF ITS DETERMINATION     **10** (1992, 1994)

Regulation of glomerular filtration occurs due to the presence of intrarenal autoregulatory mechanisms. These mechanisms basically regulate the renal blood flow and consequently glomerular capillary pressure and GFR. These mechanisms are directed towards the afferent arteriolar diametre which is the major site of vascular resistance determining blood flow, and hence glomerular filtration. So the regulation of glomerular filtration is secondary to regulation of renal blood flow. Following are the probable autoregulatory mechanisms for renal blood flow:

i. Myogenic mechanism
ii. Tubuloglomerular feedback (TG feedback)

### Myogenic Mechanism

It is similar to that present in any other autoregulatory vascular bed. Vascular smooth muscles are known to contract in response to increased stretch. An increased intra-arteriolar pressure distends the vessels, stretches the vessel wall and it contracts due to its inherent response, thereby constricting and increasing the resistance of the vessel. This leads to decreased blood flow and decreased vascular pressure and consequently decreased hydrostatic pressure in the afferent arterioles.

Kidney is able to maintain constant blood flow in spite of variation in mean arterial pressure between 80 and 150 mm Hg, with increase in pressure, resistance of arterioles increases and with decrease in pressure, resistance of arterioles decreases, thereby net filtration pressure is maintained at a constant level.

## TUBULOGLOMERULAR FEEDBACK 2.5 (2008)

It has been seen that each individual nephron can regulate the rate of glomerular filtration through tubuloglomerular feedback. There is a feedback from the tubule to regulate the flow of filtrate through proximal tubule and loop of Henle so that a constant load is delivered to the distal tubule. The sensor lies in the macula densa in distal tubule. Cells of macula densa sense the load of chloride or maybe $Na^+$ present in the filtrate and cause the release of renin and subsequently angiotensin II is formed. Angiotensin II causes the constriction of arterioles, specially the afferent arterioles and controls the vascular resistance, and subsequently glomerular filtration, so this mechanism also acts through renal arterioles.

## COMPARE MECHANISM OF WATER REABSORPTION IN THE PROXIMAL TUBULE AND COLLECTING DUCTS 2 (2004), (2011)

## COMPARE OBLIGATORY AND FACULTATIVE WATER REABSORPTION 2 (2002), 2 (2008)

In the PCT passive reabsorption of 60–70% water occurs along the osmotic gradient set by the active transport of solutes. Passive reabsorption of water in the PCT secondary to the active reabsorption of $Na^+$ is called **obligatory reabsorption of water**. **Aquaporin I** is involved in this process.

The reabsorption of water under the influence of ADH in collecting ducts is called **facultative water reabsorption**. Water is reabsorbed according to the needs of the body in the collecting ducts. In the collecting ducts the osmolality in the tubular fluid changes according to water permeability of the tubule. Antidiuretic hormone increases the permeability of the tubular epithelial cells to water and another 10–12% of filtered water is reabsorbed. **Aquaporin II** is involved in this process.

## COMPARE OSMOTIC AND WATER DIURESIS 2.5 (2006), 2 (2008), 2 (2010)

| Osmotic diuresis | Water diuresis |
|---|---|
| 1. It is produced due to presence of large quantities of unabsorbed solutes such as sodium, glucose, urea, etc. in the renal tubules when the | 1. It is produced by large amount of drinking water or hypotonic fluid. It begins 15 minutes after intake of a water load and reaches |

*Contd.*

*Contd.*

| Osmotic diuresis | Water diuresis |
|---|---|
| filtered load exceeds the maximum capacity of the tubules to reabsorb them | its maximum in 40 minutes |
| 2. The concentration of urine is that of plasma (300 mOsm/L) | 2. It is characterized by diuresis of dilute urine (50 mOsm/L) up to 20 L/day |
| 3. It is produced due to decreased water reabsorption in the PCT and loop of Henle | 3. It is produced due to inhibition of ADH secretion secondary to decrease in plasma osmolality after water is absorbed. Therefore, amount of water reabsorbed in the PCT of nephron is normal |

## DESCRIBE THE ROLE OF KIDNEY IN MAINTENANCE OF WATER BALANCE IN THE BODY     10 (1993)

## DESCRIBE THE TYPES AND MECHANISMS OF WATER REABSORPTION IN THE RENAL TUBULE. WHAT ARE THE FACTORS AFFECTING THIS MECHANISM     4 + 4 = 8 (2012)

Kidney plays an important and primary role in controlling water balance in the body. It functions by controlling daily output of urine. If body water is diminished due to less water intake, urinary load of waste metabolites is excreted in small urinary volume, i.e. more concentrated urine is passed and vice versa if water intake is large, more dilute urine is passed.

Kidney can produce a urine of osmolarity as low as 250 mOsm/L and a maximally concentrate urine of osmolarity 1400 mOsm/L.

However, a minimum volume of urine must be excreted to get rid of 600 mOsm/L of waste metabolites called the obligatory urine volume and is equal to 700 ml/day. Normally, a urine osmolarity of 700 mOsm with daily volume of 1.4 L is passed. Kidney is capable of producing a concentrated or dilute urine depending upon the body needs. Concentration of urine occurs under the effect of ADH produced from the posterior pituitary. ADH is responsible for the reabsorption of water in the collecting duct by increasing the permeability of epithelial cells to water.

For the reabsorption of water it is essential that the medullary interstitium is hyperosmolar.

Hyperosmolarity of interstitium is created by:

   i. Countercurrent multiplier system in loop of Henle.

   ii. Countercurrent exchanger present in vasa recta.

   iii. Smaller blood flow in the medulla.

**(These mechanisms have been explained earlier.)**

ADH secretion is controlled by the osmolarity of body fluids. If body fluids are hyperosmolar ADH secretion is stimulated, water reabsorption occurs and osmolarity is restored back to normal. Conversely, if body fluids become hypo-osmolar ADH is inhibited, water is not reabsorbed, osmolarity is restored and kidney produces dilute urine, i.e. water is lost in excess of solutes.

**Formation of dilute urine** Thick segment of the ascending limb of loop of Henle and first part of distal tubule are relatively impermeable to water and removal of solute in excess of water makes the fluid dilute so these are called the diluting segments of nephron.

Normally, 1.5 L of urine having osmolarity of 700 mOsm/L is passed per day and urine is not normally maximally concentrated.

## TUBULOGLOMERULAR FEEDBACK    **2 (2000, 2011)**

Feedback signals from tubules affect glomerular filtration. As flow rate through ascending limb of loop of Henle and early distal tubule increases, glomerular filtration in the same nephron decreases and vice versa. It aims at maintaining the constancy of load delivered to the distal tubule. Sensor for the response lies in macula densa. GFR is modified by changing the caliber of afferent arteriole (Fig. 3.3).

## GLOMERULOTUBULAR BALANCE    **2.5 (1993), 2 (2000)**

Proximal tubular reabsorption of solutes is adjusted so that a constant percentage rather than a constant amount is reabsorbed. Mechanism is specially prominent for $Na^+$ reabsorption. It is probably dependent on oncotic pressure in the peritubular capillaries but other factors may also be responsible (Fig. 3.3).

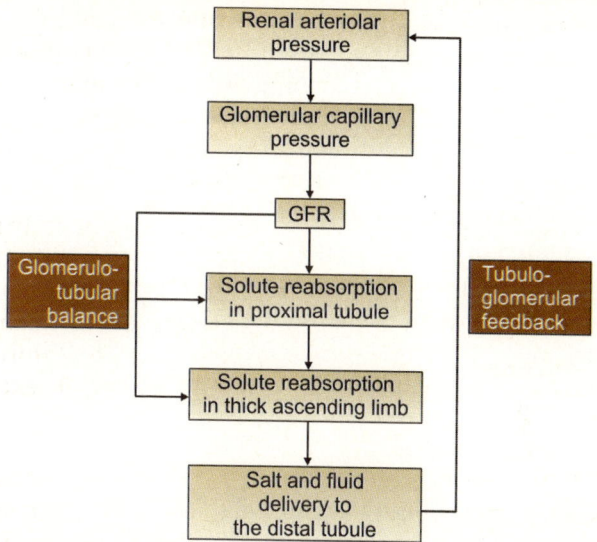

**Fig. 3.3:** Mechanism of glomerulotubular balance and tubuloglomerular feedback

## DESCRIBE THE MECHANISM OF URINE CONCENTRATION BY THE KIDNEY
**10** (1991)

## COUNTERCURRENT MECHANISM IN THE KIDNEY
**2** (2003)-IPU, **2** (2011)

Kidney has the power of producing urine of varying osmolarity. It can produce dilute or concentrated urine depending on body requirement.

Human kidneys can produce dilute urine of osmolarity between 50 mOsm/L to 1200 mOsm/L as compared to normal plasma osmolarity of 250 mOsm/L. Urine is concentrated as a result of reabsorption of water from the tubular fluid into the medullary interstitium in collecting ducts and DCT under the influence of ADH. Reabsorption of water occurs due to hyperosmolarity of the medullary interstitium.

In fact an osmotic gradient exists as we go deep from cortex to medulla. Greatest osmolarity exists in the innermost part of medulla corresponding to the site of renal papillae. Creation of medullary osmolarity is the function of loop of Henle of corticomedullary nephrons constituting the **countercurrent multiplier system**. The hyperosmolarity is maintained due to special features of vasa recta running close and parallel to the loop of Henle constituting the **countercurrent exchanger**.

Elaboration of concentrated urine thus occurs due to the presence of:

i. Countercurrent multiplier
ii. Countercurrent exchanger
iii. Relatively low medullary renal blood flow

All these operate to make the medullary interstitium hyperosmolar.

Anatomically collecting ducts are placed in close vicinity of the loop of Henle and vasa recta. Loop of Henle makes a hairpin bend at the tip of renal papillae.

## Generation of Medullary Osmolarity

This depends on the varying permeability to different substances along the loop of Henle:

1. Thick ascending limb actively transports chloride ions into the interstitium and $Na^+$ follows it.
2. Thick ascending limb is relatively impermeable to water, urea, NaCl, thereby limiting diffusion from the interstitium.
3. Descending limb is freely permeable to water, impermeable to ions and partially permeable to urea.
4. Thin ascending limb is permeable to NaCl, somewhat permeable to urea and impermeable to water.

As $Na^+$ and $Cl^-$ ions are actively transported out of thick ascending limb, hence the interstitium become hyperosmolar.

In medulla except for the ascending limb of Henle all other structures, i.e. descending limb, interstitium and collecting ducts are in osmotic equilibrium. Thus the descending limb acquires the hyperosmolarity of the interstitium. The effect is multiplied as more osmolar fluid from the proximal tubule enters the descending limb and pushes concentrated fluid down to hairpin bend, reaching maximum osmolarity at the bend.

**Role of urea:** The transport of urea occurs into the interstitium by the process of diffusion in collecting ducts as they are permeable to urea and urea concentration is high here as amount of filtrate decreases. This helps to create medullary hyperosmolarity.

## Maintenance of Hyperosmolarity of Interstitium

Medullary blood flow is relatively small in comparison to that of cortex and helps to maintain the hyperosmolarity.

Further, there exists an exchanger system in the vasa recta. Blood enters the vasa recta at osmolarity of 300 mOsm/L as it flows deeper and deeper into the medulla $Na^+$ and chloride ions diffuse into the descending limb and water moves out. After the hairpin bend is reached the process is reversed and ions move into the descending limb. Thus, ions are returned back and water is lost. Hence the water is reabsorbed from the collecting ducts into the hyperosmolar interstitium and the urine is concentrated (Fig. 3.4).

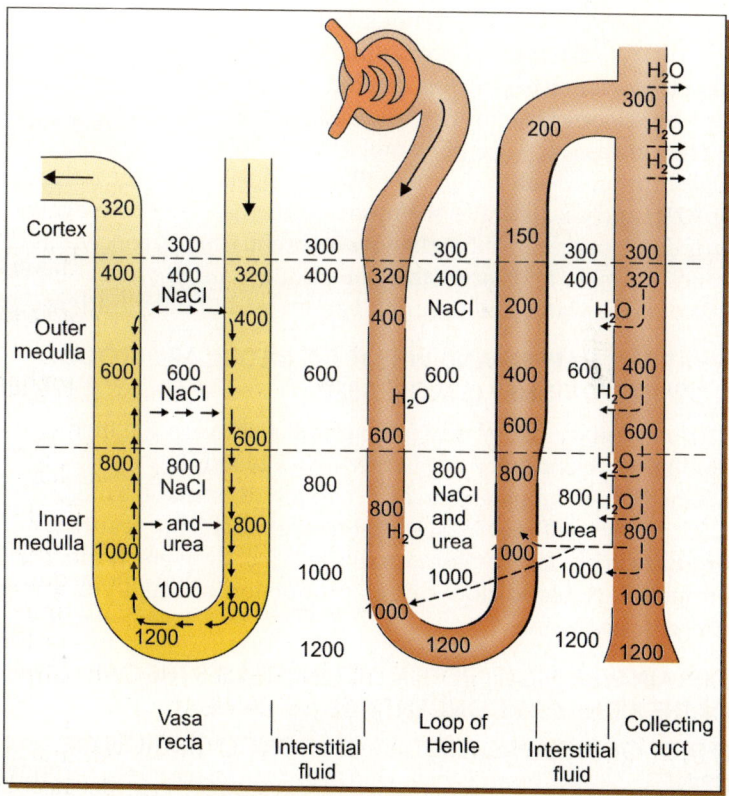

**Fig. 3.4:** The countercurrent mechanism for concentrating urine (values are in mOsm/L)

## WHAT WILL HAPPEN AND WHY IF THERE IS NO COUNTER-CURRENT EXCHANGER IN THE KIDNEY          2.5 (1991)

Countercurrent exchanger in the kidney is the function of capillary loops present in close proximity and parallel to the loop of Henle present in corticomedullary nephrons. This capillary loop is called **vasa recta**.

The two limbs of vasa recta run parallel and close to each other and lie in the hyperosmolar medullary interstitium. The two limbs of vasa recta act as countercurrent exchanger. Blood enters the vessel loop at an osmolarity of 300 mOsm/L. As it flows down deeper into medulla, $Na^+$ from the hyperosmotic interstitium diffuses into the descending limb but diffuses back into interstitium from ascending limb after the bend in the loop. As a result electrolytes are not carried into the venous circulation but diffuse back to medullary interstitium and maintain its hyperosmolar state. The hyperosmolar state which is created by countercurrent multiplier system of loop of Henle is not allowed to be dissipated by **exchange system** of vasa recta. Hyperosmolarity of interstitium facilitates the reabsorption of water from the collecting ducts under the influence of ADH and concentrates the urine, thus conserving body water.

If this countercurrent exchanger is absent, urinary concentration is not possible and large amount of dilute urine with valuable loss of body water will occur and could lead to dehydration.

## WHAT WILL HAPPEN AND WHY IF THE MEDULLARY BLOOD FLOW IN THE KIDNEY IS INCREASED          1 (2006)

The medullary osmolality is inversely related to the medullary blood flow. Hence increase in medullary blood flow either due to haemodilution or increase in ECF volume decreases the medullary osmolality and decreases water reabsorption resulting in production of a large volume of dilute urine. Conversely, decrease in medullary blood flow causes production of small volume of concentrated urine.

## EXPLAIN WHY HIGH PROTEIN DIET INCREASES THE CAPACITY OF THE KIDNEY TO CONCENTRATE THE URINE          1 (2003)-IPU

## EFFECT OF HIGH PROTEIN DIET ON CONCENTRATION OF URINE          (2001)

Urea contributes to the establishment of osmotic gradient in the medullary pyramids and to the ability to form a concentrated urine in the collecting ducts. The amount of urea in the medullary interstitium in addition to the amount of urea in the urine varies with the amount of urea filtered and this in turn depends upon the dietary intake of proteins. Therefore, a high protein intake increases the ability of the kidneys to concentrate the urine.

## ACIDIFICATION OF URINE

### CHEMICAL REACTIONS INVOLVE IN REABSORPTION OF BICARBONATE IN KIDNEY 2.5

Bicarbonate reabsorption is an active process. It is accompanied by secretion of $H^+$ ions. It occurs in proximal tubules and collecting ducts. Reactions involved are as follows:

| Tubular lumen | Tubular epithelium | Interstitial fluid | Blood |
|---|---|---|---|
| $CO_2 \longrightarrow$ | Metabolism | | |
| | $CO_2 + H_2O$ | | |
| | $\downarrow$ CA | | |
| | $H_2CO_3$ | | |
| | $\downarrow$ | | |
| $H^+ \xleftarrow[\text{Transport}]{\text{Active}}$ | $H^+ + HCO_3^- \xrightarrow{\text{Diffusion}}$ | $HCO_3^- \longrightarrow$ | $HCO_3^-$ |

### WHAT HAPPENS AND WHY TO URINE pH FOLLOWING A MEAL 1 (2005)

When gastric acid secretion is increased following a meal, sufficient $H^+$ may be secreted to raise the $HCO_3^-$ in gastric venous blood which contributes a greater amount of $HCO_3^-$ to the systemic circulation and pH of systemic blood rises. This is called **postprandial alkaline tide** which is characterized by high pH of urine.

### ANION GAP 2.5 (2008)

**Anion gap** refers to the difference between the concentration of cations other than sodium and anions other than $Cl^-$ and $HCO_3^-$ in the plasma. It includes proteins in the anionic form, $HPO_4^{2-}$, $SO_4^{2-}$ and organic acids.

   **Normal value:** 12 mEq/L

Value is increased under the following conditions:

1. When the plasma value of K $^+$, Ca$^{2+}$, Mg$^{2+}$ is decreased
2. Concentration (or charge on) plasma proteins is increased
3. Organic anions or lactate or foreign anions accumulate in the blood: Metabolic acidosis due to ketoacidosis, lactic acidosis and other forms of acidosis in which organic anions are increased.

## Value is Decreased

1. Cations are increased
2. Plasma albumin is decreased

## ROLE OF KIDNEY IN REGULATION OF pH          5 (1994)

The body remains in a steady state with respect to production of fixed acid and excretion of H$^+$ by the kidneys and the pH is thus maintained at a constant rate. Source of fixed acid in the body is mainly protein metabolism. The excretion of H$^+$ from fixed acids in the body is indirect and the kidneys play a major role. H$^+$ ions produced in the body are immediately buffered by bicarbonate ions of the blood buffer system resulting in loss of bicarbonate ions which need to be restored. Kidney regulates the body pH by increasing or decreasing bicarbonate reabsorption which is accompanied by the secretion of H$^+$ by tubular cells.

Chemical reactions involved are as follows:

| Blood | ECF | Epithelial cell | Tubular lumen |
|---|---|---|---|
| $HCO_3^- \longleftarrow$ | $HCO_3^- \longleftarrow$ | $HCO_3^- + H^+ \longrightarrow$ | $H^+$ |
| | | $\uparrow$ | |
| | | $H_2CO_3$ | |
| | | $\uparrow$ | |
| | | $CO_2 + H_2O$ | |

Hence, H$^+$ are secreted by epithelial cells and bicarbonate ions are reabsorbed in the ECF and finally to blood. $HCO_3^-$ is thus restored and pH is brought to normal.

If more bicarbonate ions increase in the ECF, more is present in the blood and more is filtered at the glomerulus and excreted. Secretion of H$^+$ by the tubules and hence reabsorption of bicarbonate ions is less and pH is restored to normal.

Hydrogen ions secretion by the kidneys, however, has a limiting value and beyond that no more secretion can occur. This limit corresponds to a urinary pH of 4.5 called the **limiting pH** which can be reached rapidly and further secretion of $H^+$ by tubular cell will stop. However, certain buffer system are present in the kidney to buffer these secreted hydrogen ions so that the process continues.

Buffer system in kidney are:

a. Bicarbonate buffer system
b. Dibasic phosphate system
c. Ammonia synthesised by tubular cells, i.e. ammonia buffer system.

## REACTION WITH VARIOUS BUFFER MECHANISMS

| Filtrate in lumen | Tubular epithelium | Blood |
|---|---|---|
| $NaHCO_3$ | | |
| $Na^+ + HCO_3^-$ | | |
| $HCO_3^- + H^+$ ⟵——— $H^+ + HCO_3^-$ ———⟶ | | $HCO_3^-$ |
| ↓ ↑ | | |
| $H_2CO_3 \leftarrow H_2O + CO_2 \leftarrow$———$CO_2 + H_2O$ | | |
| Bicarbonate buffer | | |
| $Na_2HPO_4$ | | |
| $Na^+ \ Na^+HPO^- + H^+$ ⟵——— $H^+ + HCO_3^-$ ———⟶ | | $HCO_3^-$ |
| ↓ | | |
| $NaH_2PO_4$ | | |
| Phosphate buffer | | |
| $NH_4^+$ ⟵——— $H^+ + NH_3$ ———⟶ | | $HCO_3^-$ |
| $NH_4^+ + A^-$ | | |
| Ammonia buffer | | |

## RENAL FUNCTION TESTS

### TESTS FOR GLOMERULAR FUNCTION                              2 (2005)

The tests for glomerular function include:

- **Inulin clearance:** 126 ml/min.
- **Creatinine clearance:** Although inulin clearance can be used to measure GFR but in clinical practice it is more common to determine the endogenous creatinine clearance as an estimate of GFR. Its determination does not require administration of exogenous creatinine as it is a measure of muscle metabolism. Normal range of creatinine clearance is 90–110 ml/min.
- **Measurement of renal blood flow (RBF) and renal plasma flow (RPF):** RBF can be measured by applying the Fick's principle to the kidneys, i.e. amount of substance taken up by an organ per unit time is equal to the arteriovenous difference for the substance across the organ times the blood flow. Since the kidney filters plasma, the RPF equals the amount of a substance excreted per unit time divided by the renal arteriovenous difference of the substance.

  Measurement of RPF is done by using the clearance value of **Diodrast and Para-amino hippuric acid (PAH)**.
- **Measurement of filtration fraction (FF):** This is the ratio of GFR: RPF and normal value varies between 0.16 and 0.20.

## URINARY BLADDER

### PHYSIOLOGICAL BASIS OF DIURETICS                          3 (2004)-IPU

| Agent | Mechanism of action |
|---|---|
| Water | Inhibits vasopressin secretion |
| Ethanol | Inhibits vasopressin secretion |
| Antagonists of $V_2$ vasopressin receptors such as astolvaptan | Inhibits action of vasopressin on collecting duct |
| Large quantities of osmotically active substances such as mannitol and glucose | Produce osmotic diuresis |
| Xanthines such as caffeine and theophylline | Decrease tubular reabsorption of $Na^+$ and increase GFR |
| Acidifying salts such as | Supply acid load; $H^+$ is buffered, |

*Contd.*

*Contd.*

| Agent | Mechanism of action |
|---|---|
| $CaCl_2$ and $NH_4Cl$ | but an anion is excreted with $Na^+$ when the ability of the kidney to replace $Na^+$ with $H^+$ is exceeded. |
| Carbonic anhydrase inhibitors such as acetazolamide (Diamox) | Decrease $H^+$ secretion, with resultant increase in $Na^+$ and $K^+$ excretion |
| Metolazone (Zaroxolyn), thiazides such as chloro-thiazide (Diuril) | Inhibit the $Na^+$–$Cl^-$ cotransporter in the early portion of the distal tubule |
| Loop diuretics such as fur-osemide (Lasix), ethacrynic acid (Edecrin), and bumetanide | Inhibit the $Na^+$–$K^+$–$2Cl^-$ cotransporter in the medullary thick ascending limb of the loop of Henle |
| $K^+$-retaining natriuretics such as spironolactone (Aldactone) triamterene (Dyrenium), and amiloride (Midamor) | Inhibit $Na^+$–$K^+$ exchange in the coll-ecting ducts by inhibiting the action of aldosterone (spironolactone) or by inhibiting the ENaCs (amiloride) |

## CYSTOMETROGRAM (2001)

The relationship between intravesical pressure and volume in the urinary bladder is studied. A catheter is inserted into the bladder and it is emptied. Then intravesical pressure is recorded while the bladder is filled with 50 ml increments of water **(cystometry)**.

The plot between the intravesical pressure and the volume of fluid in the bladder is called **cystometrogram**.

- The curve shows an initial slight rise in pressure when the first increments in volume are produced, a long nearly flat segment as further increments are produced and a sudden sharp rise in pressure as the micturition reflex is triggered. These three components are called $I_a$, $I_b$ and II (Fig. 3.5).
- The first urge to void is felt at about 150 ml and a marked sense of fullness is felt at about 400 ml of bladder volume.
- The flatness of segment $I_b$ is a manifestation of **law of Laplace** which states that distending pressure ($P$) in a spherical hollow viscus is equal to twice the wall tension ($T$) divided by the radius ($R$), i.e. $P = 2T/R$. In case of the bladder, the tension increases as the organ fills but so does the radius. Therefore, the pressure increase is slight until the organ is relatively full.

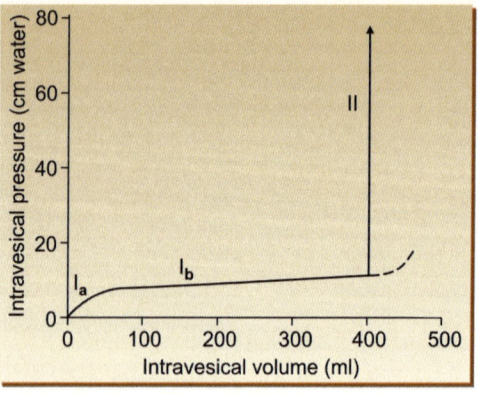

Fig. 3.5: Cystometrogram in normal human

## MICTURITION REFLEX                    2.5 (2006)

Micturition is fundamentally a spinal reflex facilitated and inhibited by higher brain centres and like defecation is subject to voluntary facilitation and inhibition.

- The bladder smooth muscles have some inherent contractile activity, however, when its nerve supply is intact stretch receptors in the bladder wall initiate a reflex contraction that has a lower threshold than the inherent contractile response of the muscle. The reflex is integrated in the sacral portion of the spinal cord. About 300–400 ml of urine in the bladder initiates reflex contraction in the bladder due to stimulation of stretch receptors located in the wall of urinary bladder (Fig. 3.6).

- Afferents from stretch receptors travel via pelvic nerves (parasympathetic) to spinal centre.

- Efferents via pelvic nerves cause contraction of detrusor muscles along with the relaxation of the internal sphincter.

- External sphincter is innervated by somatic nerves and is under voluntary control.

- The sympathetic nerves to the bladder play no role in micturition, but they do mediate contraction of the bladder muscle that prevents semen from entering the bladder at the time of ejaculation.

- Higher control of micturition reflex:

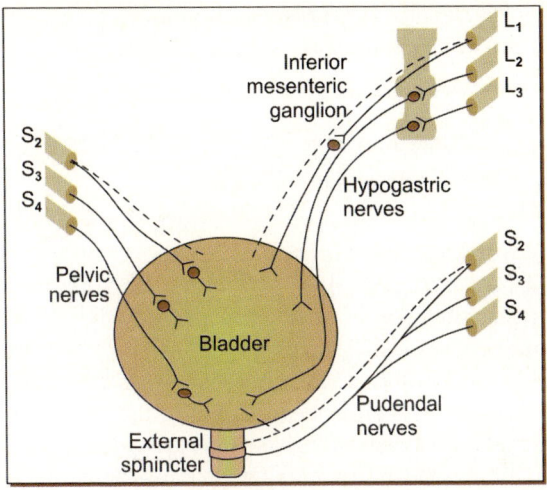

**Fig. 3.6:** Innervation of the bladder

– **Facilitatory areas:** Pontine region and posterior hypo-thalamus

– **Inhibitory area:** Midbrain

– The bladder can be made to contract by voluntary facilitation of spinal voiding reflex when it contains only a few ml of urine. Voluntary contraction of the abdominal muscles aids the expulsion of urine by increasing the intra-abdominal pressure, but voiding can be initiated without straining when the bladder is nearly full.

## WHAT WILL HAPPEN AND WHY IF URINARY BLADDER IS COMPLETELY DENERVATED                                          1 (2010)

- This is produced when both afferent and efferent nerves to the bladder are destroyed as is seen in tumours of **cauda equina** or **filum terminale**.
- The bladder is distended and flaccid for a while, gradually however the muscles of the decentralized bladder becomes active, with many contraction waves that expel dribbles of urine out of the bladder.
- The bladder wall becomes shrunken and the bladder wall hypertrophic. The hyperactive state seen in this condition

suggests the development of denervation hypersensitivity even though the neurons interrupted are preganglionic rather than postganglionic.

## WHAT WILL HAPPEN AND WHY TO MICTURITION IN COMPLETE TRANSECTION OF THE SPINAL CORD                    2 (2012)

Complete transection of the spinal cord leads to spinal shock where the bladder is flaccid and unresponsive. It becomes overfilled and urine dribbles through the sphincters leading to overflow incontinence. After spinal shock has passed, the voiding reflex returns but without any voluntary control or inhibition and facilitation from higher centres. In some cases the voiding reflex becomes hyperactive, bladder capacity is reduced and the bladder wall becomes hypertrophic **(spastic neurogenic bladder)**. This hyperactivity may be made worse by or caused by infection in the urinary bladder in some cases.

## AUTOMATIC BLADDER                    2.5 (2003)-IPU

After a few days to weeks of spinal injury that has deprived the micturition reflex of higher centres, the reflex activity starts returning. During this phase the bladder fills to a threshold and then empties to a considerable extent as a result of bladder contraction, without any voluntary control. Hence it is an automatic bladder. However, gradually the patient learns to initiate micturition by stroking the skin in genital area and can empty the bladder periodically at a desirable time and place even without voluntary control.

## ATONIC BLADDER

The bladder is flaccid and relaxed all the time. It is seen for a few days or weeks following lesion in neuraxis that interrupts the control of the brainstem and higher centres on sacral segment concerned with micturition reflex.

It is a state of "shock" when spinal cord is suddenly deprived of regulation from the higher centres. It is a more prominent feature when afferent fibres from bladder are involved and micturition reflex cannot operate. An atonic bladder keeps on filling till it cannot contain any more urine. Then it forces a little urine out of urethra passively known as **overflow incontinence**.

## NEUROGENIC BLADDER

Bladder is irritable and empties small quantities of urine at a time repeatedly. It is unable to control the onset of micturition satisfactorily. It occurs due to incomplete destruction of some of the neural pathways.

## EXPLAIN WHY IN URETERIC OBSTRUCTION GFR DECREASES
1 (2004)

Ureteric obstruction increases pressure within the capsule of the kidney that opposes filtration pressure, hence the GFR decreases.

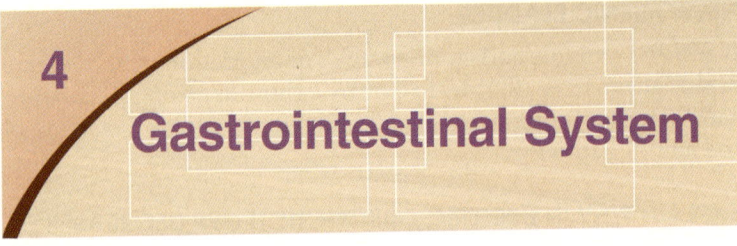

# 4 Gastrointestinal System

## FUNCTIONS OF SALIVA
2.5 (2006)

**Saliva has the following functions:**

1. It contains salivary α-amylase also called ptyalin that aids in the digestion of starch producing α-limiting dextrins and maltose. It can digest starch only after the starch granules have been burst by the process of cooking. It acts in a neutral or weakly acidic pH and can digest starch to maltose. Amylase digestion can continue in the stomach till arrested by the acidity of the gastric contents.

2. Mucin—present in saliva has the following functions:
   a. It lubricates the food helping in mastication and swallowing
   b. Protects the oral mucosa
   c. Facilitates speech by facilitating movements of the lips and tongue.

3. It keeps the mouth moist and serves as a solvent for molecules to stimulate the taste buds.

4. It protects the oral mucosa from infection and caries due to lysozymes present in saliva which kill the bacteria. IgA that provides immunological defence against bacteria and viruses and lactoferrin which binds iron and arrests the bacterial multiplication.

5. Buffers and 'prolin' rich proteins in saliva help to bind toxic tannins and maintain the oral pH at 7.0. At this pH saliva is saturated with calcium, therefore, teeth do not loose calcium to oral fluids. Hence, it protects the tooth enamel.

6. Buffers in the saliva help to neutralise the gastric acid and relieve heartburn when gastric acid is regurgitated back into the oesophagus.

7. It contains somatostatin, glucagon, and in some species renin and nerve growth factors but their function is not known.
8. It acts as a vehicle for excretion of certain drugs, alcohol, morphine and certain inorganic ions: $K^+$, $Ca^{2+}$, $HCO_3^-$, iodine and thiocyanate.

## MOUTH AND OESOPHAGUS

### DEGLUTITION
**2 (2003)-IPU**

- Swallowing also called deglutition is a reflex response that is triggered by afferent impulses in the trigeminal, glosso-pharyngeal and vagus nerves from the receptors in the oral cavity, palate and pharynx. These impulses are integrated in the nucleus of tractus solitarius and the nucleus ambiguous. The efferent fibres pass to the pharyngeal musculature and the tongue via the trigeminal, facial and hypoglossal nerves.
  - It is divided into three phases:
    1. Phase I: Oral stage (voluntary)
    2. Phase II: Pharyngeal stage (involuntary)
    3. Phase III: Oesophageal stage (involuntary)

### Phase I

Swallowing is initiated by the voluntary action of collecting the oral contents on the tongue and propelling them backwards into the pharynx.

### Phase II: (A number of reflex actions take place in this phase)

- This starts as a wave of involuntary contractions in the pharyngeal muscles that pushes the material in the oesophagus.
- Soft palate is elevated and thrown against posterior pharyngeal wall to close of the nasal cavity.
- Inhibition of respiration and glottic closure are also a part of this reflex.

### Phase III

- A peristaltic ring contraction of the oesophageal muscles forms behind the material which is then swept down the oesophagus at a speed of 4 cm.

- In the upright position in humans, liquids and semi-solid foods fall by gravity to the lower oesophagus ahead of the peristaltic wave.

## EXPLAIN WHY APNOEA OCCURS IN DEGLUTITION    1 (2007)

During the pharyngeal stage (Stage II) of swallowing larynx rises with elevation of the hyoid bone, vocal cords are approximated and breathing is temporarily stopped reflexly. This is called **deglutition apnoea**. It helps to prevent aspiration of food in the larynx and guides the food towards the oesophagus.

## FUNCTIONS OF LOWER OESOPHAGEAL SPHINCTER   2.5 (1991)

A circular smooth muscle layer at lower end of oesophagus (2.5 cm from its junction with stomach) functions as lower oesophageal sphincter. It normally remains tonically contracted and prevents acidic contents of stomach from entering the oesophagus and damaging it. However, during the act of swallowing as peristalsis passes through the oesophagus, there is receptive relaxation of this part ahead of the wave of peristalsis. A condition when this functional sphincter fails to relax as food passes through the oesophagus is called *Achalasia Cardia*. Sometimes the sphincter does not contract adequately, thereby permitting the reflux of gastric contents producing heart burn and oesophagitis.

## STOMACH

### MECHANISM OF VOMITING                          2.5 (1992)

Vomiting is a reflex phenomenon by which gastric contents are thrown out through the mouth. It is initiated by irritation of upper GIT mucosa. Vomiting centre is situated in the reticular formation of medulla at the level of the olivary nuclei. Afferent impulses are relayed by visceral afferents in vagus and sympathetic nerves. After integration efferent pathways are relayed to various visceral and somatic structures and following reflex activity is initiated:

1. The glottis closes (prevents aspiration of contents to the trachea).
2. Respiration is held in mid-inspiration (chest is held in fixed position).
3. Abdominal muscles contract and increase intra-abdominal pressure.

4. Oesophagus and gastric cardiac sphincters relax and abdominal contents are thrown into oesophagus and ejected from the mouth.

Vomiting centre can also be stimulated by emotional stimuli from higher centres, e.g. nauseating smells and sickening sights.

Head injury and increased intracranial tension causes vomiting by stimulating vomiting centre. Close to the vomiting centre is a chemosensitive area called **chemoreceptor trigger zone** which when stimulated by certain drugs and toxins causes vomiting.

Vomiting in general ejects harmful substances from the stomach and protects the body.

## MUCOSAL BARRIER IN THE STOMACH                    (2001)

The surface epithelium of the gastric mucosa consists of columnar or mucous cells that secrete mucus and $HCO_3^-$. Mucous is made up of glycoproteins (mucins). It is an alkaline gel like substance which coats the mucosa of the stomach and lubricates the food.

The mucus along with $HCO_3^-$ plus tight junctions between the mucosal cells forms the **mucosal bicarbonate barrier** that serves a protective function preventing damage to the mucosa of the stomach and duodenum by acid or peptic digestion. Any mechanical stimulation of surface mucosa and prostaglandins increases the secretion of mucus and bicarbonate ions.

## GASTRIC EMPTYING                               2.5 (1991)
## EMPTYING OF STOMACH CONTENTS                    2.5 (2004)

It is the process of transfer of gastric contents into the duodenum through the pylorus. At the junction of duodenum and pylorus of stomach, the pyloric sphincter is present which is tonically contracted.

As the stomach gets filled and hence distended, peristaltic contractions start in the midpoint of the body of the stomach and proceed towards the antrum. The contractions become stronger as chyme reaches the antrum. Antrum, pylorus and first part of duodenum function as a single unit and contract sequentially. Contractions of antrum ahead of gastric contents squeeze small amount of contents into the duodenum. This peristaltic wave is called **pyloric pump** and it relaxes the pyloric sphincter also. This

**pyloric pump** is stimulated by gastric peristalsis and gastrin and inhibited by duodenal factors:

1. Distension of the duodenum
2. Hyperacidity of duodenal contents
3. Hyperosmolarity in duodenum
4. Products of protein and fat digestion in duodenum
5. GIT hormone, viz. cholecystokinin, secretin and GIP.

Emptying is also influenced by the type of food. The rate of emptying being highest with carbohydrates followed by proteins and slowest with fatty food.

## MECHANISM OF HCl FORMATION BY THE STOMACH  10 (1985)

HCl is one of the major constituents of the gastric secretion. It is formed by oxyntic (or parietal) cells lining gastric glands. It is formed inside the intracellular canaliculi that project from the lumen of the glands deep into cells. Microvilli are present at the membrane of canaliculi increasing its surface area.

### Chemical Reactions for the Secretion of HCl (Fig. 4.1)

- Source of $H^+$ is the dissociation of carbonic acid formed in cells by hydration of $CO_2$ present in the cell in the presence of enzyme carbonic anhydrase.
- $H^+$ so generated are actively transported out of the cells against concentration gradient into the lumen of canaliculi. The energy for transport is provided by $H^+ - K^+$-ATPase present in the mucosal membrane.
- Parietal cells have abundant enzyme carbonic anhydrase which catalyzes the hydration of $CO_2$ to $H_2CO_3$ and stores of $H_2CO_3$ to provide $H^+$ are replenished.
- $HCO_3^-$ formed as a result of dissociation of carbonic acid, diffuses out of the cell into the interstitium and is replaced by $Cl^-$ which enters the cell from interstitial fluid. $Cl^-$ are actively transported into the lumen and combine with $H^+$ to form HCl.
- $HCO_3^-$ from interstitium enters the blood and hence blood leaving the stomach has high $HCO_3^-$ content and is alkaline.

As gastric secretion is stimulated after a meal, large amount $H^+$ are secreted which consequently raises the $HCO_3^-$ concentration of blood. This increased amount of $HCO_3^-$ are excreted by the kidneys making the urine highly alkaline, called

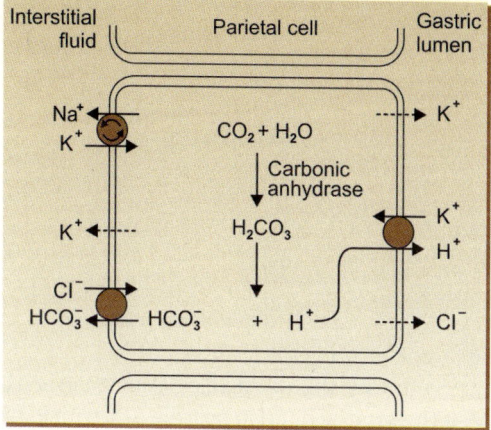

**Fig. 4.1:** HCl secretion by parietal cells in the stomach

**postprandial alkaline tide**. Acid secretion is elevated by the following factors:

i. Histamine via $H_2$ receptors
ii. ACh through $M_1$ muscarinic receptors
iii. Gastrin via gastrin receptors.

All the three types of receptors are present in the membrane of parietal cells, and act by increasing the activity of $H^+–K^+$-ATPase for transport of hydrogen ions into the gastric lumen.

Histamine is secreted by mucosal cells resembling the mast cells, ACh from postganglionic cholinergic neurons and gastrin by G cells present in the mucosa of the antrum. They interact to control HCl secretion.

## DESCRIBE THE COMPOSITION, FUNCTION AND REGULATION OF GASTRIC SECRETION                    10 (1993)
## REGULATION OF GASTRIC SECRETION  2.5 (1980), 2.5 (2003)-IPU
## NERVOUS REGULATION OF GASTRIC JUICE SECRETION (1991)
### Composition of Gastric Secretion

Gastric juice is secreted by various types of gastric glands in the stomach mucosa.

Volume – 2.5–3 L/day
Reaction – strongly acidic, pH 1–2
Water – 99.5%
Solids – 0.5%

### Electrolytes

**Cations:** $Na^+$, $K^+$, $H^+$, $Mg^{2+}$
**Anions:** $Cl^-$, $HCO_3^-$, $HPO_4^{2-}$, $SO_4^{2-}$

### Organic
### Enzymes

  i. Pepsinogens
  ii. Rennin
  iii. Gastric lipase
  iv. Mucus
  v. Intrinsic factor

- HCl secreted by the oxyntic cells of gastric glands in the body of the stomach, (also secrete—intrinsic factor)
- Pepsinogen by chief cells of gastric glands.
- Mucus is of 2 types:
  - i. Visible—secreted by surface epithelium.
  - ii. Soluble—secreted by mucus secreting cells in neck of gastric glands throughout the stomach.

### Functions of Gastric Secretion

### Digestive Functions

  i. **Pepsinogen:** Pepsinogen is converted into pepsin by HCl, which is the active form and acts as a proteolytic enzyme. It acts on the proteins and polypeptides. It acts on the linkages between aromatic and aliphatic amino acids in an acidic medium.

  ii. **Gastric lipase:** Acts only on butter fat, i.e. butyric acid.

  iii. **Hydrochloric acid:** It has the following actions
    a. Activates pepsinogen to pepsin.
    b. Provides an acidic medium for the action of pepsin.
    c. May function as a bacteriocidal agent to kill the bacteria present in food.

  iv. **Mucus:** Along with bicarbonates an unstirred layer is formed along surface of the mucosa and protects mucosal cells from damage by gastric acid and pepsin digestion. Soluble mucus helps in lubricating the food and aids in its smooth passage through the stomach.

  v. **Intrinsic factor:** Essential for the absorption of vitamin $B_{12}$ from small intestine.

## Regulation of Gastric Secretion

Neural and hormonal factors influence the gastric secretion.

  I. Neural regulation is through:
- i. Local reflexes
- ii. Parasympathetic regulation through the vagus nerve.

 II. Hormonal regulation is discussed under the different phases of gastric juice secretion, namely: Cephalic, gastric and intestinal phases.

### 1. Cephalic phase

Gastric secretions occurs not only due to the presence of food in the mouth but also at the thought, smell and sight of food. This is a vagally mediated reflex. Afferent impulses either arise in the mouth or higher centres (psychic juice). Efferent fibres arise from dorsal nucleus of vagus. Juice so produced is highly acidic and rich in pepsin. Secretion occurs after a latency of 5–7 minutes, reaches a peak after 1 hr and continues up to 3 hrs.

### 2. Gastric phase

As food reaches the stomach, further secretion of gastric juice occurs known as the gastric phase. Secretion occurs due to the stretch of the mucosa which reflexly stimulates secretion. In addition products of protein digestion cause the release of hormone gastrin from antral mucosal G cells. Gastrin in turn stimulates gastric glands and augments the secretion of HCl. Neural and hormonal stimulations are synergistic in action in this phase.

### 3. Intestinal phase

As the chyme enters small intestines, a number of hormones are secreted, namely gastrin, secretin and GIP (gastric inhibitory peptide) in response to the products of protein and fat digestion. Secretin and GIP inhibit acid and pepsin secretion.

III. Other influences
- 1. Emotions: Anger, frustration and anxiety increase secretion. Fear, grief and depression decrease the secretion. These influences act on the vagal nucleus to vary the secretion.

2. Hypoglycaemia: Stimulates acid and pepsin secretion by acting via vagal efferents.

3. Histamine: Stimulates HCl secretion by acting through $H_2$ receptors present on the parietal cells.

4. Alcohol and caffeine have a direct stimulatory effect on the gastric mucosa.

Nervous influences stimulate the release of gastric juice during cephalic phase (before food reaches the stomach) as well as during gastric phase (when food is in the stomach) of secretion.

## PEPTIC ULCER                                          3 (2004)-IPU
## PATHOPHYSIOLOGY OF PEPTIC ULCER AND ITS
## TREATMENT                                  4 (2004)-IPU, (2010)

Peptic ulcer is the term given to the condition arising due to the breakdown of mucosal barrier of the stomach and/or duodenum.

### Pathogenesis

Peptic ulceration in human is related primarily to the breakdown of the barrier that prevents irritation and autodigestion of the mucosa by the gastric secretion. Infection with the bacterium *Helicobacter pylori* disrupts this barrier as do aspirin and other nonsteroidal anti-inflammatory drugs (NSAIDs) which inhibit the production of prostaglandins, decreasing mucus and $HCO_3^-$ secretion.

Another cause of ulceration is prolonged secretion of acid as is seen in **Zollinger-Ellison syndrome**. This syndrome is seen in patients of gastrinomas. These tumours can occur in the stomach and duodenum but most of the time are found in the pancreas. The gastrin causes prolonged hypersecretion of the acid and severe ulcers are produced.

### Physiological Basis of Management of Peptic Ulcers

- Gastric and duodenal ulcers can be given a chance to heal by inhibiting acid secretion by the drugs that block the $H_2$ histamine receptors on parietal cells, e.g. cimetidine.
- Omeprazole acts by inhibiting the $H^+-K^+$-ATPase pump.
- *H. pylori* may be eradicated by giving antibiotics.

- NSAID induced ulcers can be treated by either stopping the NSAID or when this is not advisable by treatment with the prostaglandin agonist **misoprostol**.
- Gastrinomas sometimes can be removed surgically.

### EXPLAIN WHY PROTON PUMP INHIBITORS ARE USED IN PATIENTS OF PEPTIC ULCER          1 (2011)

Prolonged acid secretion as is seen in cases of **Zollinger-Ellison syndrome** is one of the causes producing peptic ulcer. This is also seen in patients having gastrinomas which can occur in the stomach or duodenum but most of them are found in pancreas. The gastrin causes prolonged hypersecretion of acid leading to ulcers. Hence, gastric and duodenal ulcers can be given a chance to heal by inhibition of acid secretion with drugs such as omeprazole and related drugs that inhibit $H^+ - K^+$-ATPase (proton pump inhibitors) responsible for the secretion of the acid.

### WHAT WILL HAPPEN AND WHY IF TOTAL GASTRECTOMY IS DONE IN PATIENTS OF PEPTIC ULCER          1 (2003)

Gastrectomy is occasionally used in the treatment of severe peptic ulcer disease or its complications. While the vast majority of peptic ulcers (gastric ulcers in the stomach or duodenal ulcers in the duodenum) are managed with medication, partial gastrectomy is sometimes required in patients who have complications. These include patients who do not respond satisfactorily to medical therapy, those who develop a bleeding or perforated ulcer, and those who develop pyloric obstruction (a blockage to the exit from the stomach). It helps to reduce gastric acid secretion in such patients.

### WHAT WILL HAPPEN AND WHY IF TOTAL GASTRECTOMY IS DONE          2.5 (1989), 1 (2008)

Total gastrectomy is complete surgical removal of the stomach. Under these circumstances food rapidly enters the small intestine. In the absence of the stomach, entry into the intestine is not regulated and consequently:

1. Glucose is rapidly absorbed in the intestine producing hyper-glycaemia and consequent release of insulin, which causes

hypoglycaemic symptoms like weakness, dizziness and sweating after meals **(dumping syndrome)**.

2. Rapid entry of hypertonic food into the duodenum causes the movements of water into the gut which may result in hypovolemia and consequent fall in cardiac output.

3. Due to absence of intrinsic factor, absorption of vitamin $B_{12}$ suffers producing pernicious anaemia.

4. Iron absorption also suffers as stomach helps in conversion of ferric iron to ferrous form for absorption. This may result in iron deficiency anaemia.

These persons should take small frequent meals supplemented with vitamin $B_{12}$ and iron injections to cope with the situation.

## WHAT WILL HAPPEN AND WHY IF INTRINSIC FACTOR SECRETED BY GASTRIC MUCOSA IS ABSENT    2.5 (1989), 1 (2000)

Intrinsic factor is a glycoprotein secreted by parietal or oxyntic cells of the gastric glands. It is essential for the absorption of vitamin $B_{12}$ from the small intestines. Vitamin $B_{12}$ combines with intrinsic factor, forms a complex and is then actively absorbed in the ileum. In the absence of intrinsic factor, absorption of vitamin $B_{12}$ suffers. Vitamin $B_{12}$ is essential for the normal maturation of RBCs. Dèrangement of DNA synthesis occurs in the absence of vitamin $B_{12}$ and leads to the formation of abnormally large precursor cells called megaloblasts, which are prone to destruction. This leads to anaemia known as pernicious anaemia. Intrinsic factor deficiency occurs after gastrectomy or due to idiopathic atrophy of gastric mucosa.

## EXPLAIN WHY GASTRECTOMY LEADS TO PERNICIOUS ANAEMIA    1 (2006)

Instrinsic factor necessary for the absorption of vitamin $B_{12}$ from the small intestine is secreted by the parietal (oxyntic) cells of gastric mucosa. In the absence of this factor which occurs following gastrectomy absorption of this vitamin suffers thus producing pernicious anaemia.

## CELL TYPES IN GASTRIC MUCOSA    2.5 (1989)

Cell types in **gastric mucosa** are:

I. **Surface epithelium:** Tall columnar cells that secrete thick mucus.

II. **Glandular cells:** Lining gastric glands in the body and fundus

   a. Parietal or oxyntic cells: Secrete HCl and intrinsic factor.

   b. Chief or zymogen cells: Secrete pepsinogen.

   c. Mucus secreting cells in neck of glands: Secrete soluble mucus.

### In Pyloric and Cardiac Region

Glandular cells secrete soluble mucus.

**In gastric antrum:** G cells in gastric glands secrete a hormone gastrin.

## DESCRIBE THE MECHANISM OF GASTRIC EMPTYING AND ITS REGULATION     10 (1993)

### Mechanism of Gastric Emptying

- When food enters the stomach it relaxes (primarily the fundus) by a reflex process to accommodate 1–2 litres of food called **receptive relaxation**. Stretch receptors in the stomach detect the presence of food and initiate vasovagal reflex producing receptive relaxation.

- Food that enters the stomach consists of a mixture of solids and liquids, while the chyme that leaves the stomach is liquid. Gastric emptying starts when a large portion of contents is in fluid form. As food enters stomach peristaltic contraction starts which mix the food and empty the chyme into the duodenum at a controlled rate.

**Gastric peristaltic waves:** They occur once the stomach is full. These are controlled by basic electrical rhythm **(BER)** of smooth muscles. Usually, it begins near the body of the stomach and moves towards the antrum and propels the contents along with it. Peristaltic waves become strong in the antrum providing powerful forces that pushes the contents towards the pylorus. Contraction of the antrum is followed by a sequential contraction of pyloric region and duodenum. Antrum, pyloric region and duodenum function as a unit in gastric emptying.

As peristaltic wave passes through the antrum, the pylorus ahead of it contracts so that only small amount of chyme can squirt into the duodenum with each peristaltic wave. This prevents the entry of solid contents into the duodenum. Thus this peristaltic activity provides a pumping action for transfer of contents into duodenum and is known as the **pyloric pump**.

Normally, regurgitation of contents from the duodenum does not occur as constriction of pyloric region persists longer than that of duodenum. This is also aided by the action of CCK and secretin on the pyloric sphincter.

**Regulation of gastric emptying:** It is regulated by the following factors:

I. **Type of food:** Emptying is fastest with carbohydrates, proteins leave slowly and fats take the longest time to leave the stomach.

II. **Duodenal factors**
   a. **Osmolarity of contents:** Gastric emptying is delayed if duodenal contents are hyperosmolar. Osmolarity is probably sensed by osmoreceptors present in the duodenum and affect is neurally mediated.
   b. **Acidity of duodenal contents:** Excess of acidity of duodenal contents inhibits emptying which is neurally mediated.
   c. **Products of protein digestions:** Presence of amino acids in duodenum reflexly reduces stomach emptying.

III. **Gastrointestinal hormones:**
   a. **Gastrin:** Stimulates gastric peristaltic waves and hence emptying.
   b. **CCK-PZ:** Inhibits gastric motility and hence emptying.
   c. **Secretin:** Also inhibits gastric motility and emptying.
   d. **GIP:** Inhibits gastric motility and emptying.

All these hormones function in an integrated manner so that gastric contents are transferred to the duodenum at a rate appropriate for proper digestion and absorption of food.

## PANCREAS

### ENUMERATE THE ENZYMES OF PANCREATIC JUICE AND DESCRIBE THE FUNCTION OF ANY ONE OF THEM   2.5 (1991)

### TRYPSINOGEN                                           3 (1985)

Pancreatic juice secreted by exocrine part of pancreas contains the following enzymes:

i. **Proteolytic enzymes**
   a. Trypsin as trypsinogen
   b. Chymotrypsin as chymotrypsinogen
   c. Carboxypeptidase A as procarboxypeptidase A
   d. Carboxypeptidase B as procarboxypeptidase B
   e. Elastase as proelastase
ii. **Lipolytic enzymes**
   a. Pancreatic lipase
   b. Pancreatic esterase (cholesterol esterase)
   c. Phospholipase $A_2$ as prophospholipase $A_2$.
iii. **Pancreatic amylase**
iv. **Nucleases**
   a. Ribonuclease
   b. Deoxyribonuclease

## Functions of Trypsin

Trypsin is an important proteolytic enzyme secreted as inactive precursor trypsinogen which is activated by an enteropeptidase or enterokinase. It acts on the proteins and polypeptides causing cleavage of peptide bonds adjacent to arginine or lysine. Proteins are hydrolyzed to polypeptides and peptones.

## CCK AND ITS FUNCTION                    5 (1990)

CCK-PZ Cholecystokinin-pancreozymin is a peptide hormone secreted from upper part of the small intestines. It is produced as a large molecule called prepro-CCK. Few amino acids are cleaved from the precursor to form CCK which is active. It is released in response to the presence of products of protein digestion, i.e. peptide, amino acids and fatty acids containing more than 10 carbon atoms.

## Actions of CCK

i. Causes contraction of the gallbladder, as a result bile is poured into the duodenum, hence it acts as a cholagogue.
ii. Stimulates the secretion of pancreatic juice rich in enzyme content.
iii. Augments the action of secretin in causing the release of pancreatic juice rich in bicarbonate content.

iv. Inhibits gastric emptying and hence regulates the entry of chyme into duodenum at an appropriate rate.

v. It is trophic to the pancreas.

vi. May stimulate motor activity of small and large intestine.

vii. Along with secretin the contraction of pyloric augments sphincter and regulates the entry of chyme into the duodenum.

viii. Increases secretion of enterokinase.

ix. Stimulates glucagon secretion along with gastrin.

CCK thus causes the entry of bile into the duodenum and secretion of pancreatic juice. This helps in the digestion of proteins and fats. End products of proteins and fat digestion stimulate further release of CCK. A type of positive feedback system operates to regulate CCK secretion. This positive feedback is terminated as chyme leaves the small intestine.

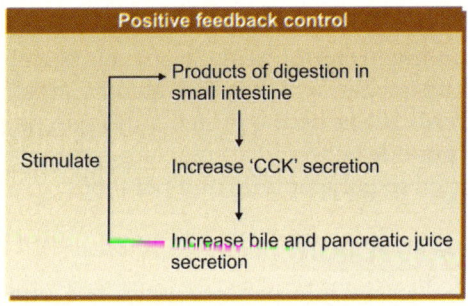

## DESCRIBE THE COMPOSITION, FUNCTIONS AND REGULATION OF PANCREATIC JUICE                10 (1992)

## LIST THE MAIN COMPONENTS OF PANCREATIC JUICE AND DESCRIBE THE VARIOUS MECHANISMS THAT REGULATE THEIR SECRETION                5 (2004)-IPU

Pancreatic juice is secreted from the exocrine portion of the pancreas.

### Composition of Pancreatic Juice

Volume – 1500 ml/day
pH      – alkaline 7.5–8.5
Water  – 99%

## Inorganic Substances

Bicarbonate and chlorides of $Na^+$ are main inorganic content. In addition small amounts of $K^+$, $Ca^{2+}$, $Mg^{2+}$ and $SO_4^{2-}$ are present.

## Organic Substances

Enzymes to hydrolyse proteins, fats and carbohydrates are present.

I. **Proteolytic enzymes**
   a. Trypsin as trypsinogen
   b. Chymotrypsin as chymotrypsinogen
   c. Carboxypeptidase A as procarboxypeptidase A
   d. Carboxypeptidase B as procarboxypeptidase B
   e. Elastase as proelastase

Trypsinogen is activated to form trypsin by enterokinase produced by the intestinal mucosa. Trypsin so formed activates more trypsinogen and other inactive enzymes to their respective active forms.

II. **Lipolytic enzymes**
   a. Pancreatic lipase
   b. Pancreatic esterase (cholesterol esterase)
   c. Phospholipase A as prophospholipase A (activated by trypsin)

III. **Nucleases**
   a. Ribonuclease
   b. Deoxyribonuclease

IV. **Pancreatic $\alpha$ amylase**

## Functions of Pancreatic Juice

Trypsin and chymotrypsin are potent protein hydrolysing enzymes. Trypsin acts on proteins and polypeptides, splitting peptide bonds adjacent to arginine or lysine and converts them to proteases and peptones. **Chymotrypsin** also acts on proteins and polypeptides cleaving the bonds adjacent to aromatic amino acids.

## Carboxypeptidase A and B

Acts on polypeptides (formed by the action of trypsin and chymotrypsin) splitting their terminal amino acids and thus releasing free amino acids as end products of protein digestion.

## Pancreatic Lipase

Hydrolyses triglycerides (neutral fats) to fatty acids and monoglycerides.

**Cholesterol esterase:** Converts cholesterol esters to cholesterol.

**Phospholipase $A_2$:** Acts on phospholipids, e.g. lecithin and splits it into smaller molecules.

**Nucleases:** Act on nucleic acids present in food converting them to nucleotides.

**Pancreatic amylase:** Acts on starch and other polysaccharides hydrolyzing them at 1:4 linkages forming disaccharide maltose. It acts on cooked as well as on raw starch.

## Bicarbonates

Present in appreciable amount in pancreatic juice and serves the following functions:

a. Neutralizes the acid of gastric juice as chyme reaches duodenum.

b. Provides an alkaline medium in duodenum (along with bile) for the enzymes in pancreatic juice to act.

## Regulation of Pancreatic Juice Secretion

Secretion of pancreatic juice is under hormonal and nervous control. Hormones play a major role in control of its secretion.

**Hormonal control:** Two hormones secretin and cholecystokinin-pancreozymin (CCK-PZ) are produced by duodenal and jejunal mucosa in response to the entry of chyme into the duodenum. Products of protein and fat digestion stimulate their release.

**Secretin** is produced by argentaffin cells in crypts of duodenal mucosa. It causes copious secretion of juice rich in bicarbonates and poor in enzyme content. It acts on the epithelium of small pancreatic ducts and stimulates the secretion of $HCO_3^-$.

## Cholecystokinin-Pancreozymin (CCK-PZ)

Stimulates the release of pancreatic juice rich in enzyme content. It acts on the cells lining pancreatic acini causing the release of enzyme containing zymogen granules.

## Nervous Control

Vagal stimulation causes the release of small amount of enzyme rich pancreatic juice. This effect is blocked by atropine and vagotomy. Vagal stimulation and CCK-PZ cause the release of zymogen granules from acinar cells.

## EXPLAIN WHY SERUM AMYLASE LEVEL IS RAISED IN CHRONIC PANCREATITIS                                                  1 (2004)

In the pancreatic juice prophospholipase $A_2$ is secreted in an inactive form and gets converted to phospholipase $A_2$ by trypsin. It can split a fatty acid off lecithin forming lysolecithin which damages the cell membrane. In acute pancreatitis phospholipase $A_2$ gets activated in the pancreatic ducts causing disruption of the pancreatic tissue and necrosis of the surrounding fat. Small amounts of pancreatic digestive enzymes normally leak into the circulation but in acute pancreatitis the circulating level of digestive enzymes rises markedly due to tissue damage. Hence, measurement of plasma amylase or lipase concentration is of value in diagnosing this disease as their concentration is more than normal.

## EXPLAIN WHY PANCREATIC PROTEOLYTIC ENZYMES DO NOT PRODUCE AUTODIGESTION                                             1 (2006)

The pancreatic juice contains a range of digestive enzymes but most of these are released in an active form and get activated only when they reach the intestinal lumen. The enzymes are activated following proteolytic cleavage by trypsin which is secreted as an inactive precursor trypsinogen. The release of even a small amount of trypsin into the pancreas results in a chain reaction that could produce active enzymes capable of digesting the pancreas. This is prevented by secretion of trypsin inhibitor by the same acinar cells and at the same time as pancreatic proenzymes which protects the pancreas from autodigestion.

## LIVER AND GALLBLADDER

## WHAT WILL HAPPEN AND WHY TO DIGESTION OF FAT IF BILE DUCT IS COMPLETELY BLOCKED                                        2.5 (1991)

When the bile duct is completely blocked, bile cannot reach the small intestine as happens normally. This will lead to impaired digestion of fats. Bile contains bile salt which are necessary for fat digestion due to the following actions:

   i. They cause emulsification of fat prior to their digestion by lipases.

   ii. They also play a part in activation of pancreatic lipase.

Due to incomplete digestion of fats, faecal matter has high content of fat, is bulky and foul smelling.

## FUNCTIONS OF BILE        3 (1993)

Bile is a digestive secretion from the liver. Main constituents of bile are bile salts and bile pigments.

### Functions

1. Bile salts are necessary for digestion and absorption of fats
   i. They produce emulsification of fats.
   ii. Activate pancreatic lipase.
   iii. They form micelles with fatty acids and help in their absorption.
2. Bile salts promote further secretion of bile and are hence **choleretics**.
3. Bile salts have mild laxative action.
4. Bicarbonates in bile help neutralize acidity of chyme as it enters the duodenum so that pancreatic enzymes can produce their action.

## COMPARE HEPATIC DUCT BILE AND GALL-BLADDER BILE       2 (2003)-IPU

| Feature | Hepatic duct bile | Gallbladder bile |
|---|---|---|
| • Colour | Light golden yellow | Almost black in colour |
| • Consistency | Like water | Thicker than liver bile due to presence of mucus and absorption of water by the gall bladder mucous membrane |
| • pH | 7.8–8.6 | 7.0–7.4 |
| • Water | 97% | 89% |
| • Percentage of solids | 2–4% | more, 10–12% |
| • Bile salts/bile acid (mg/dL) | 120–180 | more, 5–6 times the liver bile |

*Contd.*

*Contd.*

| Feature | Hepatic duct bile | Gallbladder bile |
|---|---|---|
| • Bile pigments (mg/dL) | 50 | more, 5–6 times the liver bile |
| • Cholesterol (mg/dL) | 60–170 | more, 5–6 times the liver bile |
| • Lecithin(mg/dL) | 140–810 | more, 5–6 times the liver bile |
| • Electrolytes (mEq/L) | | |
| (a) $Na^+$ | 180–220 | Increases by 2 times |
| (b) $K^+$ | 6–8 | Increases by 2 times |
| (c) $Cl^-$ | 60–70 | Decreases by 5–6 times |
| (d) $HCO_3^-$ | 60–70 | Decreases by 5–6 times |

## COMPARE CHOLERETICS AND CHOLAGOGUES

**2 (2004)-IPU, 2 (2003)**

**Choleretics** are the substances which increase biliary secretion from the liver, e.g. bile salts and bile acids.

## COMPARE BILE SALTS AND BILE PIGMENTS

**2 (2005)**

| Bile salts | Bile pigments |
|---|---|
| • These are sodium and potassium salts of bile acids (taurocholic and glycocholic acids) | • They are bilirubin and biliverdin and its derivatives. They are formed from the globin portion of haemoglobin after the destruction of old RBC's in the reticuloendothelial system |
| • Bile salts reduce surface tension and in conjunction with phospholipids and monoglycerides are responsible for the emulsification of fat preparatory to its digestion and absorption in the small intestine | • They are responsible for the golden yellow colour of liver bile. They are only excretory products and have no digestive function |

**Cholagogues:** These are substances that cause contraction of the gallbladder, e.g. fatty acids in the small intestine, products of protein digestion, $Ca^{2+}$, etc. These substances cause contraction of the gallbladder by release of CCK-PZ from the duodenum.

## BILE SALTS    2.5 (1985, 1986)

Bile salts are one of the major constituents of bile juice. Chemically, they belong to a group of steroid compounds and are $Na^+$ and $K^+$ salts of bile acids conjugated with glycine or taurine. These salts are essential for the digestion and absorption of fats.

- They reduce surface tension and cause emulsification of fats, thus increasing their surface area for lipase to act on them.
- They combine with lipids in small intestines forming micelles
- They form water soluble complexes, so that lipids can be easily absorbed.
- They stimulate the further secretion of bile and hence are choleretics.
- Bile salts keep cholesterol in solution in bile.
- Help in absorption of fat soluble vitamins A, D, E and K.
- They have a mild laxative action.

## ENTEROHEPATIC CIRCULATION OF BILE SALTS    2.5 (1990)

Bile salts are important constituents of bile. Bile is poured into the duodenum. Bile salts help in the digestion and absorption of lipids. In the terminal part of small intestines, major amounts (95%) of bile salts are reabsorbed by active processes and by way of portal blood draining the intestines and enter the liver, called *enterohepatic circulation* of bile salts. From the liver they are again secreted into bile. It is a mechanism to conserve the bile salts. It is estimated that bile salts pool recycles twice per meal and 6–8 times per minute.

When this circulation of bile salts is blocked, liver cannot produce adequate amount of bile salts, hence digestion and absorption of fats suffers.

## CHOLELITHIASIS    2 (2002)

- Presence of stones in the gallbladder or bile ducts is called *cholelithiasis*. This is a common condition whose incidence increases with age.
- The stones are of two types: Calcium bilirubinate (15%) which are radiopaque and cholesterol stones (85%) that are radiolucent.

- Three factors appear to be involved in the formation of gall-stones:

  1. **Bile stasis:** Stones form in the bile that is sequestered in the gallbladder rather than the bile that is flowing in the bile ducts.

  2. **Supersaturation of the bile with cholesterol:** Cholesterol is very insoluble in bile and it is maintained in solution in micelles only at certain concentrations of bile salts and lecithin. At concentrations above this the bile is super-saturated and contains small crystals of cholesterol in addition to micelles.

  3. Those are a mix of **nucleation factors** that favour formation of stones from the supersaturated bile. The exact nature of nucleation factors is unsettled although glycoproteins in gallbladder mucus is implicated. It is unsettled whether stones form as a result of excess production of components that favour nucleation or decreased production of anti-nucleation components that prevent stones from forming in normal individuals.

## SMALL INTESTINE

### MOTOR FUNCTIONS OF SMALL INTESTINES     5 (1989)
### COMPARE SEGMENTAL AND PERISTALTIC CONTRACTIONS
### 2 (2010)

Smooth muscles in the wall of small intestines are present as circular and longitudinal layers as well as in muscularis mucosa. These muscles show following types of contractions.

a. Segmental contractions

b. Peristaltic contractions

c. Villus contraction

These contractions are initiated in the gut wall itself and are independent of extrinsic innervation. Local intact myenteric plexus is essential for intestinal motility. Muscle contractions are co-ordinated by small intestinal slow waves, which is a wave of smooth muscle depolarization that moves from the duodenum towards the anus. Frequency of slow waves is 12/min in jejunum and 9/min in the ileum.

## Segmental Contractions

Ring-like contractions appear in a part of the intestine at fairly regular interval dividing the gut into a number of segments. As the contracted segments relax, a new set of contractions occur in the segments between previous contractions.

Segmental contractions are initiated due to stretch by chyme as it enters the duodenum. Their frequency is determined by the rate of slow waves. They move the chyme from side-to-side increasing the surface area exposed to the mucosa for absorption. They also mix chyme with intestinal secretions (Fig. 4.2).

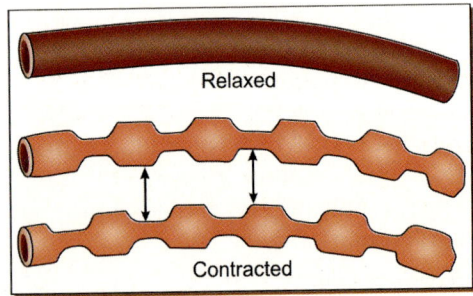

**Fig. 4.2**: Diagram of segmentation contractions of the intestine

## Peristaltic Contractions

These are propulsive contractions that push the chyme analwards. When the intestinal wall is stretched a deep circular contraction is formed proximal to a point of stretch and this wave of peristalsis (contraction) moves towards the rectum at varying rates. Peristaltic waves differ in intensity and distance travelled. Peristaltic activity of small intestines is greatly enhanced after a meal due to entry of chyme in duodenum and also by **gastroenteric reflex** (initiated by distension of the stomach). If a part of the gut is cut and re-stitched peristaltic waves can cross the stitched end but if the gut is re-stitched in reverse direction, peristaltic wave stops at the reversed part. If intestinal lumen is obstructed due to some cause very intense contractions called peristaltic rushes occur. This local response of smooth muscle to stretch is also known as **myenteric reflex**.

Parasympathetic nerve stimulation increases peristaltic activity and sympathetic stimulation has opposite effect.

**Villus movements:** Intestinal villi also show movements. They occur during the process of digestion and absorption and not at rest. They show shortening and lengthening movements due to contraction and relaxation of muscularis mucosa. They help in the movements of lymph in the lacteals and of blood in the capillaries present in the villus and thus help in the process of absorption.

## PERISTALSIS                                    2.5 (1991)

Peristalsis is a wave of contraction seen in gut and other hollow viscera, e.g. urinary bladder ureter, and due to the contraction of smooth muscles present in their wall. Whenever gut wall is stretched, it responds by contraction and a wave of contraction travels analward called **myenteric reflex** that requires an intact local myenteric nervous plexus. Whenever gut or viscera is stretched, a ring of contraction appears proximal to the stimulus (stretch) and it travels analwards propelling the contents forward.

If a part of the gut is removed and re-stitched in its original position, peristaltic waves can cross the point of stitching but if the gut is stitched in reverse direction, peristaltic waves will stop at the reversed segment.

## SHORT NOTE ON MIGRATING MOTOR COMPLEXES   5 (2007)

During fasting between periods of digestion, the pattern of electrical and motor activity in the gastrointestinal smooth muscle becomes modified so that cycles of motor activity migrate from the stomach towards the distal ileum.

These are known as the migrating motor complexes and are divided into three phases (Fig. 4.3):

**Phase I:** Quiescent period

**Phase II:** Period of irregular electrical and mechanical activity.

**Phase III:** Regular electrical and mechanical activity.

- The MMCs are initiated by motilin. The circulating level of this hormone increases at intervals of 100 min in the interdigestive state, coordinated with the contractile phase of the MMC.

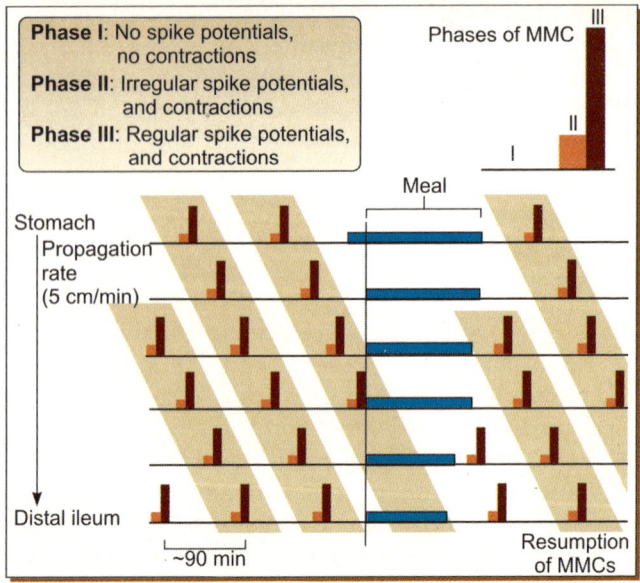

**Fig. 4.3:** Migrating motor complex

- The contractions migrate aborally at the rate of 5 cm/min and also occur at intervals of approximately 100 min.
- Gastric secretion, bile, pancreatic secretion increases during the MMCs.
- They help to clear the stomach of its luminal contents in preparation of the next meal. When a meal is ingested secretion of motilin is suppressed and the MMC is abolished until digestion and absorption are complete.

### EXPLAIN WHY ORS IS ADVISED IN INFANTS WITH DIARRHOEA                                     1 (2011)
### EXPLAIN WHY SODIUM AND GLUCOSE ARE USED IN ORS 1 (2005)

In the small intestine active transport of sodium helps in co-transport of glucose, amino acids and other substances. Similarly, the presence of glucose in intestinal lumen facilitates the reabsorption of $Na^+$. That is why for treatment of sodium and water loss in diarrhoea specially in infants, oral administration of solutions containing both NaCl and glucose as in ORS or cereals containing carbohydrates is recommended.

## LARGE INTESTINE

### AGANGLIONIC MEGACOLON                    2 (2011)

This disease is commonly seen in children and is due to congenital absence of the ganglionic cells in both the myenteric and submucous plexus or due to degeneration of myenteric plexus. It is also called **Hirschsprung disease**.

There appears to be a mutation in the receptors for endothelin B that are necessar ooedemaanormal cranial to caudal migration of neuroblast during development.

The site most commonly involved is distal colon and pelvirectal junction. This leads to blockage of both perios oedema and mass contractions, therefore, faeces pass the aganglionic segment with difficulty and accumulates in the large intestine. Children with this disease defecate as infrequently as once in three weeks.

The disease is treated by cutting the aganglionic portion of pelvirectal junction and anastomosing the cut ends. However, this is not possible if an extensive segment is involved, in which case colectomy is required.

### DIETARY FIBRE              2.5 (1990, 2000), 2 (2007)

Dietary fibre is the component of human diet, that is not acted upon by digestive enzymes and reaches the large intestines undigested. Some of constituents of dietary fibres are cellulose, hemicellulose, lignin, various gums and pectins. They serve the following functions:

1. The increased bulk of this undigested residue stimulates intestinal peristalsis which in turn facilitates the passage of food through the intestine. Thus high fibre diet plays an important role in the treatment and prevention of constipation.

2. It reduces the efficacy of absorption of digested foodstuffs by forming a mechanical barrier between the nutrients and absorptive surface. This helps to reduce the sudden increase in blood glucose level after a meal (called postprandial hyperglycemia). This helps to reduce the requirement of insulin during the postprandial phase. Therefore, this is useful in treatment and prevention of diabetes mellitus.

3. It reduces the blood cholesterol level by binding the bile salts:

Binding of bile salts → increases excretion of bile salts in the faeces → decreases the amount available for enterohepatic circulation → increases synthesis of fresh bile salts → increases utilization of cholesterol → decreases blood levels of cholesterol.

This helps to control all metabolic disorders associated with overnutrition like obesity, atherosclerosis, hypercholesterolemia and diabetes mellitus.

4. Dietary fibre decreases the incidence of cancer of the colon by:
- Dilution of carcinogens by the water held by the dietary fibre
- Reducing the duration of contact between carcinogen and mucous membrane of the colon
- Binding of carcinogens to the dietary fibre.

### EXPLAIN WHY DIETARY FIBRE INTAKE IS RECOMMENDED
1 (2011)

Individuals with low dietary fibre intake in their meals have a greater than normal capacity to breakdown cellulose and related products, thus reducing the residue in their colon. It has been claimed that there are higher incidences of constipation, cancer of the colon, diverticulitis, diabetes mellitus and coronary artery disease in such individuals.

## GIT HORMONES

### HORMONES OF GIT
2.5 (1993)

Hormones of GIT are polypeptides in nature. These are produced by specialized mucosal cells lining the stomach and intestines.

These hormone secreting cells can take up amines, similar to norepinephrine or serotonin and decarboxylate them called 'APUD' cells.

Based on their structural and to some extent functional similarity, the hormones are classified as:

I. **Gastrin family:** Gastrin and CCK

II. **Secretin family:** Secretin, glucagon, GIP and VIP

III. **Other polypeptides:** Motilin, gastrin releasing peptide, somatostatin, substance P, endorphins and enkephalins. Hormones secreted by endocrinal cells are released locally, absorbed in venous blood and reach their target cells through arterial blood and produce their actions.

## Functions of Hormones in General

i. Regulation of gastrointestinal secretion
ii. Control motility of stomach and intestine
iii. Some of the polypeptides act as neurotransmitter at local nervous plexus in gut wall.

## Functions of Some of Functionally Important Hormones

**Gastrin:** Stimulates gastrin secretion and motility.

## CCK-PZ

1. Stimulates pancreatic secretion rich in enzyme content.
2. Causes contraction of gallbladder and bile is poured in the duodenum.
3. Inhibits gastric emptying.

## Secretin

1. Stimulates secretion of pancreatic juice rich in bicarbonate content.
2. Inhibits gastric acid secretion and motility.

**GIP:** Inhibits gastric secretion and motility.

**Somatostatin:** Inhibits gastrin, secretin, GIP and VIP.

These hormones act in an integrated manner to control digestion of nutrients. Other polypeptides act as neurotransmitters at local neuronal synapses.

## GIVE AN ACCOUNT OF GASTROINTESTINAL HORMONES WITH REFERENCE TO     10 (1985)

**A. SITE OF PRODUCTION**
**B. REGULATION OF SECRETION**
**C. FUNCTION**

Gastrointestinal hormones can be grouped into three classes:

**I. Gastrin family**
   a. Gastrin
   b. CCK-PZ

## II. Secretin family
  a. Secretin
  b. Glucagon
  c. Gastric inhibitory peptide (GIP)
  d. Vasoactive intestinal peptide (VIP)

## III. Other polypeptides
  a. Motilin
  b. Substance P
  c. Gastrin releasing peptide (GRP)
  d. Somatostatin
  e. Endorphins
  f. Enkephalins

They are all polypeptide hormones. This grouping is based on their structural similarity (amino acids) and to some extent functional similarity.

**Gastrin:** It is a polypeptide produced by G cells in mucosal glands of gastric antrum. Gastrin is secreted as food reaches the stomach in response to stretch of stomach wall and presence of products of protein digestion (amino acid). These two stimuli cause stimulation of mucosal stretch and chemical receptors respectively. Afferents from receptors enter the Meissner's plexus of gut wall. Efferents from the plexus innervate gland cells and stimulate them to produce gastric secretion. Acid in antrum inhibits gastrin secretion and stops further release by a negative feedback action.

### Functions

1. Gastrin stimulates gastric glands to cause HCl and pepsin secretion.
2. Enhances gastric motility and hence gastric emptying.
3. Trophic action on gastric mucosa.
4. Stimulates insulin and glucagon secretion after protein meal.

### CCK-PZ

Cholecystokinin-pancreozymin is secreted by mucosa of upper small intestines (duodenum and jejunum).

It is secreted as chyme reaches the duodenum, in response to presence of amino acids and fatty acids.

CCK-PZ so secreted causes further digestion of proteins and fats by causing the secretion of proteolytic and lipolytic enzymes by the pancreas. As a result more of amino acids and fatty acids are released which in turn further stimulate the secretion of CCK-PZ **(positive feedback mechanism)**.

## Functions of CCK-PZ

   i. Causes contraction of gallbladder and as a result bile is poured into the duodenum.
   ii. Stimulates the release of pancreatic juice rich in digestive enzymes.
  iii. Augments the action of secretin in producing bicarbonate rich pancreatic juice.
  iv. Decreases gastric motility and hence controls emptying of gastric contents into duodenum at an appropriate rate.
   v. Exerts a trophic action on pancreas.
  vi. Stimulates motility of intestines.
 vii. Augments the action of secretin in contracting pyloric sphincter and hence regulating the entry of chyme into duodenum.
viii. Enhances the secretion of enterokinase.
  ix. Along with gastrin stimulates glucagon secretion.

## Secretin

Produced by mucosal cells in small intestines.

## Functions

   i. Enhances the secretion of bicarbonate in pancreatic secretion by acting on cells lining the duct system via cyclic AMP.
  ii. Stimulates the secretion of bicarbonates in bile juice by acting on biliary ducts.
  iii. Augments the action of CCK-PZ in secreting pancreatic juice rich in enzyme content.
  iv. Inhibits gastric HCl secretion.

**Secretion of pancreatic juice stimulated by**

   a. Products of protein digestion in chyme entering small intestines.
   b. Acid present in chyme.

Pancreatic juice so released neutralizes the acidity of chyme from the stomach. As acidity decreases further secretion of secretin is not there, thus exerting a feedback control on secretin release.

## Gastric Inhibitory Peptide (GIP)

Secreted from mucosa of duodenum and jejunum. It is secreted in response to fat and glucose in the chyme entering the duodenum.

### Functions

i. Inhibits secretion of gastric juice.

ii. Decreases gastric motility and hence helps to regulate entry of chyme into the duodenum.

iii. Stimulates insulin release. It is considered to be the physiological **gut factor** that normally stimulates the release of insulin. All these hormones, i.e. gastrin, CCK-PZ, secretin and GIP act in an integrated manner to regulate secretion of various digestive juices and also control motility of the gastrointestinal tract.

## Vasoactive Intestinal Peptides (VIP)

It is secreted throughout the mucosa of gastrointestinal tract.

### Functions

1. Stimulates intestinal secretion containing various electrolytes and water.
2. Inhibits the secretion of HCl by gastric glands.
3. Potentiates the action of acetylcholine for secretion of saliva.
4. It is a dilator of peripheral blood vessels.
5. It functions as a neurotransmitter in CNS and autonomic nerves.

**Motilin:** It is produced by duodenal mucosa and stimulates HCl secretion by the stomach.

## Gastrin Releasing Peptide (GRP)

GRP is secreted all along the GIT. It causes the release of gastric secretions. It probably functions as a neurotransmitter at vagal nerve endings in gastric gland cells and causes vagally mediated secretion of gastric juices.

**Somatostatin:** Secreted by D cells in the gastrointestinal tract (similar to D cells present in islets of Langerhans in pancreas).

Secreted in large quantities in the gastric lumen in response to the presence of acid.

## Functions

1. It inhibits the secretion of gastrin stopping further HCl secretion. It acts in a paracrine manner through gastric juice to inhibit gastrin secretion.
2. It also inhibits the release of other gastrointestinal hormones like VIP, GIP, secretin and motilin.
3. Inhibits gastric and pancreatic secretions.
4. Inhibits motility in gastrointestinal tract, e.g. gastric emptying and gallbladder contraction.

## Glucagon

It is a hormone secreted by 'α type' cells present in mucosa of stomach and duodenum.

## GASTRIN                                          3 (1991)

Gastrin is an important gastrointestinal hormone produced by G cells of gastric glands in antrum of the stomach.

It is a polypeptide that is produced as a large molecule called preprogastrin. Amino acids are cleaved from the molecule and gastrin having variable number of amino acids is produced. Three mains forms of gastrin having 34, 17 and 14 amino acids are known as G-34, G-17 and G-14 respectively. G-17 is the main form playing a role in gastric secretion and motility. It is produced as the food enters the stomach in response to (a) stretch of stomach wall, (b) presence of products of protein digestion through locally mediated reflexes.

## Functions

1. It causes the secretion of gastric juice having large amount of HCl and pepsin.
2. It also stimulates gastric motility and hence emptying.
3. Stimulates insulin and glucagon release following a protein meal.
   Presence of HCl in antrum inhibits gastrin release and thus stops further secretion of HCl. Hence, HCl regulates gastrin secretion by a negative feedback mechanism.
   If acid producing cells of stomach are damaged due to some reason, gastrin level rises.

## COMPARE SECRETIN AND CCK                    **2** (2002)

**Secretin:** It is secreted by the 'S cells' that are located deep in the glands of the mucosa of the upper portion of the small intestine.

### Functions

- It increases the secretion of bicarbonates by the duct cells of the pancreas and the biliary tract causing production of watery alkaline pancreatic juice.
- It decreases gastric acid secretion and may cause contraction of the pyloric sphincter.

### Regulation

The secretion is increases by the products of protein digestion and by acid bathing the mucosa of the upper small intestine

**Cholecystokinin:** It is secreted by the 'I cells' in the mucosa of the upper part of small intestine. It is also found in the nerves of the distal ileum and colon.

### Functions

- Stimulation of pancreatic enzyme secretion.
- Contraction of the gallbladder and relaxation of sphincter of Uddi which allows both bile and pancreatic juice to flow into the intestinal lumen.
- It is found in the brain especially the cerebral cortex. It may be involved in the regulation of food intake and in the production of anxiety and analgesia.
- It inhibits gastric emptying.
- It has a trophic action on pancreas.
- Increases the synthesis of enterokinase.
- Enhances the motility of the small intestine and colon.
- CCK along with gastrin stimulates glucagon secretion and since activation of both the hormones is increased by a protein meal, either one or both may be the 'gut factor' that stimulate glucagon secretion.

### Regulation

The secretion of CCK is increased by contact of the intestinal mucosa with the products of digestion particularly peptides and amino acids and fatty acids containing more than 10 carbon atoms.

## MISCELLANEOUS

### PROTEIN-CALORIC MALNUTRITION   4 (1991,1992), 2.5 (2010)

Protein-caloric malnutrition is the most common form of malnutrition in infants and young children between the ages of 1–3 years. It is the main cause of childhood morbidity and mortality in developing countries. Marasmus and Kwashiorkor are the two clinical forms of malnutrition. Basic reasons of malnutrition are:

   i. Inadequate diet both in quality and quantity.
  ii. Infections, e.g. diarrhoea, respiratory tract infection and parasitic infestations due to poor environmental conditions.

**Marasmus:** Diet deficient in both calories and protein content. Child is underweight, marked wasting of muscles and subcutaneous tissue occurs and has bony appearance. Mental development is usually not affected.

**Kwashiorkor:** Occurs due to severe protein deficiency. There is generalized oedema of body and not much of wasting occurs. Mental growth is usually affected. Hair is sparse and silky and skin may be depigmented.

### DEFINE BMR. HOW IS IT MEASURED IN MAN?
### NAME THE FACTORS AFFECTING IT          10 (1990)

### FACTORS AFFECTING BMR          2.5 (1986)

BMR is basal metabolic rate. BMR may be defined as energy output by an individual under certain standardized resting conditions, i.e. complete physical and mental rest, 10–12 hrs after meals (post-absorptive phase) and in comfortable environmental temperature. It is also known as resting metabolic rate. Under such conditions energy liberated is used to maintain vital body functions, i.e. heart beat, respiration, brain activity and to maintain the body temperature.

Clinically, BMR is expressed as percentage, above or below the accepted normal value for the individual taking into consideration age, sex and body surface area.

In male its value is 40 kcal (or 165 kJ) and in females it is 37 kcal (or 155 kJ) per hr per sq. metre body surface area. It is also related to body weight, being 1 kcal/ kg/hr.

## Determination of BMR

In man metabolic rate is determined from the value of $O_2$ consumption. It is known that when 1 litre of $O_2$ is consumed, 4.875 kcal are produced (calorific value of oxygen). Oxygen consumption over a period of time is calculated with a oxygen filled spirometre fitted with $CO_2$ absorbing mechanism.

$O_2$ consumed per hour is calculated and value is corrected for age, sex, surface area and ambient temperature and pressure using normograms. BMR is expressed in terms of percentage above or below normal.

Clinically, it is used as an index of thyroid functions as thyroid hormones determine the BMR.

## Factors Affecting BMR

1. **Age:** BMR per sq. metre of body surface area is greater in children than adults. There is a further gradual fall in adult with advancement of age.
2. **Surface area:** BMR is directly related to surface area. Surface area of a person can be calculated from height and weight using DuBois formula or normogram.
3. **Effect of food intake:** Food intake stimulates metabolism. This is because energy is needed for assimilation of food. Different foods increase metabolism to different extent known as specific dynamic action (SDA) of food. SDA of proteins is greater than fats and carbohydrates.
4. **Exercise:** There is an increase in oxygen consumption and metabolism proportional to severity of exercise.
5. **Body temperature:** For each degree rise in internal body temperature (in celsius) metabolic rate increases by 14%.
6. **Environmental temperature:** Exposure to cold increases metabolism. This helps in maintaining body temperature by increasing heat production.
   Exposure to heat for short duration has little effect, but on prolonged exposure a gradual fall in metabolism occurs.
7. **Starvation:** Starvation over a long period of time slows down metabolism.
8. **Emotions:** Anxiety and tension elevate BMR as they increase epinephrine secretion and increase in muscle tone. A depressed patient has lower BMR.

9. **Effect of thyroid hormones:** An excess of thyroid hormones increases BMR and deficiency decreases it.
10. **Role of catecholamines:** Epinephrine and norepinephrine stimulate metabolism and hence increases BMR.

## NUTRITIONAL REQUIREMENTS OF LACTATING MOTHER
**5 (1993), 4 (1989)**

During lactation there is an additional requirement of calories, proteins, calcium, vitamins C and D.

500 kcal/day in addition to normal requirements, i.e. 2500 kcal/day.

Proteins – 2 gm/kg/day

Calcium – 1 gm/day

Vitamin C – 80 mg/day.

Nutritional requirements of lactating mother are met with following food items supplying 2500 kcal/day:

| Food item | Quantity/day |
| --- | --- |
| Cereals | 580 gm |
| Pulses | 80 gm |
| Leafy vegetables | 40 gm |
| Other vegetables | 40 gm |
| Root and tubers | 60 gm |
| Milk | 300 gm |
| Oil and fat | 50 gm |
| Sugar | 50 gm |

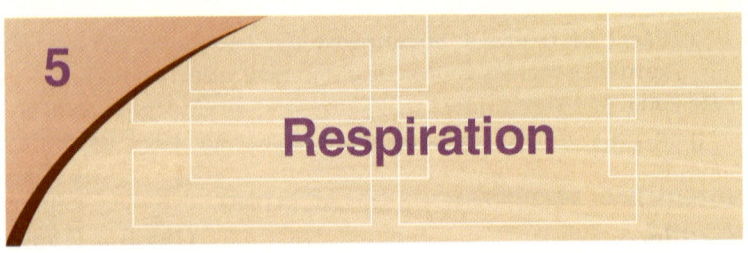

**5**

# Respiration

## COMPARE COMPOSITION OF INSPIRED AND EXPIRED AIR
**2 (2003)**

All values are expressed in mm Hg
Values in parenthesis express the percentage of the total gas

|  | Inspired air | Expired air |
|---|---|---|
| $pO_2$ | 158 (20.98%) | 116 (16%) |
| $pCO_2$ | 0.3 (0.03%) | 32 (4%) |
| $pH_2O$ | Variable depending upon the humidity of the atmosphere | 47 (6.2%) |
| $pN_2$ | 596 (78.06%) | 565 (73.8%) |

## NON-RESPIRATORY FUNCTIONS OF LUNGS
**2.5 (1986, 1989), 2 (2004), 2.5 (2007), 3 (2004)-IPU**

The non-respiratory function of lungs can be divided into three main categories:

1. Lung defense mechanisms
2. Functions of pulmonary circulation
3. Metabolic and endocrine functions of lungs.

### Lung Defense Mechanism

a. Humidify and cool or warm the inspired air.
b. Bronchial secretions contain IgA and other substances like NO that help resist infection and maintain the integrity of the mucosa.
c. Prevent foreign bodies from reaching the alveoli.

i. Particles > 10 μm—strained out by hair in the nostrils or settle down on the mucous membrane of the nose or pharynx.

ii. Particles 2–10 μm—fall on the wall of the bronchi as airflow slows in the air passages producing reflex broncho-constriction and coughing, they are moved away from the lungs by the **ciliary escalator action**.

iii. Particles < 2 μm—generally reach the alveoli where they are ingested by the macrophages called the **pulmonary alveolar macrophages (PAMs).**

## Functions of Pulmonary Circulation

a. Reservoir for left ventricle—if LV output becomes transiently greater than the venous return, it can be maintained for a few strokes by drawing out blood stored in the pulmonary circulation.

b. Pulmonary circulation acts as a filter, filtering small fibrin, blood clots, fat cells, detached cancer cells, gas bubbles, agglutinated RBCs, platelets, WBCs, debris from stored blood or intravenous solutions.

c. Fluid exchange and drug absorption:

i. Low pulmonary hydrostatic pressure tends to pull fluid from the alveoli into the pulmonary capillaries and keeps the alveolar surface free from fluids.

ii. Drugs that rapidly pass through the alveolo-capillary barrier by diffusion, rapidly enter the systemic circulation. Therefore, anaesthetic gases and other bronchodilators are administered by inhalation.

## Metabolic and Endocrine Functions

a. Substances used and synthesized in the lungs: Surfactant.

b. Substances synthesized or stored and released into the blood: Prostaglandins ($PGE_2$ and $PGF_{2\alpha}$, histamine and kallikrein).

c. Substances removed from the blood: Prostaglandins ($PGE_1$, $PGE_2$, $PGF_{2\alpha}$), bradykinin, adenine nucleotides, serotonin, norepinephrine and ACh.

d. Substances activated in the lungs: Angiotensin I is converted to angiotensin II by angiotensin converting enzyme.

e. Vasoactive hormones that pass through the lungs without being metabolized: Epinephrine, dopamine, oxytocin, vasopressin and angiotensin II.

f. Storage of hormones and certain biologically active peptides in 'APUD' cells and nerve fibres of the lungs: VIP, substance P, CCK-PZ and somatostatin.

g. Contains fibrinolytic system that lyses blood clots in the pulmonary vessels.

## EXPLAIN WHY APICAL ALVEOLI HAVE HIGHER $pO_2$ THAN BASAL ALVEOLI 1 (2010)

Gravity has a relatively marked effect on pulmonary circulation. In the upright position the upper portion of the lungs are well above the level of the heart and the bases are below it. In the upper portion, the blood flow is less and the alveoli are larger. Hence they take up more oxygen leading to a higher partial pressure of oxygen at the apex compared to the base of the lung.

## MECHANICS OF RESPIRATION

### PULMONARY SURFACTANT 5 (1985), 3 (2012), 3 (2003)-IPU

Surfactant is a lipid surface-tension lowering agent secreted by **type II epithelial cells** lining the lung alveoli. Chemically a lipoprotein complex consisting of phospholipids and two major proteins. It is present in the fluid lining the alveoli. It is made up of a hydrophilic head portion and two parallel hydrophobic fatty acid chains. The molecules are oriented parallel to air–water interface in the alveoli. Surface tension in alveolar fluid is inversely proportional to the concentration of surfactant.

It performs the following functions:

i. It **lowers the surface tension** in the alveoli, as a result lung compliance is increased and work done during respiration decreases, thereby conserving energy.

ii. **Stabilizes the size of alveoli:** As alveoli tend to become smaller, surfactant becomes concentrated and surface tension is reduced, conversely as alveoli tend to be larger, surfactant is spread more and surface tension is increased. As a consequence as radius increases, surface tension also increases. According to 'Laplace law'.

$$P = \frac{2T}{R}$$

$P$ = Pressure

$T$ = Tension

$R$ = Radius

As $R$ and $T$ change proportionately, the $P$ is kept constant and size of all alveoli tends to remains the same.

iii. **Keeps the alveoli dry:** By lowering surface tension it decreases traction of fluid towards the alveoli and prevents pulmonary oedema. If oedema occurs, it interferes with the gaseous exchange by increasing the width of the alveolar membrane. If surfactant is absent or deficient at birth, lungs fails to expand at birth and cause death leading to respiratory distress syndrome/hyaline membrane disease. Corticoids are required for the maturation of surfactant and its synthesis is influenced by thyroid hormones.

## COMPARE ALVEOLAR AND PULMONARY VENTILATION
2 (2005)

Pulmonary ventilation is the volume of air inspired or expired in one minute. Therefore, it is calculated as TV × RR. Normal value = 6 L/min.

Alveolar ventilation is the amount of air ventilating the alveoli per minute. It is calculated as (tidal volume – dead space ) × respiratory rate. Normal value is around 4.2 L/min.

In rapid shallow breathing (tachypnoea) alveolar ventilation decreases though the pulmonary ventilation remains normal, as a result, less air is available for exchange. While in slow and deep breathing, both alveolar and pulmonary ventilation are normal.

## EXPLAIN WHY FEV$_1$% REMAINS NORMAL IN RESTRICTIVE LUNG DISEASE
1 (2002)

FEV$_1$% is the volume of forced vital capacity expired in the 1st second of exhalation with a normal value of 80% of FVC. In restrictive disorders (kyphoskoliosis and ankylosing spondylitis) chest expansion is reduced while the expiratory phase is normal. Hence, the vital capacity is reduced but the FEV$_1$% is normal.

## FUNCTIONAL RESIDUAL CAPACITY AND ITS MEASUREMENT                          2.5 (1991)

Functional Residual Capacity (FRC): It is the volume of gas in the lungs at resting expiratory level. It is the sum of expiratory reserve volume and residual volume, i.e. 1 L + 1.2 L = 2.2 L in an adult male with total lung capacity of 6 L. It cannot be determined by spirometry. It is determined by finding out the $N_2$ content of expired air after a person breathes in pure oxygen for a period of 5 minutes, using open circuit method. It is assumed that normal alveolar air contains 80% $N_2$ and hence all the $N_2$ in expired air is from the alveoli.

Example:

| | | |
|---|---|---|
| Volume of expired gas | = | 40,000 ml |
| $N_2$ % | = | 5 |
| Volume of $N_2$ in expired air | = | 2000 ml |

2000 ml of $N_2$ = 80% of lung volume

Lung volume at resting expiratory level will be:

$$FRC = \frac{2000 \times 100}{80} = 2500 \text{ ml}$$

## COMPARE AND CONTRAST RESIDUAL VOLUME AND FRC 2 (2003)

**Residual volume:** This is the volume of air that remains in the lungs following maximum expiration. Normal values:1200 ml
**Functional Residual Capacity (FRC):** This is the volume of air that remains in the lungs at the end of expiration, i.e. after tidal expiration. It is computed as RV + ERV. Normal value is 2.5 litres. FRC maintains the residual volume constant. It acts as a buffer and allows the continuous exchange of gases to occur even during expiration, thereby preventing the sudden change in the partial pressure of the gases during respiration (Fig. 5.1).

## COMPARE ANATOMICAL AND PHYSIOLOGICAL DEAD SPACE                          2 (2004)

Dead space is the amount of air in the respiratory passages that do not take part in the gas exchange function of the lungs.

It is divided into two types:

1. **Anatomical dead space:** It is the volume of air contained in the conducting zone of the 'respiratory passages', i.e. from nose

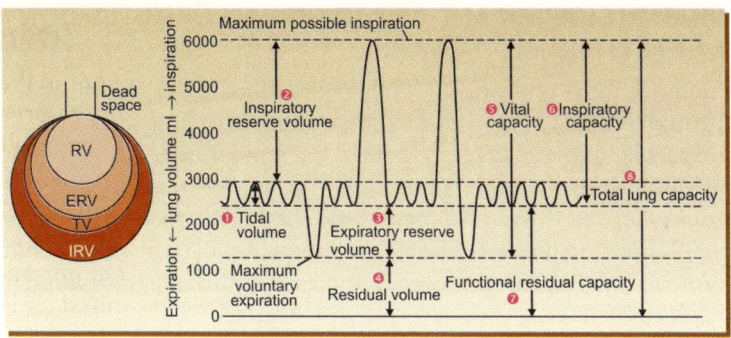

**Fig. 5.1:** Normal spirogram

and mouth up to the terminal bronchioles where exchange of gases does not take place.

**Normal value:** 150 ml (approx equal to the body weight in pounds).

2. **Physiological dead space:** It includes anatomical dead space plus volume of air in the alveoli which does not take part in the gas exchange function of the lungs.

**For example:**

a. Volume of air that ventilates the alveoli but receives no pulmonary blood flow.

b. Some of the alveoli may be overventilated.

Clinically, anatomical and physiological dead space are equal in volume. If ventilation and perfusion are not in equilibrium, then only they differ in volume.

## MEASUREMENT

Anatomical dead space is measured by two methods:

a. **Direct method:** This is based on the Bohr's equation that states expired air volume includes the alveolar air volume and inspired air volume in dead space.

$$\frac{\text{Expired air volume} \times (CO_2\% \text{ in alveolar air} - CO_2\% \text{ in expired air})}{CO_2 \text{ in alveolar air}}$$

b. **Indirect method:** Single breath oxygen technique.

*Measurement of physiological dead space.*

$$\frac{\text{Expired air volume} \times (pCO_2 \text{ in alveolar air} - pCO_2 \text{ in expired air})}{pCO_2 \text{ in alveolar air}}$$

## WHAT WILL HAPPEN AND WHY TO THE RATE OF RESPIRATION IF THERE IS PNEUMOTHORAX                    2.5 (1991)

Pneumothorax is a condition when air enters in the pleural space, through either a hole in chest wall or rupture of lungs. As a result, pressure in pleural space is same as the atmospheric pressure and not sub-atmospheric as is normally present. Lung on the affected side collapses due to its recoil tendency. This leads to uneven ventilation and normal gaseous exchange cannot occur. As a result, hypoxia and hypercapnia occur and cause marked stimulation of respiration.

In addition, due to lung collapse, pulmonary deflation receptors are stimulated, reflexly causing rapid and shallow breathing.

## PHYSIOLOGICAL /CLINICAL SIGNIFICANCE OF LAW OF LAPLACE AS APPLIED TO THE LUNGS                    3 (2012)

According to the law of Laplace in a spherical structure like alveoli, distending pressure equals two times tension divided by the radius

$$P = \frac{2T}{R}$$

$P$ = Distending pressure
$T$ = Tension in the wall due to surface tension
$R$ = Radius

Here surface tension is the inward force with $P$ constant, if $T$ is not reduced as $R$ is reduced during expiration, surface tension may overcome the distending pressure and then lungs will collapse. But in the lungs with reduction of radius, there is reduction of surface tension by a surface tension lowering agent called surfactant. The lower surface tension when the alveoli are small is due to the presence of this surfactant in the fluid lining the alveoli.

## TRANSPORT OF GASES

### OXYHAEMOGLOBIN DISSOCIATION CURVE                    (2000)

This gives the oxygen carrying capacity of Hb by relating the percentage oxygen saturation of Hb to the $pO_2$ (Fig 5.2). This has a characteristic sigmoid shape due to the **T-R interconversion**. In de-oxyhaemoglobin, the globin units are tightly bound in a tense (*T*) configuration which reduces the affinity of the molecule for oxygen. When oxygen is first bound, the bonds holding the globin units are released, producing a relaxed (*R*) configuration, that exposes more oxygen binding sites. This results in 500 fold increase in the oxygen affinity of Hb.

Factors affecting the oxygen – Hb dissociation curve (Fig 5.2a)

- **Shift to the right:** These factors reduce the oxygen affinity of Hb causing unloading of oxygen:
  a. Increase in body temperature (Fig. 5.2b)
  b. Fall in blood pH due to increased $CO_2$ or presence of any acid in the blood (Figs 5.2c and 5.2d)
  c. Increase in concentration of 2, 3 DPG

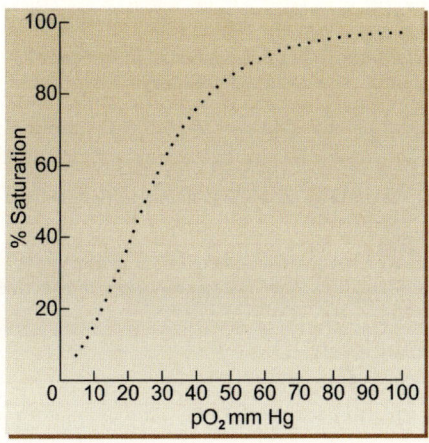

**Fig. 5.2 a:** Normal $O_2$ dissociation curve

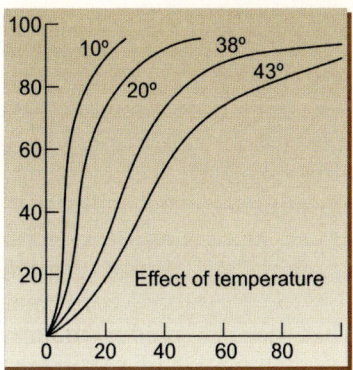

**Fig. 5.2b:** Effect of temperature on $O_2$ dissociation curve

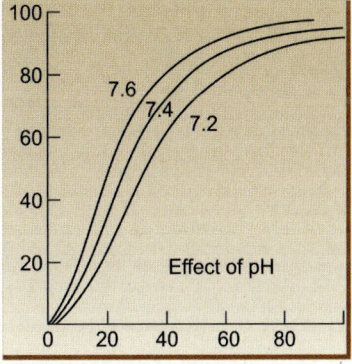

**Fig. 5.2c:** Effect of pH on $O_2$ dissociation curve

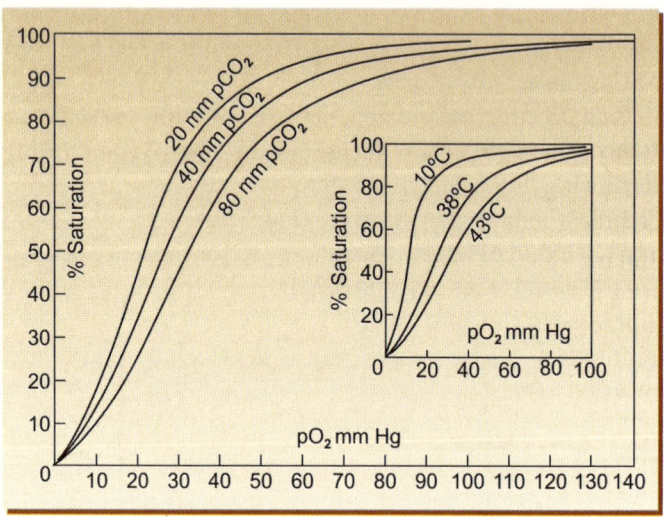

**Fig. 5.2d:** Effect of $pCO_2$ on $O_2$ dissociation curve

- **Shift to the left:** Affinity of oxygen to combine with Hb increases causing less release of oxygen to the tissues:
  a. Carbon monoxide
  b. Fetal haemoglobin
  c. Myoglobin
  d. Decrease in body temperature

## HOW DOES HYPERCAPNIA CONTROL RESPIRATION   10 (1991)

Hypercapnia is a situation when $CO_2$ tension ($pCO_2$) of arterial blood is more than the normal value of 40 mm Hg. It can occur as a result of:

i.  Increased tissue metabolism raising the $pCO_2$ in blood.

ii. When gas mixture containing excess of $CO_2$ is inhaled, it increases alveolar $CO_2$ and so diffusion of $CO_2$ from blood into alveoli will be less and as a consequence $pCO_2$ will rise in arterial blood. A raised arterial $pCO_2$ has a stimulatory effect on ventilation. As a result of this, more $CO_2$ is washed off in the expired air till $pCO_2$ of arterial blood is restored to normal. There exists a linear relationship between $pCO_2$ and pulmonary ventilation. Hypercapnia stimulates ventilation by stimulating the chemoreceptors which are sensitive to changes in arterial blood with regard to:

1. $pCO_2$
2. $pO_2$
3. $H^+$ concentration.

A rise in $pCO_2$ and $H^+$ and a fall in partial pressure of oxygen stimulate respiration. Chemoreceptors are present in:

i. Aortic and carotid bodies: Peripheral chemoreceptor.

ii. Medulla of brainstem: Central chemoreceptor.

Medullary chemoreceptors are more sensitive to hypercapnia and account for major part of the response. $CO_2$ stimulates central chemoreceptors by increasing the concentration of $H^+$ in brain interstitial fluid and CSF. It is this increase in $H^+$ to which central chemoreceptors respond. $CO_2$ can rapidly diffuse through membranes and so also through the blood brain barriers. It is soon hydrated to $H_2CO_3$ and dissociates to hydrogen and bicarbonate ions. These $H^+$ stimulate respiratory centres. Medullary chemoreceptors are situated on the ventral surface of medulla, close to respiratory centre but is separate from it.

## PERIPHERAL CHEMORECEPTORS

They have special chemosensitive glomus cells. When stimulated impulses are carried in the vagus and glossopharyngeal nerves to respiratory centres, the inspiration is modified to maintain a constant $pCO_2$ of arterial blood at 40 mm Hg.

## EFFECT OF BREATHING A GAS MIXTURE CONTAINING EXCESS OF $CO_2$

Initially there is a linear relationship between $pCO_2$ in alveolar air and degree of ventilation but there is an upper limit to this relationship. When $pCO_2$ of inspired air is close to that of alveolar air, elimination of $CO_2$ becomes difficult. As $CO_2$ content of inspired air is raised to 7% of alveolar air, arterial blood $CO_2$ begin to rise as no exchange occurs in the alveoli in spite of hyperventilation. $CO_2$ accumulates in the body fluids and depresses the nervous system along with respiration. This condition is called **$CO_2$ narcosis**.

## CO POISONING                                 2.5 (2007)

CO is formed in small amount in the body and may act as a chemical messenger in the brain and elsewhere. In larger amounts it may be poisonous causing death.

- CO is toxic because it reacts with Hb to form carbonmonoxy-haemoglobin which does not take up oxygen. It is often considered a type of anaemic hypoxia since the total amount of Hb that can carry oxygen is reduced but the total Hb content of blood remains unaffected by CO.
- The affinity of Hb for CO is 210 times more as compared to oxygen and COHb liberates CO very slowly. COHb liberates the CO very slowly, shifting the dissociation curve of the remaining $HbO_2$ to the left thus decreasing the amount of oxygen released to the tissues.
- CO is also toxic to the cytochromes in the tissues but the dose for this is 1000 times the lethal dose. Hence, tissue toxicity plays no role in clinical CO poisoning.

## Symptoms

- Symptoms are similar to any type of hypoxia specially nausea and headache but there is little stimulation of respiration because the carotid and aortic chemoreceptors are not stimulated.
- The cherry red color of COHb is visible in the skin, nail beds and mucous membranes.
- Symptoms produced by chronic exposure to sub-lethal doses of CO are those of progressive brain damage, including mental changes, and sometimes a parkinsonian like state.

## Treatment

Treatment includes immediate termination of exposure and adequate ventilation by artificial respiration, if necessary. Ventilation with oxygen is preferable to fresh air, since oxygen hastens the dissociation of COHb. Hyperbaric oxygen therapy is useful in this condition.

### EXPLAIN WHY CO POISONING CAN BE TREATED ONLY BY HYPERBARIC OXYGEN THERAPY                 1 (2003)-IPU

In CO poisoning the amount of Hb which is available to combine with oxygen is reduced since the affinity of CO to combine with Hb is 210 times higher compared to oxygen. Hence, the only way to improve oxygenation of tissues is to increase the amount of dissolved oxygen. This is done by giving 100% oxygen at 2–3 atmospheres to those suffering from CO poisoning.

## EXPLAIN WHY CO POISONING DECREASES THE OXYGEN CARRYING CAPACITY OF BLOOD     1 (2004)

The affinity of CO to combine with haemoglobin is 210 times its affinity to combine with oxygen leading to the production of carboxyhaemoglobin (COHb). COHb which is formed also liberates the CO very slowly hence both these factors reduce the oxygen carrying capacity of blood.

## HOW IS $CO_2$ TRANSPORTED FROM THE TISSUES TO THE LUNGS? DESCRIBE THE MECHANISMS INVOLVED     10 (1986)

## CARBON DIOXIDE TRANSPORT     2 (2010)

## CHLORIDE SHIFT     2.5 (2005)

### Carbon Dioxide Transport from Tissues to the Lungs

Carbon dioxide is carried from tissue to the lungs in venous blood. Large amount of $CO_2$ is produced in body as a result of tissue metabolism. It is a highly diffusible gas being 20 times as diffusible as oxygen. From tissue it diffuses into the interstitial fluid and then into the venous circulation from the venous end of the capillaries due to pressure gradient.

From the capillaries it is carried in the blood and transported to the lungs from where it is expired out.

### $CO_2$ Transport in Blood

In blood, it is transported in:

I. Plasma
II. RBCs

I. **Transport in plasma:** $CO_2$ content of venous blood is 38 ml/dL. In plasma $CO_2$ is carried in:

   a. **Dissolved form:** Responsible for $CO_2$ tension of blood, which is equal to 46 mm Hg.

   b. **Carried as $HCO_3^-$:** $CO_2$ is hydrated to $H_2CO_3$ which dissociates to hydrogen and bicarbonate ions. $H^+$ are buffered in plasma and bicarbonate ions combines with cations like $Na^+$.

   c. **Carbaminocompounds:** Carbon dioxide combines with plasma proteins forming carbaminoproteins and is transported to the lungs.

II. **Carbon dioxide transport in RBCs:** $CO_2$ from the plasma diffuses quickly into RBCs. $CO_2$ content of RBCs in venous blood is 14 ml/dL.

In RBCs, it is transported:

a. In combination with haemoglobin
b. As bicarbonate

    a. **$CO_2$ carriage by haemoglobin:** $CO_2$ forms carbamino-Hb with haemoglobin, it combines with $NH_2$ group of histidine residue present in $\alpha$ and $\beta$ chains of globin. Reduced Hb has greater capacity to form this compound. Formation of carbamino-Hb is decreased in the presence of 2, 3 DPG as they compete for the same groups in the $\beta$ chains of globin. This mode accounts for 10% of total transport.

    b. **Transport as $HCO_3^-$ in RBCs**

In RBCs, $CO_2$ is hydrated to $H_2CO_3$ in the presence of carbonic anhydrase, an enzyme which catalyses this reaction many thousand times.

Bicarbonate ions diffuse into plasma in large amount as its concentration rises in the RBCs. To maintain electrical neutrality $Cl^-$ shifts from the plasma into RBCs. This is known as **chloride shift** and is mediated by a membrane protein called **Band 3** (Fig. 5.3).

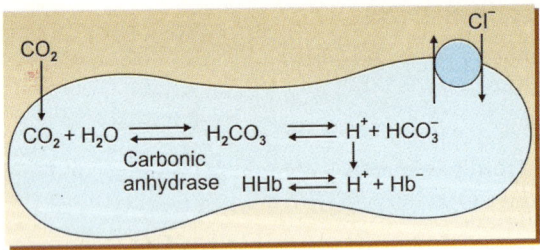

**Fig. 5.3:** Chloride shift

As chloride ions shift into RBCs, water follows it and RBCs increase in volume. So RBCs in venous blood are larger than in arterial blood. As a result haematrocit of venous blood is little more than that of arterial blood. As a result of carbon dioxide carriage, pH of venous blood is 7.36. It is less alkaline than that of arterial blood which is 7.40.

## COMPARE AND CONTRAST BOHR AND HALDANE EFFECTS
**2 (2003)-IPU, 2 (2006)**

The decrease in the oxygen affinity of Hb when the pH of blood falls is called **Bohr effect**.

Binding of oxygen to Hb reduces its affinity for carbon dioxide which is called **Haldane effect**.

## EXPLAIN WHY CARBON DIOXIDE RETENTION IS RARELY A PROBLEM IN PATIENTS WITH DEFECTIVE ALVEOLAR VENTILATION
**1 (2003)-IPU**

Carbon dioxide is a highly diffusible gas (being 20 times more diffusible than oxygen), hence carbon dioxide retention is never a problem in patients with defective alveolar ventilation.

## EXPLAIN WHY CYANOSIS IS NOT OBSERVED IN SEVERE ANAEMIA
**1 (2008)**

Cyanosis is produced when at least 5 gm of reduced haemoglobin per 100 ml of blood is there in the capillaries. Severe anaemia does not lead to cyanosis as the total haemoglobin content is low so enough reduced haemoglobin is not there to produce bluish discolouration of cyanosis.

## CYANOSIS
**2.5 (1991)**

Cyanosis is a clinical condition characterised by bluish discoloration of skin and mucous membranes due to the presence of excess reduced haemoglobin.

For cyanosis to occur it is essential that more than 5 gm/dL of reduced haemoglobin is present.

Clinically, cyanosis can be observed in the following sites:
- Nail beds
- Mucous membranes
- Ear lobes
- Lips
- Fingers (where the skin is thin)

Cyanosis may be caused by:
a. Hypoxic hypoxia
b. Stagnant hypoxia

Clinically, cyanosis is associated with lung diseases where oxygenation of blood is inadequate.

In heart diseases when pumping action of the heart is inadequate, it leads to peripheral circulatory failure and blood stays in the tissues for longer time because of which more oxygen is extracted from the blood, thereby increasing the amount of reduced Hb.

## REGULATION OF RESPIRATION

### HERING BREUER REFLEX 4 (2004)-IPU, 2 (2006)

Hering Breuer inflation reflex *(Hering E and Breuer E,* 1868) is an increase in the duration of expiration produced by steady lung inflation. The steady inflation of the lungs stimulates stretch receptors, impulses travel via the vagi to inhibit the apneustic centre thus inhibiting inspiration producing prolonged expiration. **Physiological significance:** The reflex is absent in healthy eupnoeic man with tidal volume of 500 ml. The threshold level is at a TV of approx 1–1.5 L. Therefore, this reflex may exert a considerable influence in determining the pattern of breathing when respiration is increased during exercise.

Hering Breuer deflation reflex is a decrease in the duration of expiration produced by marked deflation of the lung.

### DESCRIBE THE NEURAL REGULATION OF RESPIRATION IN MAN 10 (1993), 2.5 (2011)

#### Neural Control of Respiration (Fig. 5.4)

Two separate neural control systems exist controlling the activity of motor neurons innervating respiratory system muscles.

i. **Voluntary control:** Exerted from neurons in the cerebral cortex to motor neurons of respiratory muscles.
ii. **Involuntary autonomic control:** Exerted through spontaneously discharging neurons in medulla and pons, i.e. 'respiratory centres'. These neurons innervate the respiratory muscles.

#### Innervation of Inspiratory Muscles

i. **Diaphragm:** Fibres from respiratory centres converge on motor neurons, giving rise to phrenic nerve in cervical 3, 4 and 5 segments of the spinal cord.
ii. **External intercostal muscles:** Fibres end on motor neurons throughout the thoracic segments of the spinal cord that supply these muscles.

## Innervation of Muscles of Expiration

Fibres from respiratory centres converge on motor neurons supplying these muscles, also through thoracic segments of spinal cord.

**Respiratory centres:** These are groups of neurons in the pons and medulla.

**Medullary centres:** These are two groups of neurons:

i. **Dorsal group:** Having predominately the neurons which when stimulated excite motor neurons to inspiratory muscles and are called **I-neurons**. These are located near the tractus solitarius. They discharge during inspiration.

ii. **Ventral group:** A column of neurons extending throughout nucleus ambiguous and nucleus retroambiguous in lateral medulla and mostly contains the neurons which discharge during expiration and are called **E-neurons**. Some of these neurons probably inhibit I-neurons during expiration.

Normally there is a reciprocal innervation of inspiratory and expiratory muscles controlled by descending pathways from the respiratory centres in medulla.

**Pontine centres**

i. **Apneustic centre:** It is a group of neurons in middle and lower pons which when stimulated, inspiratory phase of respiration is prolonged and expiration is shortened called apneustic breathing. This centre stimulates inspiratory neurons of medulla and is itself inhibited by vagal afferents coming from the stretched lungs (due to inspiration) and then expiration supervenes.

ii. **Pneumotaxic centre:** A group of neurons in upper pons which normally checks the activity of the apneustic centre. It is probably having a stimulatory effect on expiratory neurons during deep breathing (Fig. 5.4).

To simplify, normal rhythmic respiration occurs as follows:

Activity of I-neurons → discharge to motor neurons to phrenic and external intercostal muscles → inspiration → stretch of lungs increase activity in vagal afferents from lung → inhibition of apneustic centre → removal of drive of I-neurons → expiration occurs passively.

During deep breathing pneumotaxic centres stimulate E-neuron during expiration.

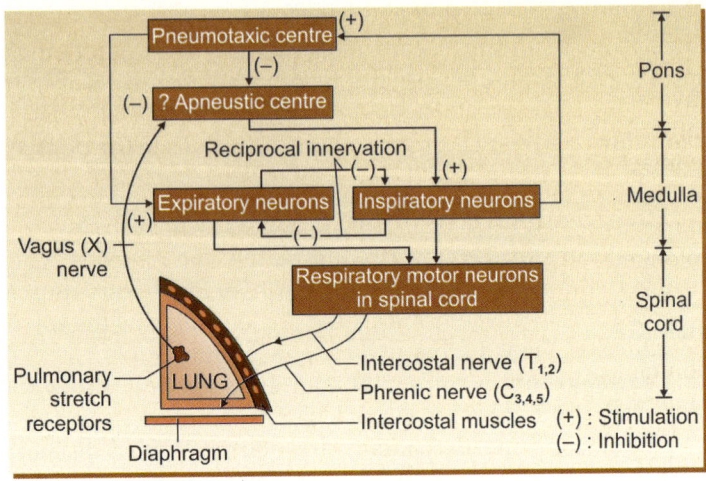

**Fig. 5.4:** Organization of respiratory centres

## Other afferents influencing the rhythm of respiration through reflex actions are:

  i. Vagal afferents from pulmonary stretch receptor → Hering Breuer reflex.
 ii. Lung irritant receptor → hyperpnoea.
iii. J-receptors from lungs → cause bronchoconstriction, apnoea, hypotension and bradycardia.
 iv. From laryngeal mucous membrane → coughing reflex causing deep inspiration followed by explosive expiration.
  v. From pharyngeal receptors → deglutition apnoea.
 vi. From peripheral chemoreceptors → modify respiration.
vii. From baroreceptors → feeble inhibitory effect.
viii. Venocaval receptors → hyperpnoea, e.g. increased venous pressure stimulates these receptors.

## WHAT WILL HAPPEN AND WHY TO RESPIRATORY PATTERN IF SECTION IS MADE BETWEEN THE PNEUMOTAXIC AND APNEUSTIC CENTRE  1 (2004)

The normal function of the pneumotaxic centre is to inhibit the apneustic centre and switch between inspiration and expiration. If a section is made between the two centres, respiration will become deep and slow and continue in the inspiratory phase.

## EXPLAIN WHY VAGOTOMY WILL LEAD TO APNEUSTIC PATTERN OF BREATHING                    1 (2003)

In lower pons there lies a respiratory centre which is tonically active and activates the inspiratory centre, called the apneustic centre. This centre is inhibited by the vagus nerve. When the vagi are intact regular rhythmic respiration continues, but on cutting the vagus nerve apneustic centre is no longer inhibited leading to an apneustic pattern of breathing characterised by deep and prolonged inspiration.

## CHEMICAL REGULATION OF RESPIRATION          5 (2003)-IPU

The main chemical factors regulating respiration include $pCO_2$, $pO_2$ and pH. These factors influence respiration in such a way that their own levels are held constant. The chemical mechanisms regulate respiration via chemoreceptors which are divided into three categories:

- Peripheral chemoreceptors
- Central chemoreceptors
- Pulmonary and myocardial chemoreceptors

**Peripheral chemoreceptors**
- They include carotid and aortic body.
- There is a carotid body near common carotid artery bifurcation and usually two or more aortic bodies near arch of aorta.
- Each contains two types of cells: Type I and type II cells.
- **Type I** cells contain catecholamines (probably dopamine). When exposed to hypoxia, they release catecholamines that stimulate the carotid sinus nerve via $D_2$ receptors.
- **Type II** cells are glial cells that surround the type I cells.
- Mechanism of action of type I cells.
  Hypoxia $\rightarrow$ decreases activity of oxygen sensitive $K^+$ channels $\rightarrow$ decreases $K^+$ efflux $\rightarrow$ increased $Ca^{2+}$ influx $\rightarrow$ depolarisation of cell membrane $\rightarrow$ release of neurotransmitter $\rightarrow$ stimulate afferent nerve endings.
- Blood flow to each carotid and aortic body is highest in the body at 2000 ml/100 gm/min, therefore, the oxygen needs are met largely by dissolved oxygen. Hence, these are not stimulated in anaemia or CO poisoning where the amount of dissolved oxygen is normal.

- **Peripheral receptors get stimulated by:**
  - **Hypoxia:** When the arterial $pO_2$ decreases, the amount of dissolved oxygen decreases.
  - **Vascular stasis:** The amount of oxygen delivered to receptors per unit of time is decreased.
  - **Asphyxia:** Combination of oxygen lack along with carbon dioxide excess.
  - **Drugs** (cyanide, nicotine, lobeline), etc. prevent oxygen utilization at tissue level.
  - Increase in **plasma $K^+$ level** such as during exercise contributes to exercise induced hyperpnoea.

## Medullary Chemoreceptors

- They are located on the ventral surface of the medulla near the respiratory centre but separate from it.
- The magnitude of stimulation is directly proportional to the concentration of $H^+$ ions in the CSF and interstitial fluid which in turn is directly proportional to the arterial $pCO_2$.

### Mechanism of $H^+$ formation

- Carbon dioxide readily penetrates the membrane, whereas $H^+$ and $HCO_3^-$ penetrate slowly. The carbon dioxide that enters the brain is readily hydrated to form carbonic acid which dissociates into $H^+$ and $HCO_3^-$. Thus local $H^+$ concentration increases.
- Central chemoreceptors get inhibited by cyanide and during sleep.

### Pulmonary and myocardial chemoreceptors

- Injection of veratidine or nicotine in the pulmonary circulation stimulates chemoreceptors in pulmonary vessels producing hypotension, bradycardia and apnoea followed by tachypnoea. This is called the pulmonary chemoreflex. A similar response is seen if these agents are introduced into the coronaries supplying the left ventricle, called the **coronary chemoreflex or Bezold Jarisch reflex.**
- This reflex has no known physiological role. It is seen only in pulmonary congestion or embolism and following **myocardial infarction.**

## COMPARE CENTRAL AND PERIPHERAL CHEMORECEPTORS
### 2.5 (2002), 2 (2007), 2 (2004)-IPU

| Central chemoreceptors | Peripheral chemoreceptors |
|---|---|
| 1. They are located on the ventral surface of the medulla near the respiratory centre | 1. There are two or more aortic bodies near the arch of aorta, and two carotid bodies, one on each side near bifurcation of common carotid artery |
| 2. Nerve fibres from here directly project over to the respiratory centre | 2. Aortic bodies are supplied by the aortic nerve (branch of X nerve), carotid body by carotid sinus nerve (branch of IX nerve) |
| 3. Increase in hydrogen ions in brain and CSF fluid causes stimulation of these receptors. They are inhibited by anaesthetics, cyanide and during sleep. | 3. They are stimulated by <br> i. Increase in arterial $pCO_2$ <br> ii. Decrease in arterial $pO_2$ <br> iii. Nicotine <br> iv. Lobeline <br> v. Cyanide |
| 4. Stimulation produces an increase in the rate and depth of respiration only. They regulate the respiration from minute to minute. About 80 to 85% of the resting respiratory drive is due to stimulatory effect of carbon dioxide on central chemoreceptors | 4. Stimulation produces an increase in rate and depth of respiration along with tachycardia and hypertension. They regulate the respiration from breath to breath. About 15–20% of the resting respiratory drive is due to stimulatory effect of carbon dioxide on peripheral chemoreceptors |

## COMPARE AORTIC AND CAROTID BODY      2 (2005)

| Carotid body | Aortic body |
|---|---|
| • They are located near the common carotid artery bifurcation on each side | • They are located near the arch of aorta |
| • They are innervated by carotid sinus branch of glosso-pharyngeal nerve | • They are innervated by aortic branch of vagus nerve |

*Contd.*

*Contd.*

| Carotid body | Aortic body |
|---|---|
| • They are 7 times more effective than aortic body in stimulating respiration increasing both the the rate and depth of respiration | • They increase only the frequency of respiration with small increase in ventilation |

## COMPARE RESPIRATORY ACIDOSIS AND ALKALOSIS   2 (2010)

| Respiratory acidosis | Respiratory alkalosis |
|---|---|
| • This is produced due to decreased pulmonary ventilation which occurs due to causes other than decrease in arterial $H^+$ concentration | • This is produced due to increased pulmonary ventilation which occurs due to causes other than increase in $H^+$ concentration |
| • Causes include inadequate ventilation as in airway obstruction and impaired gas diffusion | • This is produced due to increased gas exchange in the lungs because of increased ventilation |
| • This type of acidosis is compensated entirely by the renal mechanism. Increased $pCO_2$ supplies more $H^+$ to renal tubules for secretion which leads to increased secretion of $H^+$ as titrable acid and $NH_3$ and increased reab- sorption of $HCO_3^-$ which helps to normalize the pH | • Decreased $pCO_2$ causes a deficit of $H^+$ in the renal cells for secretion which leads to decreased secretion of $H^+$ as titrable acid and $NH_4^+$, decreased reabsorption of new $HCO_3^-$ and decreased reabsorption of filtered $HCO_3^-$ that helps to normalise the pH |

## ROLE OF RESPIRATION IN pH REGULATION       2 (2003)-IPU

Respiration forms the second line of defence against acid-base disorders which provide a short-term but rapid control. It acts via the respiratory centre, located in the medulla to regulate removal of carbon dioxide and therefore carbonic acid concentration in the blood and restores the normal pH.

## Role of Respiratory Centre

These are influenced both by the $CO_2$ as well as $H^+$ concentration through central and peripheral chemoreceptors. Respiratory response occurs in response to metabolic acid-base disorders only and consists of:

- **Hyperventilation:** This occurs in response to metabolic acidosis and results in lowering of $pCO_2$ to match the decreased $HCO_3^-$.

- **Hypoventilation:** This occurs in response to metabolic alkalosis and results in raising the $pCO_2$ to match the increased $HCO_3^-$.

### HYPOXIA

### EXPLAIN WHY PERIPHERAL CHEMORECEPTORS DO NOT RESPOND TO ANAEMIC HYPOXIA          1 (2004)

The blood flow in the chemoreceptors (carotid body) is about 2000 ml/100 g of tissue/min. Since the blood flow per unit of tissues is so enormous, the oxygen needs of the cell can be largely met by dissolved oxygen alone. Hence, these receptors are not stimulated by anaemic hypoxia where the amount of dissolved oxygen reaching the receptors is generally normal and only the combined oxygen in the blood decreases.

### EXPLAIN WHY HYPOXIA LEADS TO VASOCONSTRICTION IN PULMONARY CIRCULATION          1 (2005)

Type I glomus cells in the carotid and aortic bodies have oxygen sensitive $K^+$ channels whose conductance is reduced in proportion to the degree of hypoxia to which they are exposed. This reduces the $K^+$ efflux, depolarizing the cell and causes $Ca^{2+}$ influx via L-type of $Ca^{2+}$ channels which triggers action potential and transmitter release with consequent excitation of the afferent nerve endings. The smooth muscles of pulmonary arteries contain similar oxygen sensitive $K^+$ channels which mediate the vasoconstriction caused by hypoxia. This is in contrast to systemic arteries which contain ATP dependant $K^+$ channels that permit more potassium efflux with hypoxia and consequently cause vasodilation instead of vasoconstriction.

## COMPARE ANAEMIC AND HYPOXIC HYPOXIA  2 (2004)-IPU, 2 (2007)

| | Hypoxic hypoxia | Anaemic hypoxia | Stagnant (ischaemic) hypoxia | Histotoxic hypoxia |
|---|---|---|---|---|
| 1. Definition based on:<br>i. Arterial $pO_2$<br>ii. Haemoglobin<br>iii. Rate of blood flow of tissues | (i) ↓s; (ii) and (iii) are normal; i.e. low arterial $pO_2$ when $O_2$ carrying capacity of blood and rate of blood flow to tissues are normal | (i) ↓s; (ii) and (iii) are normal, i.e. ↓ amount of haemoglobin available to carry $O_2$ in spite of normal arterial $pO_2$ and normal rate of blood flow to tissues. | (i) ↓s; (ii) and (iii) are normal, i.e. rate of blood flow to tissues ↓s so that adequate $O_2$ is not delivered to them in spite of normal arterial $pO_2$ and haemoglobin content | (i), (ii) and (iii) are normal, i.e. normal $O_2$ delivery to tissues but they cannot make use of $O_2$ supplied to them due to action of toxic agent |
| 2. Causes | i. ↓ (↓$pO_2$)<br>ii. ↓Pulmonary ventilation<br>iii. Defective V/P ratio | Total haemoglobin ↓s due to:<br>i. Anaemia<br>ii. Haemorrhage<br>iii. Presence of haemoglobin: COHb or methaemoglobin | i. Circulatory failure<br>ii. Haemorrhage<br><br>iii. Heart failure | Cyanide poisoning |

*Contd.*

*Contd.*

| | Hypoxic hypoxia | Anaemic hypoxia | Stagnant (ischaemic) hypoxia | Histotoxic hypoxia |
|---|---|---|---|---|
| 3. Arterial $pO_2$ | ↓s (as $IpO_2$↓s) | Normal | Normal | Normal |
| 4. Arterial $O_2$ content | ↓s | Markedly reduced | Normal | Normal |
| 5. Arterial % $O_2$ saturation of haemoglobin | ↓s | ↓s | Normal | Normal |
| 6. A–V $pO_2$ difference | ↓s | Normal | More than normal | Less than normal |
| 7. Cyanosis | Present | Absent | Present | Absent (as reduced haemoglobin is produced in small amount) |
| 8. Stimulation of peripheral chemoreceptors | Present (as dissolved $O_2$ in plasma ↓s) | Absent (dissolved $O_2$ in plasma is sufficient to meet receptor demand) | Present (because arterial $pCO_2$ increases and $pO_2$ ↓s) | Present (cyanide ↓s $O_2$ utilization at tissue level) |

(↓ : decrease ↑ : increase)

## COMPARE STAGNANT AND HISTOTOXIC HYPOXIA
**2 (2003)-IPU**

## COMPARE HYPOXIC HYPOXIA AND STAGNANT HYPOXIA
**2 (2004)-IPU**

## HYPOXIA
**2.5 (2004)**

Hypoxia is defined as deficiency of oxygen at the tissue level. It is classically divided into the following four types:

1. **Hypoxic hypoxia:** $pO_2$ of arterial blood is reduced. This may be because of:
   - Low $pO_2$ in inspired air such as at high altitude.
   - Decreased pulmonary ventilation, e.g. in airway obstruction
   - Defect in exchange of gases through the alveolocapillary membrane
   - Venous-arterial shunts, e.g. cyanotic congenital heart disease.

2. **Anaemic hypoxia:** Arterial $pO_2$ is normal but the amount of haemoglobin available to carry oxygen is reduced, e.g. anaemia due to decreased RBC count, decreased haemoglobin and altered haemoglobin.

3. **Stagnant/Ischemic hypoxia:** Blood flow to the tissues is so low that adequate oxygen is not delivered to it despite a normal $pO_2$ and Hb concentration, e.g. circulatory failure and haemorrhage.

4. **Histotoxic hypoxia:** Amount of oxygen delivered to a tissue is adequate but because of the action of a toxic agent the tissue cells cannot make use of the oxygen supplied to them as the cellular oxidative enzymes are destroyed, e.g. cyanide poisoning.

### HIGH ALTITUDE PHYSIOLOGY

## WHAT ARE CARDIO-RESPIRATORY CHANGES AT AN ALTITUDE OF 18,000 FEET ABOVE SEA LEVEL
**5 (1991)**

## MOUNTAIN SICKNESS
**(2000)**

## ACCLIMATIZATION
**4 (2003)-IPU, 2 (2002), 2.5 (2003)**

A person staying at high altitude for a period gradually gets acclimatized to low $O_2$ tension in the atmosphere and in arterial blood. At an altitude of 18,000 feet, arterial $O_2$ tension is approximately 67 mm Hg and arterial blood is about 90% saturated.

## Acclimatization occurs by the following changes

i. **Increased pulmonary ventilation:** Immediately on exposure to high altitude hyperventilation occurs due to hypoxic stimulation of chemoreceptors. However, this immediate increase in ventilation blows off excess of $CO_2$ reducing $pCO_2$, hence reducing $H^+$ concentration of body fluids trying to oppose the influence of hypoxic stimulus. However, after a few days, inhibition fades away, perhaps due to transport of bicarbonate ions from CSF and interstitial fluid. Ventilation then finally increases by 3–5 times the normal value.

ii. **Increase in haemoglobin:** Hypoxia is known to stimulate erythropoiesis, thereby raising the Hb-content which is slow to begin with and takes several weeks to develop fully. Hb may rise to about 20 g/dL in a fully acclimatized individual.

iii. **Increased dissociation of oxygen from Hb:** Within a few hours of exposure, increased quantities of 2, 3 DPG are formed in the blood and oxygen dissociation curve is shifted to the right, hence more oxygen is made available to the tissues.

iv. **Increase in diffusion capacity of the lungs**

Following factors contribute towards increased diffusion capacity of lungs:

  a. Increase pulmonary blood volume.
  b. Increase in size of the surface area due to increased lung expansion.
  c. Increased pulmonary artery pressure due to hypoxic constriction of pulmonary vessels.

v. **Circulatory changes at high altitude**
  a. Increased vasculature due to increased cardiac output.
  b. Increase in number and size of blood capillaries.

vi. **Cellular acclimatization:** An increase in oxidative cellular enzymes occurs. Mitochondria also increases in number.

As a result of acclimatization, gradually the person gets used to low partial pressure of oxygen in the atmosphere. This has the following effects:

  a. Less harmful effects on body
  b. Physical performance is improved
  c. Person can ascend to higher altitude after acclimatization.

## WHAT IS MOUNTAIN SICKNESS? WHAT ARE ITS FEATURES? DESCRIBE HOW THE BODY ACCLIMATIZES ITSELF TO HIGH ALTITUDE                    10 (1989)

## EXPLAIN WHY PULMONARY OEDEMA OCCURS IN RAPID ASCENT TO HIGH ALTITUDE                    1 (2004)

### Mountain Sickness

Some symptoms occur when a person goes to high altitude called mountain sickness. These symptoms are due to hypoxia. It can be due to:

a. Acute sickness
b. Chronic sickness

### Acute Mountain Sickness

When a person ascends rapidly to high altitude symptoms of acute sickness take place. Symptoms that are produced are due to cerebral hypoxia and include:

- Confusion
- Error of judgement
- Emotional instability
- False overconfidence

If a person is not moved to lower heights it may prove to be fatal. In acute mountain sickness death results from:

i. **Cerebral oedema**

Hypoxia
↓
Cerebral vasodilatation
↓
Increased capillary pressure
↓
Leakage of fluid into tissue
↓
Cerebral oedema which compresses the brain tissues and causes brain dysfunction.

ii. **Pulmonary oedema**

Hypoxia
↓
Pulmonary vasoconstriction in some areas
↓
Other areas receive more blood flow
↓
Increased capillary pressure in these areas producing
pulmonary oedema and fatal pulmonary dysfunction.

## Chronic Mountain Sickness

In some persons after they have lived at high altitude for a long time, symptoms develop due to the acclimatization process as follows:

Increased RBC
↓
Haematocrit of blood rises
↓
Increases viscosity
↓
Increased pulmonary arterial pressure
(pulmonary hypertension)
↓
Hypertrophy of right side of heart
↓
Congestive heart failure occurs

It may cause death unless the person is moved to lower heights.
**(Process of acclimatization already discussed)**

## CHANGES IN BLOOD AT HIGH ALTITUDE     **2** (2011)

1. **Decreased affinity of Hb for oxygen:** Within a few hours after exposure to hypoxia at high altitude, there is increased amount of 2, 3-DPG in RBCs secondary to rise in blood pH. This shifts the oxygen Hb dissociation curve to the right releasing more oxygen from Hb.

2. **Rise in Hb concentration:** Hypoxia is a powerful stimulant for erythropoietin secretion thus activating erythropoiesis and oxygen carrying capacity of Hb increases. This process starts

only after 2–3 weeks, reaching a peak after several months. Therefore, the haematocrit (PCV) increases to 60%, Hb to 20 gm/dL and RBC count to 7.5–8 million/μL.

## EFFECTS OF HIGH ATMOSPHERIC PRESSURE

**CAISSON'S DISEASE AND ITS TREATMENT**      **3 (2004)-IPU**

**DECOMPRESSION SICKNESS**      **2.5 (2005)**

**WHAT WILL HAPPEN AND WHY WHEN A DEEP-SEA DIVER RAPIDLY ASCENDS TO THE SURFACE**      **1 (2007)**

Caisson's disease or decompression sickness is due to the effects of a pressure difference between the ambient pressure and the pressure of dissolved and free gases in the body. It is caused by increase $pN_2$ in blood that has two characteristic features:

- It passes through cell membranes very slowly
- Five times more soluble in fat than water.

Therefore, when a person breathes air under high pressure for a long time, the amount of $N_2$ dissolved in body fluids increase that leads to nitrogen narcosis. This is characterised by:

- Euphoria
- Impairment of mental functions and intelligence
- Symptoms similar to alcohol intoxication.

When divers suddenly come to the surface, dissolved nitrogen comes out of the fluid and forms bubbles in the tissues and blood due to sudden reduction of pressure. These bubbles are primarily of nitrogen since the body can get rid of other gases easily. These bubbles may have the following effects:

1. In the fat depot, press the nerves producing sensory and motor deficits.
2. Press myelin sheath of sensory nerves producing disturbance or loss of sensation, paraesthesia and itching, etc. whereas pressure on motor nerves produce motor paralysis which is called **Diver's palsy**.
3. Bubbles can block capillaries in brain which may lead to sensory and motor disturbances.
4. In lungs bubbles may produce dyspnoea (chokes), myocardial infarction in the heart or joint pains if lodged in joints (bends).

## Treatment and Prevention

- Subject should come to the surface slowly. If he complaints of pain in the muscles and joints he should be put into a compression chamber. Recompression is done first to dissolve the nitrogen bubbles, then slow decompression is done, so the body can get rid of $N_2$ slowly.

- Nitrogen narcosis can be avoided by breathing **oxygen-helium mixture** instead of air containing nitrogen because helium being a lower density gas is less soluble in fat compared to nitrogen.

## OXYGEN THERAPY                                          2 (2005)

Oxygen therapy is of great value in certain types of hypoxia and almost of no value in other types of hypoxia. In general simple oxygen therapy is not of much value in hypoxia because diffusion across respiratory membrane depends upon partial pressure of gases, therefore, alveolar $pO_2$ can be increased by two methods:

1. Inhalation of 100% pure oxygen.
2. Inhalation of 100% oxygen at high barometric pressure called hyperbaric oxygen therapy.

### Oxygen therapy with 100% pure oxygen at atmospheric pressure

- This is useful in most types of hypoxic hypoxia which may be due to atmospheric hypoxia, hypoventilation or hypoxia due to impaired respiratory membrane diffusion.

- This is of little value in anaemic, stagnant hypoxia or hypoxic hypoxia due to physiological or anatomical shunts, because in all these conditions oxygen is already available in the alveoli.

- It is of no value in histotoxic hypoxia.

### Oxygen therapy with 100% pure oxygen at high barometric pressure

- Advantage of hyperbaric oxygen therapy over oxygen at atmospheric pressure is that the former increases the amount of dissolved oxygen in plasma and is therefore unaffected by haemoglobin concentration.

- **Indications include:** CO poisoning, anaemic hypoxia, decompression sickness, air embolism, wounds with poor blood supply and stagnant hypoxia.

## PHYSIOLOGY OF EXERCISE

### DESCRIBE CARDIOPULMONARY CHANGE DURING MODERATE EXERCISE, SPECIALLY HIGHLIGHTING THE UNDERLYING MECHANISMS                                       10 (1992)

Cardiac change during exercise have been discussed in cardio-vascular system.

### PULMONARY CHANGES DURING MODERATE EXERCISE

During exercise there is increase in pulmonary ventilation, proportional to the severity of exercise. The increase is both in rate and depth of respiration. In moderate exercise, e.g. walking at rate of 8 km/hour, when $O_2$ consumption is 2.5 L/minute pulmonary ventilation is increased to 60 L/min from the resting value of 7 L/min.

**Mechanism of increased ventilation:** Various factors may be contributing to this increase in ventilation:

i. Impulse from higher centre constituting the emotional concomitant of physical exercise—stimulating the respiratory centres.

ii. Impulses from moving joints and muscles reflexly stimulate respiration, through higher centres.

iii. A slight fall in the $pO_2$ of arterial blood stimulates respiration and also sensitizes the respiratory centre to raised $pCO_2$ of blood, through respiratory chemoreceptors.

iv. Raised $pCO_2$ of blood stimulates respiration and increases the ventilation through chemoreceptor.

v. A rise in body temperature also has a stimulatory effect on respiration.

vi. Impulses descending in pyramidal tract to exercising muscles sends collateral to respiratory centres and stimulate them.

All these factors contribute towards increased pulmonary ventilation during exercise to:

a. Meet the increased $O_2$ demand

b. Remove excess $CO_2$ generated due to increased metabolic rate.

## OXYGEN DEBT                              2 (2004)

The extra amount of oxygen which is consumed following a period of exercise is called the oxygen debt. This extra oxygen is used to:

- Regenerate depleted stores of ATP and creatine phosphate
- To resupply oxygen to myoglobin in muscles
- To resupply dissolved oxygen in tissue fluids and blood.
- To remove the excess lactate.

This is measured experimentally by determining the oxygen consumption after exercise until a constant, basal consumption is reached and subtracting the basal consumption from total. This may be 6 times the basal oxygen consumption which indicates that the subject is capable of 6 times the exertion that would have been possible without it.

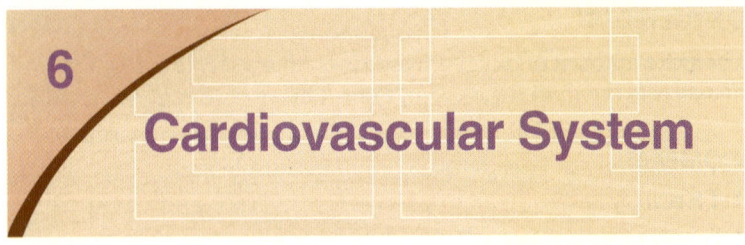

# 6

# Cardiovascular System

### EXPLAIN WHY CARDIAC MUSCLE CANNOT BE TETANISED
1 (2011)

During phases 0 to 2 and about half of phase 3 of the action potential of the cardiac muscle, it remains in the absolute refractory period (ARP), after that it remains relatively refractory until phase 4 (Fig. 6.1). As the contractile response is more than half over during ARP, the summation of contractile response is not possible because of which cardiac muscle cannot be tetanised. This is a protective mechanism that is essential for survival.

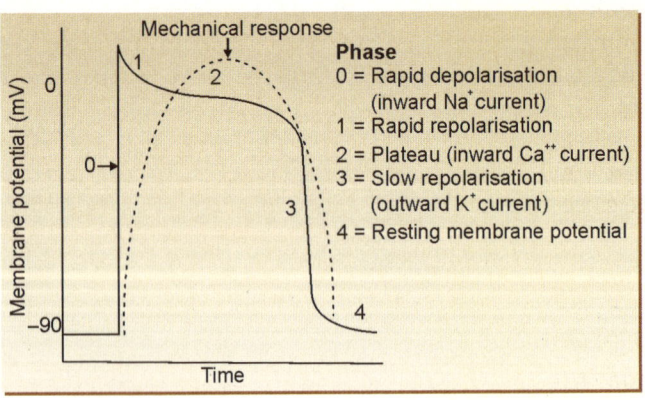

**Fig. 6.1:** Action potential in cardiac muscle

## CARDIAC CYCLE

### WRITE SHORT NOTES ON 1ST AND 2ND HEART SOUND
**2.5 (1985)**

### COMPARE FIRST AND SECOND HEART SOUND    **2 (2002)**

### 1st Heart Sound

It is the sound produced at the onset of ventricular systole during a cardiac cycle. It can be heard clinically with a stethoscope all over the precordium. At the same time it can be heard best over the mitral area, i.e. 5th intercostal space on left side just medial to midclavicular line and tricuspid area, i.e. left 5th intercostal space near sternal border.

This sound is produced due to the closure of A-V valves at the beginning of ventricular systole. Closure of these valves sets up vibrations in the walls of the heart and contained blood, thus producing the sound. It is a low pitched and prolonged sound, heard over 0.15 sec duration and sounds as 'Lubb'.

### 2nd Heart Sound

It is a sound produced at the end of ventricular systole during the cardiac cycle. Like the first heart sound it can be heard all over the precordium with a stethoscope. It is produced due to the closure of semilunar valves, i.e. aortic and pulmonary valves at the end of ventricular systole. It sounds like 'Dubb' and is of high pitch and of short duration of 0.12 sec as compared to the first heart sound.

It is heard best over the aortic and pulmonary areas of the precordium in 2nd right intercostal space and 2nd left intercostal space close to the sternal border, respectively.

## ELECTROCARDIOGRAM

### ECG IN LEAD II    **(2001)**

Standard (or classical) limb lead II is often used for cardiac monitoring as positioning of the electrodes most commonly resembles the pathway of current flow in normal atrial and ventricular depolarisation. On analysis it can be shown that at any given instant the sum of potentials in lead I and lead III equals the potential in lead II as can be seen by **Einthoven's law**.

$$Lead\ II = Lead\ I + Lead\ III$$
$$V_F - V_R = (V_L - V_R) + (V_F - V_L)$$
$$= V_F - V_R$$

In lead II, the electrodes are on the right arm and left leg with the leg positive. By convention an upward deflection is written when the active electrode becomes positive in relation to the indifferent electrode and a downward deflection is written when the active electrode becomes negative. There are four waves in a normal lead II ECG (Fig. 6.2).

- **P wave:** Atrial depolarisation
- **QRS complex:** Ventricular depolarisation
- **T:** Ventricular repolarisation

The U wave is an inconsistent finding that may be due to ventricular myocytes with long action potentials.

## THE NORMAL VALUES OF SOME OF THE IMPORTANT COMPONENTS OF ECG ARE AS UNDER

| Intervals | Normal durations Average range (sec) | Events in the heart during interval |
|---|---|---|
| **PR interval** | 0.12–0.20 | Atrioventricular conduction |
| **QRS duration** | 0.08 0.10 | Ventricular depolarisation |
| **QT interval** | 0.40–0.43 | Ventricular action potential |
| **ST interval** | 0.32 | Plateau part of the ventricular action potential |

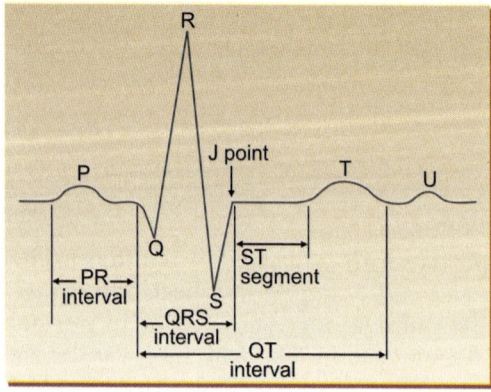

**Fig. 6.2:** Normal electrocardiogram

## SIGNIFICANCE OF PR INTERVAL IN ECG. NAME A CONDITION WHERE PR INTERVAL IS PROLONGED
### 2.5 (1985), 3 (1986)

In an ECG record PR interval is the time interval from the beginning of P wave to the beginning of R wave or Q wave if it is present, of QRS complex.

It signifies the process of atrial depolarisation and conduction of impulse through AV node.

Average PR interval is 0.18 sec when heart rate is 70/minute.

Normal range is 0.12–0.2 sec.

PR interval is prolonged and is more than 0.2 sec. when conduction from atria to ventricles is slowed but not completely interrupted. This is known as incomplete or 1st degree heart block.

## EXPLAIN WHY MOST OF THE ECG WAVES ARE NEGATIVE IN LEAD aVR
### 1 (2006, 2008)

aVR looks at the cavities of the ventricles. Atrial depolarisation, ventricular depolarisation and ventricular repolarisation, move away from the exploring electrode, therefore P wave, QRS complex and T waves are all negative (downward) deflection.

## MEAN CARDIAC VECTOR IN LEFT VENTRICULAR HYPERTROPHY AND RIGHT VENTRICULAR HYPERTROPHY
### (2001)

The normal direction of the cardiac vector lies between –30° and +110°.

- –30° to +30° is normal left axis deviation that represents horizontal position of the heart
- +75° to +110° is normal right axis deviation that represents the vertical position of the heart
- +30° to + 75° represents oblique position of the heart.

If the calculated axis falls to the left of –30° or to the right of +110°, then abnormal left or right axis deviation is said to be present as is seen in left and right ventricular hypertrophy, respectively.

## GENERAL PRINCIPLES OF CIRCULATION

### COMPARE PULMONARY AND SYSTEMIC CIRCULATION
2 (2004)-IPU, 2 (2011)

| Pulmonary circulation | Systemic circulation |
|---|---|
| • This constitutes the low pressure system (pressure < 25 mm Hg) | • This constitutes the high pressure system (pressure > 25 mm Hg) |
| • Pulmonary artery is thin walled, highly distensible structure. Branches have thin walls, large lumen, rich sympathetic innervations but lack resting vasoconstrictor tone | • Aorta is thick walled and elastic. Branches have thicker walls, narrower lumen, rich sympathetic innervations and high vasoconstrictor tone |
| • Pulmonary arteries are thin walled, have larger lumen and lower peripheral resistance | • Arterioles have thick wall, small lumen and they are the main sites of peripheral resistance |
| • There is vasoconstriction in response to hypoxia | • There is vasodilation in response to hypoxia |
| • Pulmonary capillaries are shorter and wider hence the resistance is lower. Capillary blood flow is pulsatile | • Capillaries are narrower and longer, hence the resistance is higher. Capillaries blood flow is continuous |
| • Pulmonary veins carry oxygenated blood and have minor reservoir function | • Veins carry oxygenated blood and have major reservoir function |
| • Lymphatics are abundant in pulmonary circulation | • There are fewer lymphatics |
| • There is a low pressure gradient and high velocity of blood flow. Hence, kinetic energy is an important component in the energy of blood flow | • There is higher pressure gradient and low velocity of blood flow. Hence, the major component is potential energy |

## COMPARE LOW AND HIGH PRESSURE SYSTEM    2 (2008)

| Low pressure system | High pressure system |
|---|---|
| • The pressure changes in this system are up to 25 mm Hg | • The pressure changes are more than 25 mm Hg |
| • This is responsible for control of blood volume and venous return | • This is responsible for control of systemic arterial blood pressure and distribution of blood flow |

**(See also the difference between systemic and pulmonary circulation)**

## POISEUILLE LAW AS APPLICABLE TO HUMAN CIRCULATION    4 (1994)

Poiseuille law is a mathematical expression of relationship between flow in a long narrow tube, viscosity of fluid and radius of the tube. According to the law

$$Q = \frac{\pi}{8} \times \frac{(P_1 - P_2)\, r^4}{L_\eta}$$

$P_1 - P_2$ = Pressure difference between the two ends of the tube
$r$ = Radius of the tube
$L$ = Length of the tube
$\eta$ (eta) = Viscosity of fluid
$\pi/8$ = Derived from the mathematical deduction of the volume passing per unit time.

Resistance to flow in vessels is the peripheral resistance and is a determinant of diastolic blood pressure. *In vivo* viscosity depends on PCV or the haematocrit, which does not change normally.

Length of vessels also does not change. Hence, the resistance to flow, i.e. peripheral resistance varies inversely with fourth power of radius of the blood vessels. Therefore, a small change in the radius of vessels will bring about a marked change in the peripheral resistance. Peripheral resistance in the body primarily depends upon the size of arterioles. Arterioles are normally under the tonic influence of sympathetic nerves. Hence, increase sympathetic discharge causes arteriolar constriction, a rise in peripheral resistance and a rise in DBP.

Large changes in haematocrit, e.g. in polycythemia increases peripheral resistance and increases the work of heart.

Increase in viscosity occurs due to increase in plasma proteins, e.g. increased immunoglobulins.

In severe anaemia since viscosity is decreased, peripheral resistance decreases. This will increase the velocity of blood flow, producing turbulence and heart murmurs will be produced.

## WINDKESSEL VESSELS                                         2.5 (2001)

These are highly elastic vessels and include the aorta, pulmonary artery and their large branches.

As the heart beats intermittently at the rate of 70–80 beats per minute, therefore, pressure and blood flow in the arteries and their large branches are pulsatile that must be converted to a steady flow through the capillaries to ensure maximum exchange between the capillaries and the tissues. This is achieved by two factors:

- **Windkessel effect:** Elastic recoil of the arterial system, i.e. the stretch produced on the elastic tissue of the aorta and the branches during cardiac contraction comes back to regain its original position during the diastolic phase. This is called windkessel effect.

- Resistance to outflow offered by the peripheral arterioles.

### Applied

The degenerative changes that take place in the tunica media of these vessels with aging cause loss of arterial wall elasticity, hence the windkessel effect decreases. Thus with aging the systolic blood pressure rises and the diastolic pressure falls, as extra blood leaves the aorta very rapidly. This results in an increase in the pulse pressure (which is the difference between the systolic and the diastolic pressure) resulting in defective diffusion at the periphery.

## COMPARE WINDKESSEL VESSELS AND
## RESISTANCE VESSELS                                         2 (2007)

**Resistance vessels:** These are vessels that offer resistance to blood flow towards the capillaries, therefore, also called pre-capillary resistance vessels.

- Examples include—arterioles, metarterioles and pre-capillary sphincters.

- These are the main sites of peripheral resistance. Skin and skeletal muscle  blood vessels offer the maximum peripheral resistance.

- They decrease the hydrostatic pressure across the capillaries, therefore, when the arterioles get damaged, marked transudation of fluid occurs across the capillary wall causing a decrease in the blood volume.

- They show an efficient local myogenic control of their own vascular radius.

- The radius of metarterioles and pre-capillary sphincters is controlled by two main factors:

  - **Local constrictors:** Serotonin and fall in body temperature

  - **Local dilators:** Hypoxia, hypercapnia, acidemial (fall in pH) and increase in body temperature, $K^+$, lactic acid and adenosine.

  **(For windkessel vessels *see* short note)**

## CARDIOVASCULAR REGULATORY MECHANISMS

### COMPARE AND CONTRAST EFFECTS OF SYMPATHETIC AND PARASYMPATHETIC NERVE STIMULATION OF THE HEART                                    2 (2004)

#### Sympathetic Innervation

Sympathetic supply to the heart is by sympathetic nerve cells which lie in the intermediolateral horn of the spinal cord extending from $T_1$ to $T_5$ spinal segments. The sympathetic supply goes to the nodal tissue (SA node, AV node), to the atria and the ventricles. It has the following effects on the heart:

- Increase in heart rate due to increased rhythmicity of the SA node **(positive chronotropic effect)**.

- Increased speed and force of myocardial contraction **(positive inotropic action)**.

- Increased conductivity in the conducting tissue **(positive dromotropic action)**.

- Increased excitability of the heart **(positive bathmotropic effect)**.

## Parasympathetic Innervation

Parasympathetic supply is via the vagus nerve with their cell bodies located in the medulla in the nucleus ambiguous. The parasympathetic supply goes to the SA node, AV node and to the atria, whereas there is no vagal innervations of the ventricles. Stimulation of the parasympathetic supply to the heart has the following effects:

- Decreased rate of impulse generation in the SA node causing a decrease in the heart rate **(negative chronotropic effect)**. It may cause stoppage of the heart.
- Decreased conductivity in the conducting tissue **(negative dromotropic action)**.
- Decreased speed and force of contraction **(negative inotropic action)**.
- There is no influence on the contractility of the ventricles by parasympathetic stimulation.

## EXPLAIN WHY ADMINISTRATION OF ADRENALINE CAUSES ADRENALINE APNOEA                    1 (2010)

In small doses adrenaline stimulates respiration by stimulation of the peripheral chemoreceptors, whereas injection of adrenaline in high doses raises the systemic arterial blood pressure which stimulates the baroreceptors that in turn inhibits respiration by inhibiting respiratory centre called *adrenaline apnoea*.

## SYMPATHETIC VASODILATOR SYSTEM                    3 (2004)

Sympathetic nerve endings where epinephrine or norepinephrine is the transmitter are called adrenergic nerves, whereas where acetylcholine is the transmitter are called the sympathetic cholinergic nerves  and their activation leads to vasodilation.

Sympathetic noradrenergic fibres end on blood vessels in all parts of the body to mediate vasoconstriction. In addition to the vasoconstrictor innervations resistance vessels in the organs like the skeletal muscle, heart, lungs, liver, kidney and uterus are innervated by vasodilator fibres which are cholinergic **(sympathetic cholinergic vasodilator system)**. Sympathetic constrictor supply to blood vessels of these organs is tonically active but the vasodilator fibres get activated only in biological emergencies like exercise and parturition thus helping to increase the blood flow through these organs in these situations.

## LOCAL CVS REGULATORY MECHANISM          2.5 (2008)

### Autoregulation

The capacity of the tissues to regulate their own blood flow is referred to as autoregulation. Most vascular beds have an intrinsic capacity to compensate for moderate changes in the perfusion pressure by changing the vascular resistance so that blood flow remains relatively constant. This is best developed in the kidneys but is also seen in mesentery, skeletal muscles, brain, liver and myocardium. This is a response of contractile mechanism of smooth muscle in the wall of blood vessels to stretch **(Myogenic theory of autoregulation)**.

Vasodilator substances tend to accumulate in active tissues and these also contribute to autoregulation **(Metabolic theory of autoregulation)**. When blood flow decreases they accumulate and the vessels dilate, when blood flow increases they tend to be washed away.

The metabolic changes producing **vasodilation:**

1. Hypoxia
2. Acidemia
3. Hypercapnia
4. Increased blood osmolality
5. Increased body temperature
6. $K^+$
7. Lactic acid accumulation
8. Adenosine accumulation

Local **vasoconstrictors:**

- Serotonin released from platelets secondary to injury
- Decrease in body temperature

### Role of endothelial cells

Endothelium of blood vessels secrete a variety of substances that respond to stretch, increase in inflammatory mediators and increase in blood flow. These substances include:

- Various growth factors that help in formation of blood vessels
- Vasoactive substances like prostaglandins, thromboxanes, NO and endothelins.

## PHYSIOLOGICAL/CLINICAL SIGNIFICANCE OF ENDOTHELINS          3 (2012)

Endothelins are produced by endothelial cells and are of three types: Endothelin 1, 2 and 3. Endothelin 1 is one of the most important vasoconstrictors known which acts via $ET_A$ receptors and produces vasoconstriction in many body tissues.

**Endothelin 1:** Brain, kidney and endothelial cells
**Endothelin 2:** Kidney and intestine
**Endothelin 3:** Blood, brain, kidneys and gastrointestinal tract.

## Functions

- **CVS:** Primarily a paracrine regulator of vascular tone. Its concentration is elevated in congestive heart failure and after myocardial infarction so it may play a role in the pathophysiology of these diseases.
- **CNS:** Produced both by astrocytes and neurons. They are found in the dorsal root ganglion, ventral horn cells, cortex, hypothalamus and cerebellar Purkinje cells. They play a role in regulating transport across blood brain barrier.
- **Kidneys:** There are endothelial cells among mesangial cells which participate in tubuloglomerular feedback.
- **Endocrines:** Increase plasma level of renin, aldosterone, catecholamine and ANP.
- **Respiration:** Bronchoconstriction.
- **GIT:** Regulates GIT blood flow.
- They play a role in the closure of ductus arteriosus.

## EFFECTS OF CAROTID BARORECEPTOR STIMULATION 2.5 (1985)

Carotid baroreceptors are stretch receptors located in the wall of carotid sinus. These receptors are stimulated when the pressure rises in carotid sinus causing its distension and hence stretching of its wall.

Afferent impulses are carried by the vagus nerve to medulla oblongata of brain. In medulla fibres end in nucleus of tractus solitarius (NTS) and some also pass to cardioinhibitory area. From NTS fibres project to vasomotor area of the medulla. When these receptors are stimulated they (i) inhibit vasomotor area and hence inhibit sympathetic discharge to blood vessels, (ii) stimulate cardioinhibitory area.

Thus baroreceptor stimulation causes:

1. Vasodilatation
2. Venodilatation
3. Fall in blood pressure
4. Bradycardia
5. Reduction in cardiac output.

## HEART RATE

### FACTORS AFFECTING HEART RATE       **2 (2003)**

The factors that affect heart rate are:

- **Age:** As age increases vagal tone increases and heart rate decreases but in old age heart rate is slightly higher due to fall in the vagal tone.

- **Sex:** Heart rate is slightly higher in females compared to males.

- **Body temperature:** Heart rate increases by 10 beats per minute for every 1°F rise in body temperature due to its direct effect on the SA node.

- **Catecholamines:** Epinephrine increases the heart rate due to its direct action on the heart, whereas norepinephrine leads to bradycardia due to its indirect effect via reflex increase in vagal tone.

- **Bainbridge reflex:** Rapid perfusion of blood or saline in anaesthetised animal produces an increase in heart rate if the initial heart rate is low. Atrial receptors of both sides of the heart are responsible for this. This is called **Bainbridge reflex**.

- **Diseases**
  - Increase in intracranial tension reduces the blood supply to the medulla producing local hypoxia and hypercapnia. This directly stimulates the vasomotor centre which tends to increase the blood pressure to restore the blood supply to the medulla. Increase in BP via baroreceptor mechanism stimulates the vagal outflow to the heart causing a decrease in HR and respiration. This increased intracranial tension is associated with bradycardia, a reflex called **Cushing reflex**.
  - **Thyrotoxicosis:** This leads to an increase in the resting heart rate due to its direct positive chronotropic effect and because thyroxine potentiates the action of circulating catecholamines.
  - **Hypoxia** via stimulation of chemoreceptors produces an increase in the heart rate and blood pressure.

- **Emotions:** Excitement, fear, anger increase the heart rate, whereas sudden shock, grief, apprehension lead to bradycardia, and hypotension.

- **Exercise:** Heart rate increases in linearity with the severity of exercise.
- **Painful stimuli:** Superficial pain causes sympathetic stimulation causing an increase in the heart rate, whereas deep pain leads to bradycardia.
- **Respiration:** Heart rate increases with inspiration and decreases with expiration **(sinus arrhythmia)**.

## EFFECT OF INTRACRANIAL TENSION ON HEART RATE      (2001)

Increase in intracranial tension reduces the blood supply to the medulla producing hypoxia and hypercapnia. This directly stimulates the vasomotor centre which tries to restore the blood supply to the medulla by increasing the systemic arterial blood pressure. Increase in the BP via baroreceptors stimulates the vagal outflow to the heart causing a decrease in the HR and respiration. Thus increase in intracranial tension is associated with bradycardia. This is called **Cushing reflex**.

## EXPLAIN WHY HEART RATE INCREASES WITH INCREASE IN BODY TEMPERATURE      1 (2010)

The heart rate rises by 10 beats per minute for every 1°F rise in body temperature. This is due to a direct effect on the SA node.

## WHAT WILL HAPPEN AND WHY IF BOTH SYMPATHETIC AND PARASYMPATHETIC NERVE SUPPLY TO THE HEART IS CUT    1 (2002)

There is a moderate amount of tonic discharge in the cardiac sympathetic nerves at rest, but there is considerable tonic vagal discharge (vagal tone) in humans as well. In humans in whom both the noradrenergic and the cholinergic systems are blocked, the heart rate is approximately 100 beats/minute because it beats under the influence of the rate of discharge of the SA node, the natural pacemaker of the heart.

## WHAT AND WHY WILL HAPPEN TO HEART RATE DURING INSPIRATION AND EXPIRATION      1 (2011)

The heart rate will increase during inspiration and decrease during expiration. This phenomenon is called **sinus arrhythmia**. This is a normal phenomenon and is primarily due to fluctuations in the parasympathetic innervations to the heart. During inspiration, impulses in the vagi from the stretch receptors in the lungs inhibit the cardioinhibitory area in the medulla oblongata. The tonic vagal discharge that keeps the heart rate slow decreases, hence the heart rate increases during inspiration and decreases during expiration due to increase in the vagal discharge to the heart.

## WHAT WILL HAPPEN AND WHY IF BOTH VAGI ARE CUT (ON HR AND RESPIRATION)                     2.5 (1991)

## WHAT WILL HAPPEN AND WHY TO HEART RATE IF RIGHT VAGUS IS CUT                     1 (2003)-IPU

If both the vagi are cut, it will lead to increased heart rate. Normally heart is under the influence of vagal stimulation called vagal tone. Vagal impulses have inhibitory action on heart and cause a decrease in heart rate. On cutting both vagi this effect is abolished and heart rate increases.

As far as respiration is concerned, this will cause prolonged inspiration called apneustic breathing. This is because normally vagi carry impulses from stretch receptors as lungs expand during inspiration and reflexly inhibit inspiratory drive. This is known as Hering Breuer reflex. This reflex causes inspiration to stop and expiration supervenes. That is why if vagi are cut, inspiration is prolonged.

## CARDIAC OUTPUT

## DEFINE CARDIAC OUTPUT. DESCRIBE BRIEFLY THE FACTORS AFFECTING CARDIAC OUTPUT. OUTLINE THE PRINCIPLE UNDERLYING A METHOD FOR ITS DETERMINATION     10 (1993)

## CARDIAC OUTPUT AND ITS REGULATION                     2.5 (2011)

Cardiac output may be defined as the quantity of blood pumped out by each ventricle per minute. Their output is equal in each stroke of heart.

It is equal to the product of stroke volume and heart rate, i.e.

$$CO = SV \times HR$$

For normal young adult man, it is 5.5 L/min and for a woman it is 10–20% less. It is also the quantity of blood that flows through the circulation each minute.

**Factors affecting cardiac output (CO)** can be considered as the factors effecting:

i. Stroke volume (SV)
ii. Heart rate (HR)

## Factors Effecting SV

A. Myocardial contractility  has major effect on SV. Increase in contractility increases the stroke volume. Factors increasing force of contraction  are called **positive inotropic agents**.

   i. Circulating epinephrine and norepinephrine increase force of contraction.
   ii. Sympathetic stimulation increases contractility
   iii. Parasympathetic stimulation decreases force of contraction of myocardium.
   iv. Drugs like caffeine and theophylline also increase contractility of myocardium.
   v. Glucagon  and digitalis also have a positive inotropic action.

   **Negative inotropic agents**
   i. Hypercapnia, hypoxia, acidosis and certain drugs depress myocardial contractility.
   ii. Damage to myocardium will depress its contractile power.

B. **Length of cardiac muscle:** Stroke volume varies with **(Frank-Starling law)** length of cardiac muscle fibres. According to law of heart—force of contraction is proportional to the initial length of the cardiac muscle fibre. This is known as preloading of the heart and regulation of stroke volume due to change in length of muscle fibres is known as heterometric regulation.

   Length of the muscle fibre is determined by the ventricular filling during diastole and is determined by:

C. **Venous return (VR):** This in turn depends on:
   a. Pumping action of skeletal muscle: Muscle pump.
   b. Tone in veins: Venoconstriction increases VR.
   c. Body posture: On standing venous pooling occurs, hence VR decreases.
   d. Intrathoracic pressure: Negative pressure increases VR.

D. **Intrapericardial pressure:** An increase in intrapericardial pressure will reduce contractility of myocardium.

E. Force of atrial contraction contributes to ventricular filling.

F. Total blood volume.

**Regulation of heart rate:** Heart rate is mainly controlled by its autonomic innervation. Sympathetic innervation of heart is by first and second lumbar segments of spinal cord and parasympathetic supply is by vagus nerve.

Sympathetic stimulation increases heart rate known as a positive chronotropic effect.

Parasympathetic stimulation has an opposite effect on heart rate called negative chronotropic effect.

## Method of Determining Cardiac Output—Indicator Dilution Technique

**Principle:** A known amount of a dye, e.g. indocyanine is injected into an arm vein which should have the following properties:

i. Should not be toxic to the body

ii. Should stay in circulation during the test

iii. Should not have an effect on haemodynamics of circulation.

After injection serial samples of blood are drawn from an artery and concentration of the dye is determined in each sample.

$$CO = \frac{\text{Amount of dye injected}}{\text{Avg. concentration in arterial blood after a single circulation through the heart}}$$

To get average concentration of dye log of concentration in serial samples is plotted against the time. The curve is extrapolated as the concentration rises, falls and rises again as the dye circulates again (Fig. 6.3).

## Cardiac Output

Flow during single circulation = $\dfrac{I}{c.t}$

$I$ = Total amount of dye injected

$c$ = Mean concentration of the dye

$t$ = Duration in sec of the first passage of the dye through the artery.

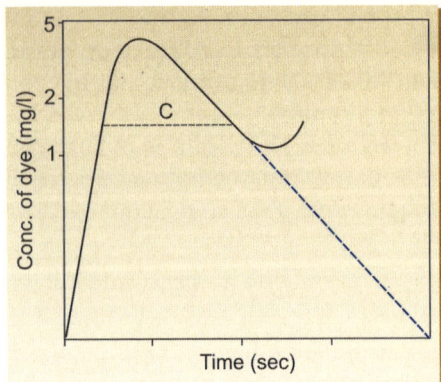

**Fig. 6.3:** Indicator dilution (or dye dilution) method of determination of cardiac output

## DEFINE CARDIAC OUTPUT AND CARDIAC INDEX. MENTION THE METHODS OF MEASURING CARDIAC OUTPUT. DESCRIBE ANY ONE OF THE METHODS APPLICABLE IN MAN. ENUMERATE VARIOUS CONDITIONS AFFECTING CARDIAC OUTPUT          10 (1989)

Cardiac output may be defined as the quantity of blood pumped out by each ventricle per minute.

It is determined by the product of stoke volume and heart rate.

It is 5.5 L/minute in normal adult male and in females, it is 10–20% less.

**Cardiac index:** It is defined as cardiac output per square metre of body surface area. On an average it is 3.2 L/m².

## METHODS OF MEASURING CARDIAC OUTPUT

I. **Direct:** used in experimental animals using electromagnetic flow metres.

II. Indirect methods applicable in human beings:

   i. Direct application of the Fick principle: The principle states that the amount of substance taken by an organ or whole body per unit time is equal to arteriovenous difference in level multiplied by the blood flow, or

$$\text{Blood flow} = \frac{\text{Amount of substance taken / minute}}{\text{A-V difference of the substance}}$$

ii. Dye dilution method

iii. Thermal dilution method

**(See previous question for details of dye dilution method)**

## Conditions Affecting Cardiac Output

1. **Exercise:** Producing an increase in CO proportional to severity of exercise.
2. **Anxiety and excitement:** Increases CO due to sympathetic stimulation.
3. **Food:** CO is elevated on eating.
4. **High environment temperature:** Increases CO.
5. **Pregnancy:** An increase in CO occurs due to increased blood volume.
6. **Epinephrine:** Increases CO by increasing SV.
7. Cardiac arrhythmia and myocardial damage decreases CO by decreasing the force of contraction of the heart.

## COMPARE HOMOMETRIC AND HETEROMETRIC REGULATION OF CARDIAC OUTPUT                    2 (2004)

| Homometric regulation | Heterometric regulation |
|---|---|
| • Changes in myocardial contractility are independent of the resting length of the cardiac muscle fibres | • Changes in myocardial contractility vary with the resting length of the cardiac muscle fibres. Thus force of ventricular contraction is directly proportional to the initial length of the cardiac muscle fibres **(Frank-Starling law of the heart)** |
| • This type of regulation depends upon the cardiac innervations: Sympathetic stimulation increases, whereas parasympathetic stimulation decreases myocardial contractility | • This type of regulation is independent of cardiac innervations |

## FACTORS AFFECTING VENOUS RETURN        2 (2007), 2 (2010)

Factors that affect venous return include the following:

• **Thoracic pump/respiratory pump**

The normal intrathoracic pressure at the end of expiration is subatmospheric (–2 mm Hg). During inspiration:

- Intrathoracic pressure decreases to –5 mm Hg causing less pressure over large veins and arteries
- Descent of diaphragm increases intra-abdominal pressure to squeeze blood out of the abdomen.

These two factors combine to favour venous return to the heart during inspiration.

- **Cardiac pump:**
  - *Vis-a-tergo* – force from behind which drives the blood forward. This is imparted by the contraction of the heart to the blood during its passage through the heart and assisted by the windkessel effect of the large vessels.
  - *Vis-a-fronte* – force acting from front to attract blood in the veins towards the heart. It is exerted by the contraction of the ventricles.
- **Muscle pump:** This is responsible for the flow of blood from the veins of the limbs to the heart.
- **Total blood volume:** Increase in total blood volume increases the venous return.
- **Capacity of the venous system:** Veins are the capacitance vessels. Increase sympathetic activity increases venous tone that increases venous return.
- **Body position:** In standing position peripheral pooling of blood occurs that decreases venous return.
- **Ventricular compliance:** Following myocardial infarction, the myocardium becomes fibrotic and nonfunctional and ventricular compliance decreases. This decreases the venous return.

## ARTERIAL BLOOD PRESSURE

### RADIAL PULSE                                           2.5 (1985)

During left ventricular systole, blood is pumped into the aorta. As it moves forwards into big arteries, it produces a pressure wave, which travels along the arteries and expands the arterial wall. This expansion of radial artery is easily palpable at the wrist and is called *radial pulse*. It is felt 0.1 sec after the peak ejection into the aorta.

Clinically, pulse is felt at radial artery and its rate and character is helpful in diagnosing certain conditions of heart and blood vessels.

Strength of pulse is related to pulse pressure which is the difference between systolic and diastolic BP. Pulse is strong when stroke volume is large, e.g. during exercise.

Radial pulse is examined with respect to:

i. Rate

ii. Rhythm–regular or not

iii. Character

iv. Volume

v. Whether synchronous on both sides

vi. Whether vessel wall is palpable or not

vii. Radiofemoral delay.

## ENUMERATE THE DETERMINANTS OF BLOOD PRESSURE. DESCRIBE THE IMMEDIATE RESPONSE OF BODY TO A SUDDEN FALL OF BLOOD PRESSURE        2.5

### Determinants of Blood Pressure

i. Determinant of systolic blood pressure is cardiac output which in turn depends upon:

a. Stroke volume

b. Heart rate

ii. Determinant of diastolic BP is peripheral resistance.

### Response of Body to Sudden Fall of BP

As the blood pressure falls suddenly, pressure also falls in carotid sinus. There is less stretching of walls of carotid sinus. This leads to decrease rate of discharge from the carotid sinus and also aortic baroreceptors. There is less inhibition of vasomotor centre through baroreceptor afferent impulses. Hence, vasomotor discharge on heart and blood vessels through sympathetic nerves increases, thereby producing the following effects on heart and blood vessels:

i. Increase force of contraction → increases cardiac output → increases SBP

ii. Vasoconstriction → increases peripheral resistance → increases DBP

iii. Venoconstriction → increases venous return → increases SV

All these factors raise the blood pressure immediately through the abovementioned baroreceptor reflexes.

## WHAT IS BLOOD PRESSURE. HOW IS IT REGULATED   **10** (1991)
## WHAT ARE THE DETERMINANTS OF BLOOD PRESSURE. DISCUSS ITS REGULATION   **10** (1986)
## ROLE OF BARORECEPTORS IN THE REGULATION OF BLOOD PRESSURE   **2** (2004)

Blood pressure is the lateral pressure exerted on walls of large arteries (like brachial and femoral) by the blood flowing through them.

This pressure rises to a peak value of about 120 mm Hg in normal adult during a cardiac cycle called systolic BP and falls to a minimum value of about 70 mm Hg called diastolic BP.

### Determinants of BP

1. Determinant of systolic BP is cardiac output which is in turn determined by:
   a. Stroke volume
   b. Heart rate.
2. Determinant of diastolic BP is peripheral resistance which is determined by:
   a. Velocity of blood
   b. Viscosity of blood
   c. Total quantity of blood in the arterial system
   d. Elasticity of the vessel wall.

### Regulation of Blood Pressure

BP is regulated by:
   i. Neural mechanism
   ii. Blood volume control mechanisms.
   iii. Neural mechanism: It is also known as short-term control as it operates immediately and is reflex in nature. It is mediated by:
      a. Baroreceptors present in carotid sinus and aortic arch. These receptors respond to the stretch of the vessels wall which depends on the blood pressure. From these receptors (via glossopharyngeal nerves from carotid sinus and vagus nerves from aortic arch) inhibitory impulses pass to vasomotor centre, which in turn decreases sympathetic discharge to heart and blood vessels. Whenever BP increases, frequency of inhibitory impulses to vasomotor centre increases from baroreceptors thereby producing:

– Vasodilatation

– Venodilatation (Fig. 6.4).

These nerves in addition stimulate the cardioinhibitory area and bring about a decrease in heart rate and thereby decrease CO. As a result there is a fall in BP and it is restored to normal level. Conversely, if BP falls, there is less stretching of vessel wall, less number of impulses pass from baroreceptors to vasomotor area and cardiac inhibitory centre, BP rises and normal level is restored. Glossopharyngeal and vagal nerves arising from these receptors are known as **buffer nerves** as they restore the blood pressure to a normal value.

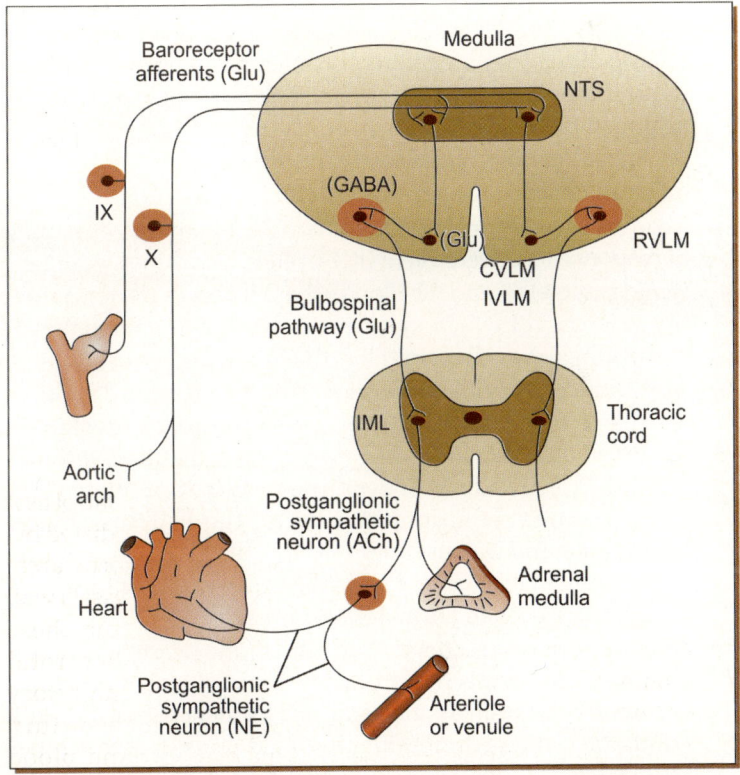

**Fig. 6.4:** Basic pathway involved in the medullary regulation of blood pressure

b. In addition, atrial and ventricular receptors might play a role in normal regulation of BP, but sinoaortic mechanism mentioned above is the primary short-term mechanism for maintaining BP.

c. Another type of receptors present in atria called atrial volume receptors may also participate in BP regulation in the following way: An increase in total blood volume also increases BP. This hypervolemia stimulates volume receptors in atria, causing a reflex decrease in ADH secretion which will cause diuresis with loss of extracellular fluid volume leading to restoration of blood volume and hence the BP.

## Blood Volume Control Mechanism

i. This is also known as long-term regulation as it takes time to be effective. This mechanism basically operates by maintaining a normal blood volume. This type of regulation is achieved by:
   a. Renin-angiotensin-aldosterone system
   b. Atrial natriuretic peptide (ANP).

ii. Renin is secreted from juxtaglomerular apparatus of kidney in response to a decrease in ECF volume and blood volume. Renin is secreted into the blood where it causes the formation of angiotensin I which in turn is converted to angiotensin II in the lungs. Angiotensin II has the following actions:
   a. Produces arteriolar constriction and hence a rise in BP.
   b. It acts directly on adrenal cortex to cause aldosterone secretion. Aldosterone in turn acts on the distal tubules and collective ducts of nephrons of kidney producing salt and water retention, increasing the ECF and blood volume and a consequent rise in BP. It is a slow but a prolonged mechanism and takes days to adjust the blood pressure back to normal.

iii. ANP: A hormone secreted from atria of the heart. When ECF volume increases, secretion of ANP is stimulated. It promotes excretion of sodium by the nephrons by increasing GFR, ECF volume and hence decreasing the blood pressure. It has other actions like:
   a. Decreases responsiveness of vascular smooth muscles to vasoconstrictor agents.

b. Decreases responsiveness of adrenal cortex to secrete aldosterone.

c. Inhibits renin and vasopressin secretion. Hence it plays an important role in regulating blood volume and blood pressure.

## REGIONAL CIRCULATION

### DESCRIBE THE CORONARY CIRCULATION IN MAN AND THE FACTORS INFLUENCING IT                    10 (1991)
### CORONARY BLOOD FLOW                        4 (2004)-IPU

#### Physiological Anatomy

Myocardium receives its arterial supply through coronary arteries which arise directly from root of aorta behind the cusps of aortic valves. These cusps are kept away from the orifices of arteries, so that they are patent throughout the cardiac cycle. In majority of people right artery is bigger and supplies myocardium of right atrium, right ventricle and a part of left ventricle. The left coronary mainly supplies anterior and lateral portions of left ventricle.

Venous blood is drained through a superficial and deep venous system. Superficial one ends in coronary sinus and anterior cardiac veins. Deep system is constituted by arteriosinusoidal vessels that empty into cardiac chambers.

Coronary arteries are end arteries there being very few anastomoses in young people between coronary and extracardiac but collaterals are found to grow in old people and young adults if partial occlusion of coronary vessels occur for a long time.

Main coronary arteries lie on the surface of heart and small arteries penetrate into the myocardium at right angle.

#### Special Features of Coronary Blood Flow

**Phasic flow**

As heart contracts during systole, the blood vessels are occluded and blood flow to myocardium is obstructed and flow occurs freely only during the diastole called **phasic flow**. Subepicardial portions are better supplied than subendocardial part.

There is regional variation in blood supply to the various parts of heart. Blood flow to left ventricle during systole is minimal as the pressure inside left ventricle is slightly more than aortic pressure. On the other hand, pressure difference between right ventricle and aorta and between atria and aorta are greater during systole, hence, blood flow is not much compromised even during systole to these regions. As practically no blood flow occurs during systole in the subendocardial portion of left ventricle, this region is prone to ischaemic damage and hence is the most common site of myocardial infarction (Fig. 6.5).

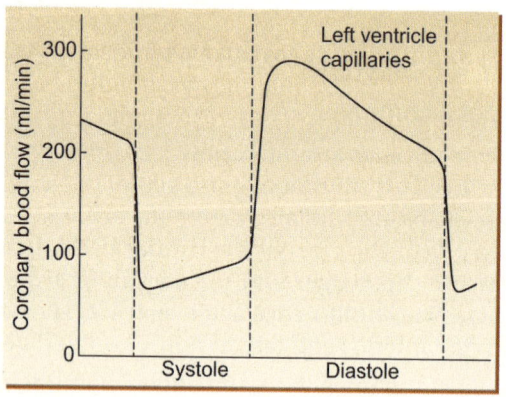

**Fig. 6.5:** Phasic flow of blood through the coronary capillaries of the human left ventricle

## Regulation of Coronary Blood Flow

Myocardium even at rest extracts 70–80% of $O_2$ from coronary blood, due to high capillary density. So increased $O_2$ demand of the heart muscle can only be met by increasing the blood flow. Factors regulating blood flow are:

  i. Pressure changes in aorta, i.e. phasic flow
  ii. Autoregulation
iii. Chemical factors
iv. Neural factors

  i. **Phasic flow** (*see* above)

  ii. **Autoregulation:** Blood flow in coronary vessels is practically unchanged between BP of 60 and 150 mm Hg in aorta. It is a myogenic mechanism independent of nerves.

iii. **Chemical factors:** Blood flow increases in direct proportion to increase in myocardial metabolism. Various factors responsible for the dilatation of coronary vessels are as follows:

1. Hypoxia
2. Increased concentration of $CO_2$
3. Increased $H^+$ concentration
4. $K^+$
5. Lactate
6. ADP and adenosine accumulation
7. Prostaglandins

iv. **Neural regulation:** Coronary arterioles contain both alpha and beta adrenergic receptors which cause vasoconstrictions and vasodilatation respectively. Sympathetic stimulation causes dilatation of coronary vessels. This effect is secondary to increase in HR and force of contraction of heart producing increase in metabolism of myocardium that causes the release of vasodilator metabolites locally.

## WHAT WILL HAPPEN IF CORONARY BLOOD FLOW TO PART OF HEART IS REDUCED                     2.5 (1989)

The extent of damage to myocardium due to reduced blood flow is determined by the degree of collateral circulation already present. In a normal heart no collateral circulation exists between larger coronary arteries but it does exist between very small branches. When sudden stoppage of blood flow occurs, small anastomoses dilate within seconds but it cannot keep up the myocardial demand and their diametre does not increase for the next 24 hours. By the 2nd or 3rd day collateral circulation starts increasing and flow is restored to almost normal level. Hence this time interval is crucial in a patient of coronary occlusion. If the area of occlusion is not very large, the patient can recover because of development of collateral circulation.

When coronary occlusion is a slow process due to atherosclerotic constriction, collaterals develop at the same time and person will not get an acute attack, but eventually atherosclerotic changes progress beyond its limits and collateral circulation cannot sustain the myocardium anymore, hence the collaterals also develop atherosclerosis. When this happens, heart muscle cannot pump adequately and eventually heart failure occurs as happens in old people.

Immediately after an acute coronary occlusion, blood flow ceases in the area of muscle beyond the occlusion and it becomes infarcted. As collateral circulation is established blood seeps into the infarct and progressive dilatation of blood vessels overfills the area of infarct. Heart muscle simultaneously extracts more oxygen from blood, haemoglobin becomes more reduced and infarcted area appears blue with surrounding engorged blood vessels. Later on blood vessels become more permeable and the area becomes oedematous and myocardial fibres swell up due to decreased cellular metabolism and loose their function.

## DESCRIBE THE SPECIAL FEATURES AND REGULATIONS OF BLOOD FLOW TO

(A)  Brain

(B)  Skin                                                                    10 (1992)

### (A) BLOOD FLOW TO BRAIN

Adult human brain receives approximately 750 ml of blood flow per minute. The amount is high being 50–60 ml/100 gm of tissues. Large blood supply is required to fulfil the high oxygen demand of brain tissue.

Internal carotid and basilar arteries supply the brain tissue. The basilar artery supplies occipital lobes, cerebellum, pons and medulla, whereas internal carotid supplies upper brainstem and rest of the cerebrum. Cerebral veins drain into venous sinuses which lie between dura mater and skull. The final drainage is mainly into internal jugular veins. Cerebral veins do not have valves and are kept open by the dura mater attached around their orifices.

Cerebral capillaries are non-fenestrated and do not allow the passage of substances across their membrane called blood brain barrier. This barrier maintains constancy of environment of neurons and protects the brain tissue from harmful effects of circulating toxins.

### Special Features of Cerebral Blood Flow

1. Blood flow is kept constant  by the process of autoregulation even in circumstances like physical exercise.

2. In adult brain, CSF and cerebral vessels are contained in rigid bony skull having a constant volume. As the brain tissue and CSF are incompressible, vessels are compressed if CSF pressure rises called **Monro-Kellie doctrine**.

A fall or rise in venous pressure produces a fall or rise in CSF pressure. This relationship between CSF pressure, venous pressure and cerebral vessels helps to regulate cerebral blood flow when arterial pressure changes at head level, e.g. as body accelerates upward, blood moves towards the feet and arterial pressure at the head level decreases, this causes a fall in venous pressure and corresponding fall in intracranial pressure with less compression of cerebral blood vessels and increased blood flow.

## Factors Regulating Cerebral Blood Flow

- Arterial blood pressure at head level
- Venous pressure at head level
- Intracranial pressure
- Viscosity of blood
- Degree of constriction or dilatation of cerebral arterioles.

1. Arterial BP: Between 60 and 150 mm Hg perfusion pressure blood flow is kept constant, this is autoregulation and is probably a myogenic response.

2. Venous pressure: A rise in venous pressure decreases blood flow by (i) decreasing effective perfusion pressure and (ii) compressing cerebral vessels due to increased CSF pressure.

3. Intracranial pressure: A rise in intracranial pressure decreases cerebral blood flow by compressing the vessels, but the cerebral ischaemia thus produced stimulates vasomotor centre, arterial BP rises and blood flow is thus increased and maintained. This is called *Cushing reflex*.

4. Viscosity of blood: Lowering of blood viscosity (by giving plasma) reduces cerebral oedema and reduces compression of brain tissue.

5. Caliber of cerebral vessels: It is controlled by local vasodilator metabolites, circulating vasoactive substances and vasomotor nerves to some extent.

$$\left.\begin{array}{l} \text{H}^+ \text{ increase} \\ \text{Adenosine, low pO}_2 \end{array}\right\} \longrightarrow \text{Vasodilation}$$

Fall in $pCO_2$: Vasoconstriction (responsible for cerebral symptoms during voluntary hyperventilation).

## (B) SKIN CIRCULATION

### Functional Anatomy

Arterioles supplying the skin give rise to metarterioles which give rise to capillaries. Capillaries are U-shaped, they rise towards the superficial layer, make a bend and go deeper and finally drain into venules and veins. Venules form a subpapillary venous plexus in subcutaneous tissues, which runs parallel to the skin surface and can hold large amounts of blood. In the skin of hands and feet large number of arteriovenous anastomosis are present which are under the tonic influence of sympathetic activity. In the limbs arteries are accompanied by venae-comitantes serving as counter-current exchange vessels for temperature regulation.

### Other Special Features

I. **Functions**
1. Supply of nutrition and oxygen and removal of waste products as usual.
2. Regulation of body temperature: Along with cutaneous receptors, autonomic nervous system and hypothalamus skin vessels participate in regulating body temperature. An environmental temperature of 27°C is comfortable for man. At lower temperature skin blood vessels are constricted through a reflex mediated via the hypothalamus and blood flow is directed to deeper structures and heat loss from body surface is prevented.
   A-V anastomosis of hand and feet are under the influence of sympathetic nerve supply. In hot environment sympathetic activity is abolished through hypothalamic control. These vessels are dilated, blood flow through them increases and heat is lost through the body surface.
3. Reservoir of blood: During circulatory stress, e.g. exercise and severe haemorrhage, strong venoconstriction occurs and blood from subcutaneous venous plexus is shifted to general circulation to make up the blood volume.

II. **Colour of skin depends upon the blood flow in**
   a. Capillary loops
   b. Sub-papillary plexus: During extreme arteriolar constriction skin becomes pale. If A-V channels are dilated, skin is red and hot.
III. **Determination of blood flow:** Blood flow depends upon the following factors:
   a. Degree of sympathetic constrictor tone
   b. Local metabolites (local vasodilator like bradykinins)
   c. Skin vessels show reactive hyperaemia
   d. Skin blood vessels show a response to injury called the **triple response**.

## Regulation of Blood Flow

   i. Temperature: Already discussed
   ii. Cardiovascular stress, e.g. exercise, haemorrhage and fight or flight reaction
   iii. Emotions, e.g. panic produces vasoconstriction and pallor, whereas rage causes reddening of the face.

## SPECIAL FEATURES OF PULMONARY CIRCULATION
### 3 (1994), 2.5 (2002)

Pulmonary arteries carrying deoxygenated blood from the right ventricle, enter the lungs and divide giving rise to arterioles and capillaries and in turn form venules and finally pulmonary veins carrying oxygenated blood to the left atrium.

## Special Features

1. All the vessels are thin walled as compared to the vessels in systemic circulation.
2. Capillaries surrounding the alveoli are so numerous that flow appears like a sheet.
3. It is a low pressure distensible system and so acts as venous reservoir.
4. Low hydrostatic pressure in capillaries prevents pulmonary oedema and keeps the alveoli dry essential for gaseous exchange in the lungs.
5. Pulmonary blood flow is mainly influenced by local $O_2$ content. Hypoxia produces local vasoconstriction.

## REACTIVE HYPERAEMIA                                    **2 (2004)**

This is a response seen in the blood vessels of many organs but is visible in the skin. Reactive hyperaemia is an increase in the amount of blood in a region when its circulation is re-established after a period of occlusion. When the blood supply to a limb is occluded, the cutaneous arterioles below the occlusion dilate. When the circulation is re-established, blood flowing in the dilated vessels makes the skin go fiery red. This arteriolar dilation is apparently due to a local effect of hypoxia.

A similar increase in blood flow is produced in the area supplied by a coronary artery if the artery is occluded and then released. This may be due to the release of adenosine.

## TRIPLE RESPONSE                          **3, 2.5 (1990, 1993, 2003)**

It is a response of the cutaneous blood vessels to injury. When a blunt firm stroke is applied across the skin, following series of responses known as triple response is observed:

1. Red reaction
2. Flare
3. Wheal

1. **Red reaction:** Redness occurs along the path of stroke called the red line. It occurs due to dilatation of pre-capillary sphincter produced by the local release of histamine due to injury inflicted by the stroke.

2. **Flare:** An irregular red area appears surrounding the red line. This occurs as a result of dilatation of arterioles, terminal arterioles and pre-capillary sphincter. The temperature of skin overlying the area is also increased due to arteriolar dilatation. The response is mediated by local axon reflex and is hence abolished by local anaesthetization. This is the only reflex which does not involve the CNS (Fig. 6.6).

3. **Wheal:** If the stimulus is strong enough, a swelling occurs spreading from the red line towards the flare area. This is due to exudation of fluid due to the following reasons.

   i. Increased capillary permeability as a result of damage

   ii. Increased capillary pressure as a consequence of dilatation of pre-capillary resistance vessels.

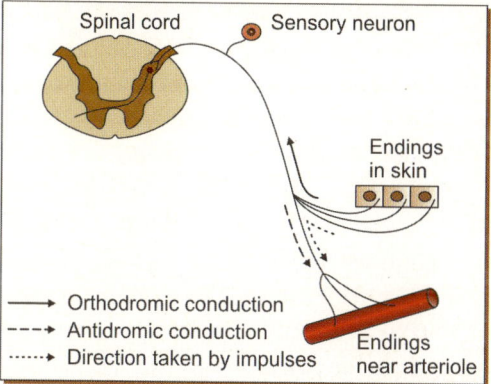

**Fig. 6.6:** The axon reflex (the afferent impulse arises from the skin and is converted into an efferent impulse (to reach to blood vessel) without reaching the spinal cord)

## CARDIOVASCULAR HOMEOSTASIS IN HEALTH AND DISEASE

### GIVE AN ACCOUNT OF CARDIOVASCULAR ADJUSTMENT DURING MUSCULAR EXERCISE                    10 (1985)

### WHAT WILL HAPPEN AND WHY TO BLOOD PRESSURE IN ISOMETRIC EXERCISE                    1 (2007)

Muscular exercise is a physiological situation when adjustments take place in cardiovascular system to increase blood flow to exercising muscles to fulfil their increase oxygen demand.

  I. Adjustment in cardiac activity

    a. Heart rate

    b. Cardiac output

    c. Coronary blood flow

  II. Adjustment in vascular system or peripheral circulation

    a. Blood pressure

    b. Regional circulation, i.e. muscle blood flow

    c. Other circulations, i.e. splanchnic and cutaneous circulation

    d. Venous return

## Heart Rate

There is an increase in the heart rate proportional to the severity of exercise. Based on increase in heart rate, muscular exercise is classified as:

| | |
|---|---|
| 1. Increase up to 100 beats/min | Mild |
| 2. Heart rate 100–125 | Moderate |
| 3. Heart rate 126–150 | Heavy or severe |
| 4. Heart rate above 150 | Very heavy or very severe |

**Causes of increased heart rate**

a. Increased sympathetic discharge
b. Adrenaline secretion
c. Decreased vagal tone
d. Raised body temperature
e. Accumulation of lactic acid leading to acidosis (only in severe exercise).

Increase in heart rate occurs both in trained and untrained individuals though increase is less prominent in trained individuals subject to higher vagal tone.

## Effect on Cardiac Output

Cardiac output increases with exercise and the increase is proportional to severity of exercise and related to increase in oxygen demand of the body.

## Causes of Increased Output

a. Increase in heart rate
b. Increase in force of contraction of heart, thereby increasing the stroke volume.

(a) and (b) together increase the cardiac output. Effect is produced due to increased sympathetic stimulation. Consequent to increase in stroke volume, end systolic volume decreases.

## Coronary Circulation

Dilatation of coronary vessels occurs due to increased cardiac activity which leads to accumulation of vasodilator metabolites locally. This is the indirect effect of sympathetic stimulation of the heart. Accumulation of local metabolites like $CO_2$ also contributes to coronary vasodilation.

## Effects on Peripheral Vascular System

### Blood pressure

**SBP:** SBP increases during exercise secondary to increase in cardiac output.

**DBP:** Depends on change in peripheral resistance. DBP change is determined by the balance between increased peripheral resistance due to sympathetic stimulation and degree of vasodilatation due to accumulation of metabolites locally.

In mild and moderate exercise, DBP generally does not vary appreciably. In severe exercise DBP may fall.

Pulse pressure will increase during exercise.

## Muscle Blood Flow

An increase in muscle blood flow even up to 30 times the resting flow occurs depending on severity of exercise.

Initial increase is neurally mediated through cholinergic sympathetic vasodilator nerves originating in cerebral cortex and projecting through hypothalamus, medulla and lateral columns of spinal cord to nerves supplying the blood vessels of skeletal muscle.

Later on local factors, i.e. accumulation of metabolites and increased temperature maintain the increase blood flow through active muscles.

## Other Circulations

Depending on the severity of exercise, varied degree of vaso-constriction due to sympathetic stimulation occurs in splanchnic and cutaneous vessels, thereby transferring blood to systemic circulation and ultimately to muscles.

**Venous return:** Venous return increases due to the following reasons:

i. Increased activity in muscle
ii. Activity of thoracic pump
iii. Mobilization of blood from viscera
iv. Vasodilatation of arterioles transferring blood to venous circulation.

Increased venous return is no more considered the primary cause of increased stroke volume.

## DESCRIBE CIRCULATORY SHOCK AND COMPENSATORY MECHANISM     10

## DEFINE SHOCK. SUMMARISE THE SHORT-TERM AND LONG-TERM COMPENSATORY MECHANISMS     5 (2004)-IPU

## HAEMORRHAGIC SHOCK     2 (2003)-IPU

Circulatory shock is a clinical condition when circulatory system fails to maintain adequate tissue perfusion. As a result tissue damage occurs due to:

   i. Hypoxia

   ii. Inadequate nutrition

   iii. Accumulation of metabolites

The condition arises due to disparity between capacity of circulatory system and available blood volume to fill the circulatory space.

### Causes of Circulatory Shock

1. Inadequate cardiac output: Cardiogenic
2. Increased circulatory capacity: Low resistance
3. Decreased circulating blood volume: Hypovolemic

Perfusion pressure is decreased as BP cannot be maintained due to the abovementioned reasons and blood supply to tissues is inadequate.

### Clinical Features

1. Patient is anxious and apprehensive
2. Skin is pale and cold
3. Pulse is fast and feeble
4. BP is low
5. Respiration may be fast
6. Cyanosis may be present
7. Intense thirst is present

### COMPENSATORY MECHANISMS

   I. **Baroreceptor mechanisms (Flow chart 6.1):** Due to a fall in BP, number of impulses from arterial baroreceptors to VMC decrease. As a result sympathetic tone to blood vessels increases producing:

**Flow chart 6.1**

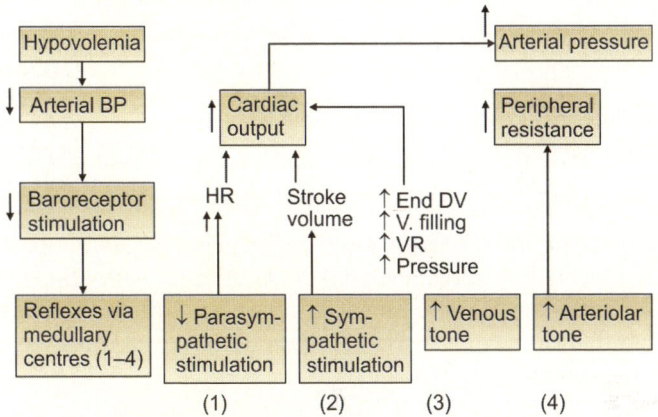

a. Generalised arteriolar constriction in the body except in heart and brain tissues is an effort to raise BP.

b. Reflex venoconstriction occurs specially in splanchnic, pulmonary and cutaneous regions and blood from these venous reservoirs is transferred to general circulation to increase circulating blood volume.

c. Stimulation of adrenal medulla with the secretion of epinephrine and norepinephrine to produce further vasoconstriction.

There is stimulation of ascending reticular formation also producing anxiety and apprehension.

II. **Chemoreceptor mechanisms:** Hypoxia due to low BP (70 mm Hg) stimulate respiratory chemoreceptors. This has:

a. Direct stimulating effect on vasomotor centre and it tends to raise the BP

b. Stimulates respiration also

III. **Increase in circulating angiotensin-II:** A fall in BP stimulates the release of renin from kidney and consequently raises the levels of angiotensin II in plasma. This acts in two ways to restore the BP:

i. Stimulates aldosterone secretion causing sodium and water retention, which increases the blood volume and hence the blood pressure.

ii. It is a potent vasoconstrictor.

IV. **Vasopressin:** Large amount of vasopressin is secreted which causes vasoconstriction and thus helps to restore BP.

V. **Fluid shift mechanism:** Fluid shifts from interstitial space to blood capillaries in an effort to increase the blood volume and restore BP. The mechanism is as follows:

Fall in BP decreases capillary hydrostatic pressure causing a shift of fluid to capillaries and restores blood volume.

VI. **Shift of blood from venous reservoirs:** As a result of venoconstriction due to generalised sympathetic stimulation and release of epinephrine from adrenal medulla, blood is shifted from veins to the circulation to increase blood volume and blood pressure.

Thus all compensatory mechanisms are directed to raise the arterial BP to maintain tissue perfusion and save tissues from the damaging effects of hypoxia.

## IRREVERSIBLE SHOCK                                    3 (2011)

When the shock is in progressive stage and is not treated adequately a vicious cycle of positive feedback mechanisms develop and patient passes into third stage of shock which is called refractory shock, earlier also called irreversible shock. In this stage all therapeutic interventions are usually ineffective and patient dies eventually.

The main factor that is responsible is the depletion of high energy phosphate compounds particularly in the liver and heart. Slow necrosis of cells of the body sets in leading to:

1. **Acute tubular necrosis** in the kidneys leading to acute renal failure and uremic death.

2. Deterioration of the lungs often leads to respiratory distress called **shock lung syndrome**.

### Mechanism of Development

Refractory shock is the manifestation of late effects of sympathetic vasoconstriction → long sustained decrease of regional circulation → operation of positive feedback mechanisms.

## EXPLAIN WHY ASPIRIN IS GIVEN IN ISCHAEMIC HEART DISEASE                                     1 (2007)

Prostacyclin is produced by endothelial cells and thromboxane $A_2$ by platelets from a common precursor arachidonic acid by the cyclooxygenase pathway. Thromboxane $A_2$ promotes platelet aggregation and vasoconstriction, whereas prostacyclins inhibit platelet aggregation and promotes vasodilation. This balance can be shifted towards prostacyclin by administration of low doses of aspirin. Aspirin produces irreversible inhibition of cyclooxygenase which inhibits production of both thromboxane and prostacyclin. However, endothelial cells manufacture new prostacyclins in a matter of hours, whereas platelets cannot manufacture the enzyme, and the level rises only as new platelets enter the circulation. Therefore, administration of low doses of aspirin for long periods reduces clot formation and has been shown to be of value in preventing myocardial infarction, unstable angina, ischaemic heart disease and stroke.

## COMPARE PRIMARY AND SECONDARY HYPERTENSION                                     (2001)

**Primary hypertension:** This is also called essential hypertension where the cause of hypertension is not known.

- This is seen in 90% of total hypertensive individuals.

- The rise in blood pressure is persistently more than 150/90 mm Hg.

- **This is divided into two forms:** Benign and malignant and the benign form is further divided into an early and late stage.

- In early stage hypertension is moderate and BP increases up to 210/110 mm Hg. It is also called labile hypertension where there is fluctuation in the SBP and this stage may continue indefinitely.

- In the late stage no fluctuation is seen in the SBP and hypertension becomes fixed in this range and cannot be relieved by rest or sedatives.

- In the malignant form of essential hypertension, death may occur from 6 months to 2 years of diagnosis.

- The blood pressure may rise up to 260/150 mm Hg and is associated with complications.

**Secondary hypertension:** This is always seen secondary to some underlying cause and accounts for 10% of all hypertensive cases. The common causes of secondary hypertension are:

- **Renal disorders** (most common cause): Nephritis, cystic renal disease, polynephritis, renal artery stenosis that cause increased 'renin' release. This via activation of the renin-angiotensin system causes hypertension.

- **Thyrotoxicosis:** The blood pressure rises secondary to increase in the cardiac output.

- **Pill hypertension:** Long-term use of oral contraceptive pills containing oestrogen and progesterone causes hypertension due to the following reasons:
  - Retention of fluid and electrolytes
  - Increased angiotensin II formation especially due to oestrogen

- **Adrenal medullary tumours:** Pheochromocytoma increases release of NE to produce hypertension.

- **Adrenal cortical tumours**
  - Primary aldosteronism (**Conn's syndrome**): Hypertension is produced due to excess production of aldosterone that causes retention of sodium and water.
  - **Cushing syndrome:** This produces hypertension due to the salt-retaining properties of glucocorticoids.

- **Coarctation of aorta:** A congenital narrowing of the thoracic aorta produces hypertension above the aortic constriction due to increase in the peripheral vascular resistance.

- **Severe polycythemia:** There is increase in the peripheral resistance secondary to an increase in the viscosity of blood.

## EXPLAIN WHY A 'g' SUIT PREVENTS VENOUS POOLING DURING SPACE FLIGHT                                   1 (2002)

During exposure to positive 'g' for the first few seconds blood is thrown into the lower part of the body, therefore, venous return to the heart decreases resulting in fall in cardiac output. SBP and

DBP also decrease because of intense vasodilation. However, recovery occurs in 10–15 secs by activation of baroreceptor reflexes. Use of antigravity '*g*' suits, i.e. double walled pressure suits containing water or compressed air compresses the abdomen and legs with a force proportionate to the positive '*g*'. This decreases the venous pooling and helps to maintain the venous return.

## EXPLAIN WHY RED OUT OCCURS ON EXPOSURE TO NEGATIVE '*g*' FORCE                                                   1 (2010)

Negative '*g*' is the force due to acceleration acting in the opposite direction, either deceleration into the earth's atmosphere or deceleration into the atmosphere. This results in intense congestion of the head and neck vessels and ecchymoses around the eyes because the eyes are not protected by the cranium. As a result the eyes become temporarily blind which is called **red out**.

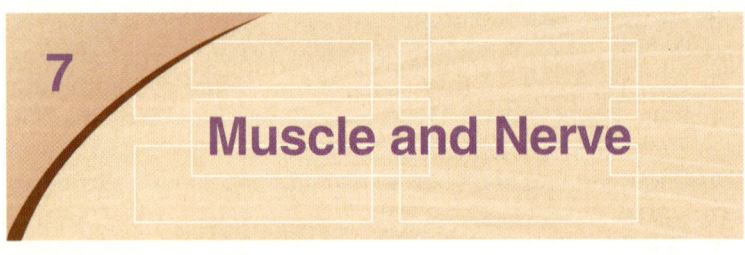

# 7

# Muscle and Nerve

**SODIUM-POTASSIUM PUMP**                                    **2.5** (1993)

**PHYSIOLOGICAL SIGNIFICANCE OF SODIUM-POTASSIUM PUMP**                    (2000), **2** (2011), **2.5** (2003)-IPU

Sodium-potassium pump is an enzyme present in the cell membrane having ATPase activity. As a result of this action, ATP is hydrolyzed to ADP and energy so released is utilized for transport of $Na^+$ out of cell and $K^+$ into the cell against electrical and chemical gradients. The pump is inhibited by ouabain and digitalis glycosides. It is made up of $\alpha$ and $\beta$ subunits. The $\alpha$ subunit has the binding sites for ATP and ouabain and the $\beta$ subunit is a glycoprotein. The pump presumably exists in two conformational states (i) it binds with $3Na^+$ accessible from inside, (ii) it binds to $2K^+$ accessible from outside of the membrane (Fig. 7.1).

It is known as an electrogenic pump as it causes passage of positive charges out of cell and has a coupling ratio of 3:2. It is present in all body cells performing different functions like:

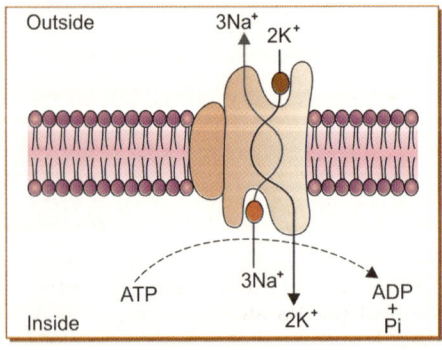

**Fig. 7.1:** Structure of $Na^+ - K^+$ pump

i. It is responsible for maintaining the high $K^+$ and low $Na^+$ concentration inside the cell.

ii. Active transport of sodium and potassium ions is one of the most important energy-using processes in the body that accounts for a large part of the basal metabolism.

iii. It helps in regulation of cell volume and pressure.

iv. Uptake of neurotransmitters.

v. Transport of $Ca^{2+}$ across cardiac muscle.

## CHRONAXIE-RHEOBASE      2.5 (1993), 2 (2003)

These terms are used in relation to excitable tissues, i.e. nerve and muscles. The relationship between the strength of the stimulating current and the duration for which it must be applied to produce a response is called **strength–duration curve** (Fig. 7.2).

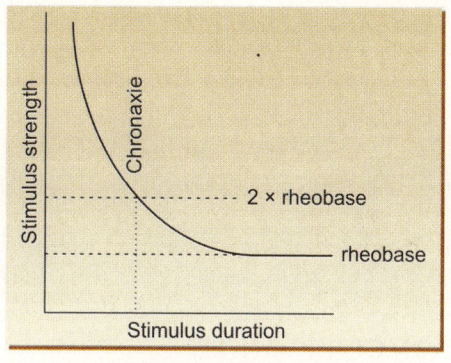

**Fig. 7.2:** Strength–duration curve

**Rheobase:** The weakest current strength that can excite a tissue if allowed to flow through it for an adequate time is called **Rheobase**. The time for which it must be applied is called **utilization time**. A still weak current fails to produce a response no matter how long is the duration of current flow.

**Chronaxie:** The length of time for which a current twice rheobase intensity must be applied to produce a response is called **chronaxie**. It is a measure of excitability of a tissue. More excitable a tissue, shorter will be the chronaxie. Chronaxie of muscles is longer than nerve, hence it is less excitable.

Clinically, chronaxie is measured to diagnose nerve injury in a suspected case. In case of a nerve injury chronaxie will be prolonged and will return to normal as the nerve regenerates.

## COMPARE GENERATOR/GRADED POTENTIAL AND ACTION POTENTIAL                                    2 (2003)-IPU, 2 (2004)-IPU

| Graded potential | Action potential |
|---|---|
| 1. It is confined to a relatively small region of the membrane and is non-propagating in nature | 1. It spreads over the membrane covering relatively a much larger area and is propagating in nature |
| 2. It is initiated either spontaneously or by a neurotransmitter or by environmental stimulus | 2. It is initiated by membrane depolarisation |
| 3. It shows a graded response and does not obey 'all-or-none law' | 3. Summation of action potential is not possible, therefore, it obeys 'all-or-none law' |
| 4. It can either be a depolarising or hyperpolarising response | 4. It is always a depolarisation with an overshoot |
| 5. It has no threshold | 5. It has a threshold that is usually 10–15 mV of depolarisation |
| 6. It has no refractory period | 6. It has a refractory period |
| 7. It is important in signalling over short distances | 7. It is a long distance signal of nerve and muscle membrane |

## CLASSIFICATION OF NERVE FIBRES                                    2.5 (1991)

I. Nerve fibres may be classified as given by Gasser and Erlanger

| Fibre type | Function | Fibre diametre (µm) | Conduction velocity (m/s) | Spike duration (ms) | Absolute refractory period (ms) |
|---|---|---|---|---|---|
| **A** | | | | | |
| α | Proprioception, somatic motor | 12–20 | 70–120 | 0.4–0.5 | 0.4–1 |
| β | Touch, pressure | 5–12 | 30–70 | | |

*Contd.*

*Contd.*

| Fibre type | Function | Fibre diametre (µm) | Conduction velocity (m/s) | Spike duration (ms) | Absolute refractory period (ms) |
|---|---|---|---|---|---|
| γ ⎫ ⎬ δ ⎭ | Motor to muscle spindle | 3–6 | 15–30 | 0.4–0.5 | 0.4–1 |
| | Pain, cold, touch | 2–5 | 12–30 | | |
| B | Pregang-lionic, autonomic | <3 | 3–15 | 1.2 | 1.2 |
| **C** | | | | | |
| Dorsal root | Pain, temp-erature, some mech-anoreceptors | 0.4–1.2 | 0.5–2 | 2 | 2 |
| Sym-pathetic | Postgang-lionic sym-pathetic | 0.3–1.3 | 0.7–2.3 | 2 | 2 |

## II Numerical classification for sensory neurons

| Number | Origin | Fibre type |
|---|---|---|
| $I_a$ | Muscle spindle, annulospiral ending | A α |
| $I_b$ | Golgi tendon organ | A α |
| II | Muscle spindle, flower spray ending, touch, pressure | A β |
| III | Pain and temperature receptors, some touch | A δ |
| IV | Pain and other receptors | Dorsal root 'C' fibres |

## III Physioclinical classification

| | Most susceptible | Intermediate | Least susceptible |
|---|---|---|---|
| Sensitivity to hypoxia | B | A | C |
| Sensitivity to pressure | A | B | C |
| Sensitivity to local anaesthesia | C | B | A |

## WALLERIAN DEGENERATION OF NERVES          2.5 (1990)
## CHANGES IN NEURON WHEN ITS AXON IS CUT     2.5 (1988)

Wallerian degeneration of nerves are the changes in the nerve cell body and its axon following injury to a nerve. Injury may be due to crushing, cutting or ischaemia of the nerve fibre.

**Changes in nerve cell body:** Within 48 hrs of the section, following degenerative changes take place:

1. Nissl granules disintegrate into fine dust-like structure. This process is known as chromatolysis.
2. Fragmentation of golgi apparatus occurs.
3. Cells swell up due to increased fluid content.
4. Neurofibrils disappear.
5. Nucleus is displaced towards cell margin.

### Changes in Axon

Within 24 hrs following changes occur in nerve fibre distal to the site of injury, called peripheral part:

1. The axis cylinder breaks into small segments.
2. Myelin sheath begins to disintegrate and is slowly replaced by fat droplets. These droplets result from hydrolysis of fats constituting the myelin. Myelin degeneration starts about the 8th day and is complete by 32 days of injury.
3. Neurolemma remains intact.
4. Schwann cells multiply mitotically forming cord of cells within endoneurial tubes.
5. Phagocytes invade from endoneurium and remove debris of axis cylinder and myelin sheath.

These hollow tubes of neurolemma containing large number of phagocytes, are called ghost tubes.

**Proximal part of the nerve:** Similar changes take place in proximal stump up to the nearest node of Ranvier.

### ACTION POTENTIAL IN SINGLE NERVE FIBRE  2.5 (1985, 1989, 1991)

When a nerve fibre is stimulated and a signal is transmitted along it, a series of potential changes take place, known as action potential (Fig. 7.3).

1. As a stimulus is applied, there is a brief irregular deflection of the base line due to current leakage from stimulating to recording electrodes. This is called **stimulus artifact**.

2. Following stimulus artifact is an isoelectric **latent period**. It is time taken for the impulse to travel along the axon and is proportional to distance between stimulating and recording electrodes and velocity of conduction across the nerve fibre.

3. Initial slow depolarisation of 15 mV from resting level of –70 mV.

4. Rapid depolarization and the point where it occurs is the **firing level**. A sharp rise to +35 mV and rapid fall is called the **spike potential**.

5. A slow fall in potential to resting level of –70 mV is called **afterdepolarisation**.

6. Overshoot after resting levels towards hyperpolarised state which is small in magnitude but prolonged in duration is called **afterhyperpolarisation**. Total time for action potential is 35–40 msec.

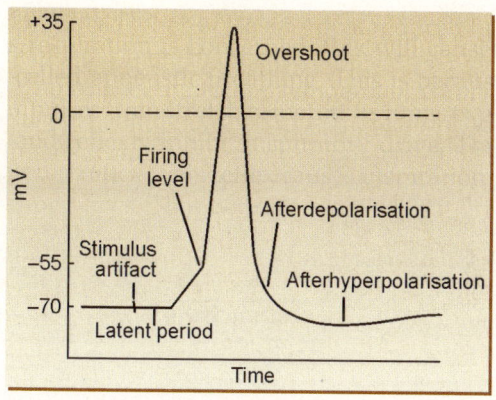

**Fig. 7.3:** Action potential in a neuron

## IONIC BASIS OF EXCITATION AND CONDUCTION IN A NERVE
**2 (2009)**

1. **Resting state or polarised state:** Inside of the membrane is negative and outside it is positive. Since potassium permeability is more than sodium permeability at rest, hence $K^+$ maintain the RMP.

2. **Depolarisation:** At the point of stimulation, a slight redistribution of ions leads to increased $K^+$ and $Cl^-$ influx restoring the RMP. However, when the depolarisation exceeds 7 mV,

Na⁺ channel activation occurs and when the firing level is reached, influx of sodium along its electrical and concentration gradient is so great that it overcomes the repolarising forces and run away depolarisation occurs.

The membrane potential fails to reach +60mV during the action potential because the increase in sodium permeability is short lived. Factors that limit Na⁺ permeability include (Fig. 7.4):

  i. Inactivation of Na⁺ channels

  ii. The direction of electrical gradient for Na⁺ is reversed during overshoot because the membrane potential is reversed

  iii. Opening of voltage-gated K⁺ channels because of which K⁺ leaves along the concentration gradient.

3. **Repolarisation:** It starts with K⁺ efflux due to opening of voltage-gated K⁺ channels and decrease in further Na⁺ influx.

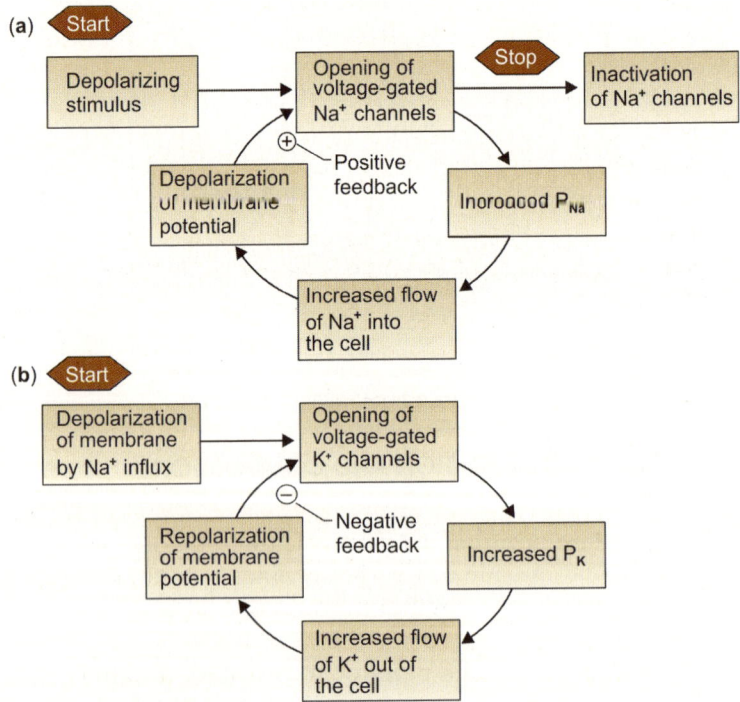

**Fig. 7.4:** Ionic basis of excitation and conduction in a nerve

The opening of voltage-gated potassium channels is much slower and more prolonged than the opening of Na$^+$ channels.

4. **Afterdepolarisation:** At the termination of spike potential, K$^+$ conduction is slowed down and thus a few msec are delay in restoring the membrane potential. This last phase of slow K$^+$ efflux is called afterdepolarisation.

5. **Afterhyperpolarisation:** With the disappearance of after-depolarisation although the membrane potential is achieved but the resting ionic status is not achieved. It is achieved by the slow return of the K$^+$ channel to the closed state.

## SALTATORY CONDUCTION　　　2.5 (1987,1990)

Saltatory conduction is the mode of transmission of impulses along a myelinated nerve. In a myelinated nerve depolarisation jumps from one node of Ranvier to the next. This is because the intervening myelin between the two nodes acts as an insulator so no ions can flow across it. Action potential is propagated from node-to-node. The electric current flows through surrounding extracellular fluid and axoplasm from node-to-node excites successive nodes one after another. Saltatory conduction has the following advantages:

i. Velocity of conduction is faster than unmyelinated nerve of the same diametre.

ii. It requires little energy for conduction of impulse. As only the nodes are depolarised and repolarised, it requires movement of ions in small amounts during conduction (Fig. 7.5).

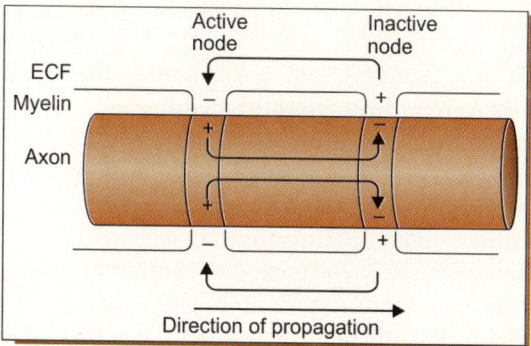

**Fig. 7.5:** Local current flow (movement of positive charges) around an impulse in axon

## CONDUCTION OF NERVE IMPULSE IN MYELINATED AND UNMYELINATED FIBRES                    2.5 (1988)

In a myelinated nerve the depolarisation process jumps from node-to-node as the myelin acts as an insulator not allowing the movement of ions across it. This is known as **saltatory conduction**. In a non-myelinated nerve, action potential is propagated all along the nerve to its end.

Velocity of conduction is much faster in a myelinated as compared to non-myelinated nerves as action potential jumps from one node to the next. This mode of propagation, also consumes less energy as transport of ions during action potential propagation occurs only at the nodes of Ranvier and not across the myelin sheath.

## NEUROMUSCULAR JUNCTION

### NEUROMUSCULAR TRANSMISSION          2 (2009), 4 (2004)-IPU

### MECHANISM OF RELEASE OF NEUROTRANSMITTER AT N-M JUNCTION                           2.5 (2010)

The neuromuscular junction transmits the impulses from the nerve to muscle. The sequence of events which cause transmission through N-M junction can be seen in Fig. 7.6:

1. **Release of Ach by the nerve terminals:** When the nerve impulse travelling in the nerve fibre reaches the terminal buttons, the voltage-gated calcium channels present on the presynaptic membrane open up increasing its permeability to calcium ions. $Ca^{2+}$ present in the ECF of synaptic cleft enters the terminal buttons. The elevated $Ca^{2+}$ triggers a marked exocytosis of vesicles releasing Ach in the synaptic cleft.

2. **Effects of Ach on postsynaptic membrane:** The Ach diffuses in the synaptic cleft and binds to the nicotinic-Ach receptors located mainly on the junctional folds of the motor end plate (postsynaptic membrane).

3. **Development of end plate potential:** Due to the opening of the Ach-gated channels in the end plate membrane, a large number of sodium ions from the ECF enter inside the muscle fibre following the electrochemical gradient. The resting membrane potential at the postsynaptic membrane is –80 mV to –90 mV. When sodium ions enter inside, there occurs depolarisation

causing a local positive potential change inside the muscle fibre membrane called end plate potential.

When a critical level of –60 mV is reached, it triggers the development of action potential in the muscle fibre. The action potentials are generated on either side of the end plate and conducted away from the end plate in both the directions along the muscle fibres thus causing muscle contraction.

4. **Miniature end plate potential:** Even at rest, small quanta of Ach are released randomly from the nerve terminal. Each quanta of Ach produces a weak end plate potential about 0.5 mV called miniature end plate potential (MEPP).

5. **Removal of Ach by cholinesterase:** The Ach released in the synaptic cleft stays for a short period and is removed within one msec by one of the two methods:

   a. By enzyme acetylcholinesterase which is present in the matrix of synaptic cleft.

   b. A small amount of Ach diffuses out of the synaptic space.

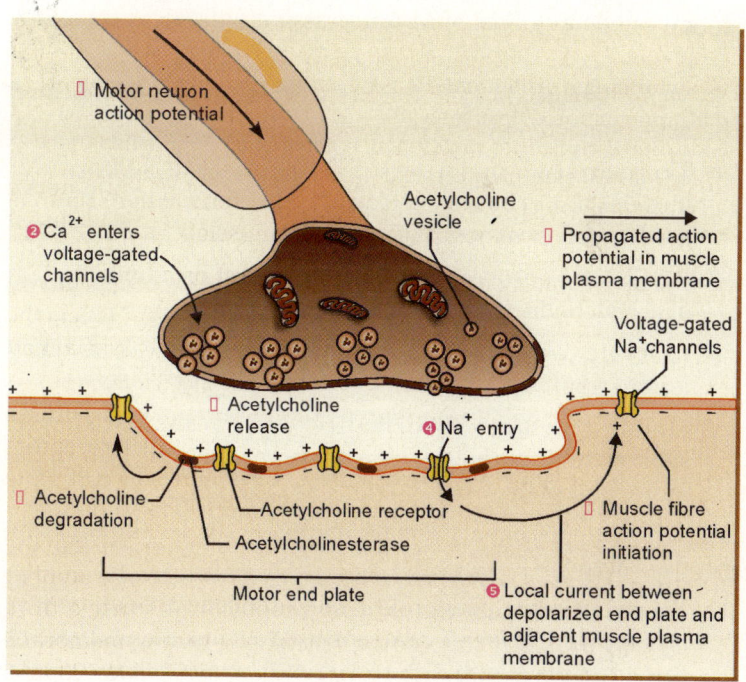

**Fig. 7.6:** Events at the neuromuscular junction

The rapid removal of Ach prevents the repeated excitation of the muscle fibre.

## MYASTHENIA GRAVIS        2.5 (1993), 4 (2004)-IPU, 2.5 (2007)
## EXPLAIN WHY MUSCULAR WEAKNESS
## OCCURS IN MYASTHENIA GRAVIS        1 (2004), 1 (2010)

1. This is a serious and sometimes fatal disease in which the skeletal muscles tire easily.

2. This has a bimodal distribution: Which peaks in 20s (women) and 60s (men).

3. Circulating antibodies are formed against nicotinic Ach receptors. They either destroy the receptor or bind others to neighbouring receptors, triggering their removal by endocytosis.

4. Normally, the number of quanta released on each motor nerve terminal will decline with repetitive stimuli. In myasthenia gravis, N-M transmission will fail at these low levels.

5. Major feature: Muscle fatigue with sustained or repeated muscular activity.

6. There are two major forms of the disease: Extraocular muscles are primarily affected and second where there is generalised weakness of the skeletal muscle.

7. Weakness improves after a period of rest or administration of acetylcholinesterase inhibitors.

8. In severe cases, the diaphragm can become weak and may lead to respiratory failure.

9. Major structural abnormality: Appearance of sparse, shallow or abnormally wide or absent synaptic cleft in the motor end plate.

10. 30% patients have a female relative with an autoimmune disorder.

11. The thymus may play a role in the pathogenesis of the disease by supplying helper-T cells sensitised against thymic proteins that cross react with Ach receptors. Thymus is hyperplastic and 10–15% people have thymomas.

## SKELETAL AND SMOOTH MUSCLES

### SARCOMERE                                                    2.5 (1985)

Sarcomere is the part of muscle fibre between two Z-lines (Fig. 7.7).
Muscle fibre under the microscope shows alternating dark A bands
and light I bands. In the middle of the I-band is a dark Z-line.
Actin filaments present in I-band are attached to the Z-line.
During muscle contraction as actin filaments slide over the myosin
filaments length of the sarcomere shortens.

   When a muscle is at rest sacromere length is 2 µm. At this stage
actin filaments completely overlap the myosin filaments. At resting
length sacromere can generate maximum force during muscle
contraction as maximum cross-bridges are formed between actin
and myosin molecules.

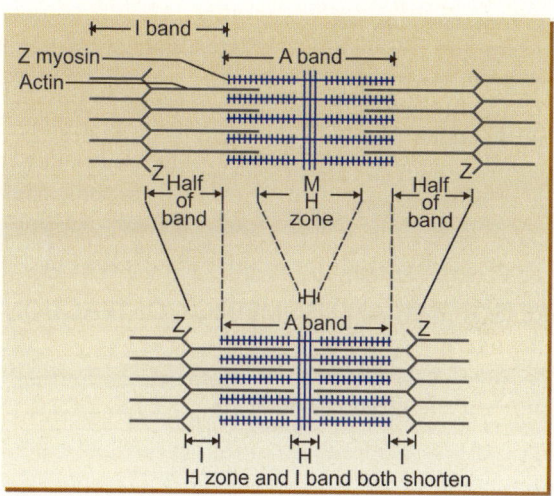

**Fig. 7.7:** Arrangement of thin (actin) and thick (myosin) filaments in
sarcomere

### COMPARE WHITE AND RED MUSCLE FIBRES          2 (2008)
### COMPARE RED AND PALE MUSCLE FIBRES          2 (2004)-IPU

| White muscle fibres | Red muscle fibres |
| --- | --- |
| 1. Muscle fibres are large in diametre with high glycogen | 1. They are of moderate diametre and moderate glycogen capacity |

*(Contd.)*

*(Contd.)*

| White muscle fibres | Red muscle fibres |
|---|---|
| capacity and ATPase activity, because they are pale therefore called white muscle fibres | with low ATPase activity. They are darker than other muscle fibres, therefore called 'red muscle fibres' |
| 2. They are innervated by large, fast conducting motor neurons, therefore also called fast muscle fibres | 2. They are innervated by small, slow conducting motor neurons, therefore also called slow muscle fibres |
| 3. These muscles have short twitch durations and are specialised for fine, rapid and skilled movements, e.g. extraocular movements and muscles of the hand | 3. These muscles have long latency and slow twitch durations. They are adapted for slow, posture maintaining contractions, e.g. long muscles of the limbs and muscles of the back |
| 4. These muscles get fatigued easily | 4. These muscles are resistant to fatigue and most used muscles |
| 5. They are particularly suited for high intensity workouts that can be sustained for only short periods of time | 5. They are required to perform work when endurance type activities are performed, i.e. to perform low-intensity work over long periods of time such as athletes, bicyclists and swimmers |

## COMPARE ISOTONIC AND ISOMETRIC CONTRACTIONS

**2 (2004)-IPU**

| Isotonic contraction | Isometric contraction |
|---|---|
| 1. Tension of the muscle remains the same, whereas the length decreases during contraction | 1. Length of the muscle remains the same, whereas tension is developed |
| 2. External work is done | 2. Since work done = force × distance, no external work is done |
| 3. The contractile component and parallel elastic component are shortened but the series elastic component does not stretch further, producing a visible shortening of the muscle | 3. Shortening produced by contractile component of the muscle is compensated by stretching of the series elastic component |

*(Contd.)*

(*Contd.*)

| Isotonic contraction | Isometric contraction |
|---|---|
| 4. **Examples:** Contraction of leg muscles while running and walking, contraction of muscles during flexion of arm | 4. **Examples:** Contraction of anti-gravity muscles, contraction of arm muscles while trying to push a wall |

## SARCOTUBULAR SYSTEM                    2.5 (1989)

In muscles myofibrils are surrounded by a network of vesicles and tubules, visible in electron photomicrographs, as sarcotubular system. It is made up of the following components:

1. **T-system:** Tubules that run transverse to the myofibrils. These are extensions of the sarcolemma going deep into the muscle surrounding the fibrils. Space between the two layers of T-tubule is the extension of ECF.

2. **Sarcoplasmic reticulum:** Form longitudinal tubes that run parallel to the fibrils in between them and give numerous interconnecting branches. These longitudinal tubes have expanded terminal sac like ends called terminal cisternae or sacs.

Terminal sacs come in close contact with T-tubules in skeletal muscles at the site of junction of the A and I band. At this junction one terminal sac is present on either side of T-tube constituting a triad. So there are two triads per sarcomere in the skeletal muscle.

### Function of Sarcotubular System

T-system being continues with sarcolemma brings about rapid transmission of action potential to all the myofibrils.

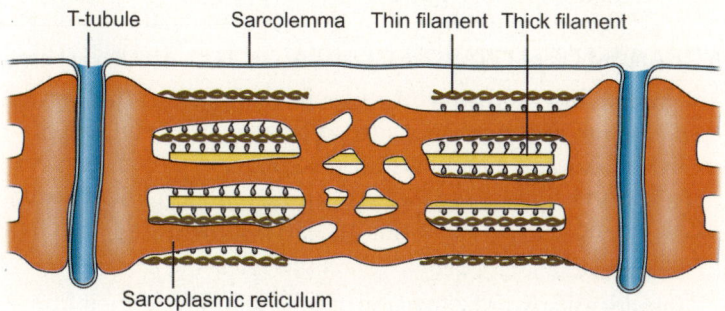

**Fig. 7.8:** Sarcotubular system

Sarcoplasmic reticulum provides $Ca^{2+}$ to fibrils and helps to initiate muscle contraction. Their close association with T-tubules forming triads causes rapid muscle contraction (Fig. 7.8).

## COMPARE SARCOTUBULAR SYSTEM IN
## SKELETAL AND CARDIAC MUSCLE                    2 (2010)

| Skeletal muscle | Cardiac muscle |
| --- | --- |
| 1. It is better developed compared to the cardiac muscle where the terminal cistern is more prominent | 1. It is present with poorly developed terminal cistern |
| 2. T system is present at the A-I junction | 2. T system is present at the Z-line |
| 3. There are 2 triads per sarcomere | 3. There is one triad per sarcomere |

## EXCITATION-CONTRACTION COUPLING
### 2.5 (1985, 1986), (2000), 2.5 (2002)

A muscle when excited by a stimulus given through its nerve responds by contracting known as **excitation-contraction coupling**. As impulse travels along the nerve, acetylcholine is released at nerve terminals. Acetylcholine (Ach) passes across the neuromuscular junctions and combines with specialised receptors at the motor end plate. Binding of Ach to receptors increases the sodium permeability of the membrane, depolarising it and setting up action potentials. This action potential is propagated along the muscle, thereby producing muscle contraction by releasing calcium from the sarcoplasmic reticulum. Hence, the process by which depolarisation of muscle fibre produces contraction is called **excitation-contraction coupling**. $Ca^{2+}$ is responsible for this process.

## MECHANISM OF EXCITATION-CONTRACTION COUPLING (1989)

Excitation-contraction coupling is the process by which depolarisation of the muscle fibre initiates contraction. Calcium acts as the coupling agent in this process.

The link between excitation and contraction in skeletal muscle is because of presence of highly specialised sarcotubular system of T-tubules and sarcoplasmic reticulum releasing $Ca^{2+}$.

- T-tubules are inward extension of sarcolemma and their lumen is in continuity with ECF surrounding the muscle fibres.

- Sarcoplasmic reticulum forms a network around the tubules and have expanded ends known as terminal sacs or cisternae.

- At the junction of A and I band, each T-tubule has a terminal sac on its either side forming what is called the triads which have a special role in muscle contraction.

- Depolarization of sarcolemma is transmitted to all fibrils via the T-tubules.

- As a result $Ca^{2+}$ is released from terminal cisternae lying close to T-tubules and diffuses around the filaments.

- Calcium binds to troponin C which weakens the bond between troponin I to actin, as a result tropomyosin moves laterally and uncovers binding sites on actin for myosin.

- There is formation of cross-bridges between myosin heads and actin resulting in sliding of actin filaments over myosin filements and the muscle shortens.

## COMPARE EXCITATION-CONTRACTION COUPLING IN SKELETAL AND SMOOTH MUSCLES 2 (2009), 2 (2011)

It is difficult to study the relationship between electrical and mechanical activity in the smooth muscle because of its continuous activity. The excitation contraction coupling can occur with as much as 500 msec delay. Hence, it is a very slow process compared to the skeletal muscle, in which the time from initial depolarisation to initiation of contraction is less than 10 msec.

## EXPLAIN WHY RIGOR MORTIS DEVELOPS AFTER DEATH
## 1 (2004)

After death, the muscle fibres are depleted of ATP and phosphocreatine. In rigor mortis almost all the myosin heads are attached to actin but in an abnormal, fixed and resistant way since ATP which is required for pumping back calcium for relaxation is not available.

## EXPLAIN WHY MOST OF THE MUSCLES IN THE BODY AT REST ARE AT OPTIMAL LENGTH 1 (2005) DU

At optimum length the muscles develop active tension, hence velocity of contraction of muscles is maximum at rest.

## ELECTROMYOGRAPHY     2.5 (1987, 1991)

Electromyography is a process by which electrical activity of the muscle, i.e. action potential are recorded on its stimulation. The record so obtained is electromyogram and the machine is electromyograph. Muscle can be stimulated through motor nerve or by its voluntary contraction.

Action potentials can be recorded by placing disc electrodes on the skin overlying the muscle or by hypodermic needle electrodes.

Activity can be recorded by ink-writing pens over a moving paper or on cathode ray oscilloscope or can be heard over a microphone.

Electromyography is useful for diagnosis of motor neuron diseases, myopathies and peripheral neuritis.

## VISCERAL AND MULTIUNIT SMOOTH MUSCLE     2.5 (1986)
## TYPES OF SMOOTH MUSCLES     3 (2004)-IPU
## COMPARE AND CONTRAST SINGLE- AND MULTI-UNIT SMOOTH MUSCLES     2 (2004), 2 (2006)

| Single-unit smooth muscles | Multi-unit smooth muscles |
|---|---|
| 1. It occurs in large sheets and has low resistance bridges between individual muscle cells, functioning in a syncytial fashion that is why called single unit smooth muscles | 1. It is made up of individual units without inter-connecting bridges |
| 2. Sites: Walls of hollow viscera, e.g. GIT, ureters, bronchi, uterus and urinary bladder | 2. Sites: Iris, ciliary muscles of the eye, pilomotor muscles of the skin, muscles of the blood vessels |
| 3. The muscles are characterised by spontaneous activity in certain areas called pacemakers | 3. These muscle fibres are richly innervated and each muscle fibre has its own nerve supply. |
| 4. Rhythmic contraction and relaxation of these muscles is independent of innervations. The nervous influence only modulates their activity | 4. These muscles only contract in response to a stimulus through their nerves by releasing chemical mediators at their endings (Ach or NE) to which |

*(Contd.)*

(*Contd.*)

| Single-unit smooth muscles | Multi-unit smooth muscles |
|---|---|
| | they are very sensitive. Here single stimulus to a nerve results in repeated firing of the action potential which produces irregular tetanic contractions rather than a single muscle twitch |
| 5. If these muscles are stretched, there is production of active tension | 5. These muscles do not respond to stretch |

## MECHANISM OF CONTRACTION OF SMOOTH MUSCLE   3 (1992)

The basic process of muscle contraction is sliding of actin filaments over the myosin filaments. However, the two filaments are not regularly arranged unlike in skeletal muscles. The different steps involved are as follows:

1. Mechanism is initiated as the muscle is stimulated by stretch, through its nerves or chemicals by an increase in intracellular calcium ions which enter via voltage-gated $Ca^{2+}$ channels.

2. Binding of $Ca^{2+}$ with **calmodulin**, a binding protein present in smooth muscle.

3. Calcium-calmodulin complex activates myosin-light chain kinase.

4. Phosphorylation of myosin by the above kinase.

5. Phosphorylation of myosin head is accompanied by ATPase activity due to which energy is released.

6. Cycles of attachment, swiveling and detachment of myosin heads to actin occur causing actin filament to slide over the myosin filaments thus bringing about muscle contraction.

In smooth muscle compared to skeletal muscle process of muscle contraction is slow, requires little energy and is sustained. The cycles of attachment and detachment of cross bridges are slow. Prolonged attachment of cross-bridges to actin is responsible for sustained contraction and is known as the **Latch-bridge phenomenon**.

## Mechanism of Contraction

Binding of Ach to muscarinic receptors
↓
Increased calcium influx into the cell
↓
Activation of calmodulin dependent light chain kinase enzyme
↓
Phosphorylation of myosin
↓
Activation of myosin ATPase
↓
Binding of myosin to actin
↓
Actin slides on myosin

## Mechanism of Relaxation

Dephosphorylation of myosin by myosin–light chain kinase
↓
Dissociation of calcium-calmodulin complex
↓
Muscle relaxation

or

Sustained muscle contraction (due to myosin remaining attached to actin even after decrease in the level of intracellular calcium ions **(Latch-bridge mechanism)**

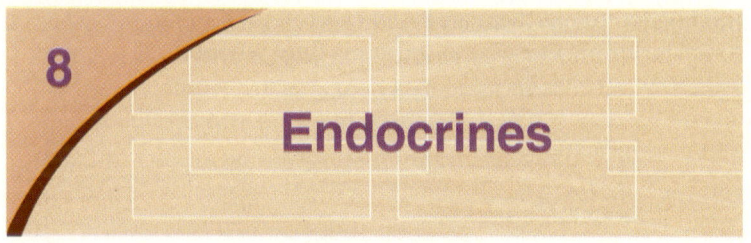

# 8

# Endocrines

## HYPOTHALAMO-HYPOPHYSEAL RELATIONSHIP (Fig. 8.1)

Hypothalamus controls the functions of hypophysis, i.e. pituitary gland. For the hypothalamic control there are connections between the hypothalamus and the pituitary.

**Hypothalamo-hypophyseal vessels** Connections between hypothalamus and anterior pituitary are vascular through **hypothalamo-hypophyseal vessels.**

Nervous connection exist between hypothalamus and posterior pituitary called **hypothalamo-hypophyseal tract.**

### Hypothalamo-hypophyseal Circulation

Branches from circle of Willis and internal carotid arteries form a capillary network on the ventral surface of the hypothalamus called the primary capillary plexus. Capillaries also enter the median eminence in the hypothalamus. Capillaries drain into portal hypophyseal vessels running in pituitary stalk. From portal vessels arise another set of capillary network called the secondary capillary plexus. As this system of vessels begins and ends in capillaries without passing through the heart, it is a portal system called hypothalamo-hypophyseal portal system.

**Hypothalamo-hypophyseal tract** It is a neural tract arising from supraoptic and paraventricular nuclei of hypothalamus. It carries the hormones oxytocin and ADH secreted by the hypothalamus to posterior pituitary by axoplasmic flow where these are stored.

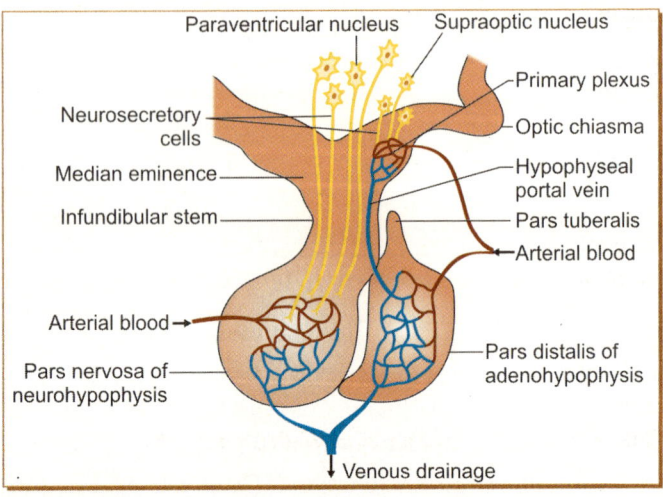

**Fig. 8.1:** Hypothalamo-hypophyseal relationship

**Hypothalamic releasing factors** A number of releasing factors are produced by the various nuclei of the hypothalamus, which exert a control on the anterior pituitary for the secretion of hormones. These factors are released by the neurons and enter the hypothalamo-hypophyseal vessels at the median eminence and are carried to the anterior pituitary where they exert their control.

Following factors are released:

1. Corticotropin releasing hormone **(CRH)**—stimulates ACTH secretion.

2. Thyrotropin releasing hormone **(TRH)**—stimulates TSH secretion.

3. Gonadotropin hormone releasing hormone **(GnRH)**—stimulates FSH and LH.

4. Growth hormone releasing hormone **(GHRH)**—causes secretion of growth hormone.

5. Prolactin releasing hormone **(PRH)**—stimulates prolactin secretion.

6. Growth hormone inhibiting hormone **(GHIH)** also called somatostatin inhibits growth hormone secretion.

7. Prolactin inhibiting hormone **(PIH)**—inhibits prolactin secretion.

Through these factors hypothalamus controls the pituitary function.

## ACROMEGALY       2.5 (1986, 1990), 2.5 (2006)
## COMPARE ACROMEGALY AND GIGANTISM      2 (2007)

Acromegaly is a clinical syndrome occurring due to excessive secretion of growth hormone by the anterior pituitary in adults. It usually occurs due to tumour of growth hormone producing acidophil cells of the pituitary.

In 20–40% of cases it is accompanied by the hypersecretion of prolactin. It causes growth in those areas where the cartilage persists. Acromegaly means enlargement of the peripheral region.

### Clinical Features

i. There is enlargement of hands and feet. As the condition occurs in adults after the fusion of epiphysis of the long bones, linear growth cannot occur, so hands and feet are bigger as bones grow in thickness.

ii. Elongation and widening of the mandible (**prognathism**) resulting in an underbite and increased interdental spaces.

iii. Enlargement of the frontal, maxillary, ethmoid and mastoid sinuses causing a prominent brow.

iv. Thickening of the skin and coarsening of facial features which are due mainly to the proliferation of connective tissue and lead to oedema (**acromegalic facies**).

v. Periosteal growth of the vertebra causes bowing of the spine (**kyphosis**) and that of metacarpals and metatarsals (**acral parts**).

vi. Hyperglycemia may be present.

vii. Hypertrophy of soft tissues of the body: Heart (cardiomegaly), liver (hepatomegaly), kidney (renomegaly), intestine and spleen (splenomegaly), tongue and muscles. There is increase in urinary excretion of creatinine.

**Gigantism / Giantism:** It is due to overproduction of GH during adolescence (before epiphyseal closure) and is characterized by excessive growth of long bones.

## Characteristic Features

  i. Tall stature (may be as tall as 8 feet)
 ii. Bilateral gynaecomastia: It may be due to increase in plasma oestrogen:androgen ratio in males
iii. Large hands and feet
 iv. Associated features: Coarse facial features and loss of libido/ impotence.

## COMPARE AND CONTRAST—ANTERIOR AND POSTERIOR PITUITARY GLAND                 2 (2011)

| Anterior lobe of pituitary gland | Posterior lobe of pituitary gland |
|---|---|
| 1. The glandular anterior lobe of the pituitary is called the **adenohypophysis** and constitutes 80% of the pituitary gland | 1. This constitutes about 20% of the pituitary and is called **neurohypophysis** |
| 2. This is divided into three parts:<br>• Pars distalis<br>• Pars intermedia<br>• Pars tuberalis | 2. This is divided into three components:<br>a. Median eminence<br>b. Infundibular stem<br>c. Infundibular process (pars nervosa) |
| 3. Adenohypophysis is influenced by hormones that come from the hypothalamus via portal vessels (hypothalamo-hypophyseal vessels) | 3. Neurohypophysis is influenced by neurons via the hypothalamo-hypophyseal neural tract that conveys hormones directly from the hypothalamic nuclei for storage in the posterior lobe. These unmyelinated nerve tracts arise from the supraoptic and paraventricular nuclei within the hypothalamus |
| 4. The hormones secreted by the anterior pituitary include: | 4. The hormones secreted by the posterior pituitary include vasopressin (ADH) and oxytocin |

*Contd.*

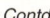

*Contd.*

| Anterior lobe of pituitary gland | Posterior lobe of pituitary gland |
|---|---|
| • TSH<br>• ACTH<br>• Growth hormone<br>• FSH<br>• LH<br>• Prolactin<br>• β-lipotropin | |

## COMPARE PITUITARY AND THYROID DWARF  2 (2004), 2 (2009)

### Pituitary Dwarf

This is produced due to growth hormone deficiency secondary to decrease in GHRH. The characteristic features include:

• Plumpness
• Immature facies
• Small genitalia
• Delicate extremities, body proportion according to chronological age
• Delayed skeletal and dental development
• Low circulating growth hormone level.

### Hypothyroid Dwarf

This is produced due to deficiency of thyroid hormone and has the following features:

• Gross retardation of physical and mental development.
• Body proportions remain infantile.
• Bone age is retarded more than height.
• Associated features of hypothyroidism.
• Earlier is the onset, more severe is the delay in growth and skeletal maturation.

## NAME THE HORMONES SECRETED BY ADENOHYPOPHYSIS
## HOW IS THEIR SECRETION REGULATED          10 (1985)

Anterior pituitary has a number of cell types, based on staining characters by immunocytochemistry technique. Each cell type secretes a different hormone.

1. Somatotropes secrete growth hormone
2. Corticotropes – ACTH and β-LPH
3. Thyrotropes – TSH
3. Gonadotropes – FSH and LH
5. Lactotropes – prolactin

## REGULATION OF SECRETION

- Discuss hypothalamo-hypophyseal portal system.
- Pouring of releasing factors from hypothalamus at the median eminence.
- Releasing and inhibitory factors.

**(Please refer to previous question on hypothalamo-hypophyseal system)**

## CIRCADIAN RHYTHM OF ACTH RELEASE                    2.5 (1990)

### Circadian Rhythm of ACTH

In humans secretion of ACTH is not continuous throughout the day. ACTH is secreted in irregular burst, i.e. the secretion is pulsatile. There are fluctuations in the levels of glucocorticoids in response to the pulsatile secretion of ACTH.

The ACTH bursts are more frequent in the morning and are minimum in the evening. This diurnal variation in ACTH secretion is called the circadian rhythm. It is somehow not related to the stress of waking up in the morning. ACTH circadian rhythm is controlled by the suprachiasmatic nucleus of the hypothalamus.

## NAME THE HORMONES SECRETED BY PITUITARY AND DESCRIBE THE HORMONAL CORRELATES OF PUBERTY IN FEMALES                    5 (1991)

### Hormones Secreted by Pituitary

Pituitary hormones can be grouped into three categories.

    I. Hormones of anterior pituitary:

        1. Growth hormone or somatotropin

        2. Thyroid stimulating hormone–TSH

        3. Adernocorticotropic hormone–ACTH

        4. Prolactin

        5. Follicle-stimulating hormone–FSH

6. Luteinising hormone–LH

7. β-lipotropin

II. Hormones of posterior pituitary

1. Oxytocin

2. Antidiuretic hormone (ADH) or vasopressin

III. Intermediate lobe hormones

1. Melanotropin or α and β MSH.

2. γ-lipotropin

3. Corticotropin like intermediate lobe peptide, i.e. CLIP

4. β-endorphin

## Hormonal Correlates of Puberty in Females

Puberty may be defined as the period when the endocrinal and gametogenic function of gonads have first developed to an extent that reproduction is possible. In females the main changes at puberty are:

i. Breast development–**thelarche**

ii. Appearance of axillary and pubic hair–**pubarche**

iii. Onset of menstruation–**menarche**

Proceeding puberty there is increased secretion of androgen by the adrenal gland called **adrenarche** and is believed to occur under the influence of adrenal androgen stimulating hormone (AASH) from the pituitary gland.

**Onset of puberty:** What actually causes the activity in gonads at puberty is not known clearly.

- As such infantile gonads in children can be stimulated by gonadotropins.

- Pituitary can also be stimulated to secrete gonadotropins.

- Hence before the onset of puberty, most probably gonado-tropin releasing hormone (GnRH) is not being secreted in an appropriate manner to cause the release of gonadotropins, i.e. FSH and LH from the pituitary. One view is that before puberty GnRH is very sensitive to negative feedback action of gonadal hormone oestrogen which is present in minute quantities, so GnRH is not secreted. At puberty threshold for this negative feedback rises and GnRH secretion also rises, thereby causing the release of FSH and LH. So female reproductive cycles begin under the influence of LH and FSH.

Another factor inhibiting the secretion of GnRH from the hypothalamus is believed to be melatonin secreted from the pineal gland. Activity of pineal gland decreases at puberty.

Hence activity of hormones from hypothalamus, pineal gland and pituitary gland is integrated to bring in the onset of puberty through secretion of GnRH, melatonin, FSH and LH sequentially. This hormonal activity is preceded by the activity of adrenal cortex under the influence of AASH from the pituitary.

## ENUMERATE THE HORMONES SECRETED BY ANTERIOR PITUITARY. DESCRIBE THE FUNCTIONS OF GROWTH HORMONE AND EFFECTS OF ITS HYPERSECRETION  10

## GROWTH HORMONE  2 (2008)

(For hormones secreted by the anterior pituitary refer to previous question)

### Functions of growth hormone

Growth hormone promotes growth and metabolism in the body. Growth promoting actions of GH are either exerted directly or indirectly through certain growth promoting factors known as Somatomedins. Somatomedins are produced in the liver mainly. In humans principle somatomedins are insulin-like growth factor-I (IGF-I) and insulin-like growth factor-II (IGF-II).

I. **Functions of GH through somatomedins**
   i. Growth of skeletal tissue and viscera
   ii. Effects on protein metabolism
   iii. Effects on electrolytes metabolism

II. **Direct actions of GH**
   i. Action on carbohydrate metabolism
   ii. Fat metabolism
   iii. Erythropoiesis

### Growth of Skeletal Tissue

GH increases linear growth of bones before the fusion of epiphysis by causing:
   i. Chondrogenesis
   ii. Widening of cartilage of epiphyseal plate
   iii. Laying down of matrix at ends of long bones
   iv. GH also causes the growth of soft tissue and viscera.

### Effects on Protein Metabolism (Protein Anabolic Hormone)

GH promotes protein synthesis by producing a positive nitrogen balance. It also promotes cell division and causes growth. It promotes amino acid uptake by the tissues specially the liver and promotes protein synthesis.

### Effects on Carbohydrate Metabolism

GH increases blood glucose level and helps to maintain normal glucose level by:

i. Increasing glucose output by the liver
ii. Decreasing peripheral utilization of glucose especially by muscle tissue, by inhibiting phosphorylation of glucose.

### Effects on Lipid Metabolism

It promotes lipolysis and is ketogenic, thereby increasing plasma free fatty acid levels. Free fatty acids are a source of energy during hypoglycemic and stress.

### Effects on Electrolyte Metabolism

• Increase calcium absorption from the intestine
• Decrease excretion of sodium and potassium from the kidney. These electrolytes are diverted to the growing tissues.

### Erythropoiesis

GH stimulates erythropoiesis

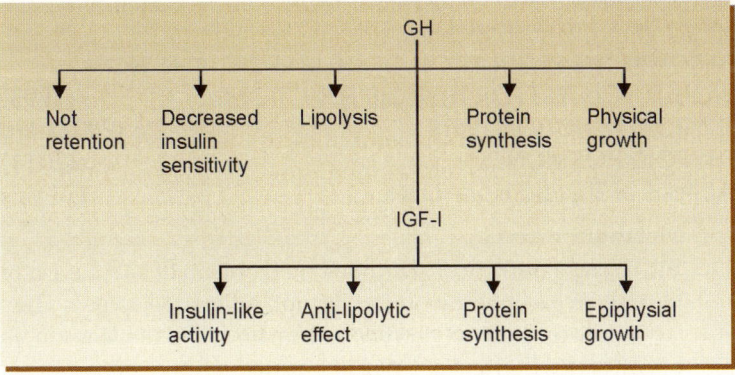

## Effect of Hypersecretion of GH

**Before fusion of epiphysis:** Increase in length of bones and person is tall and well built called **giagantism** in children.

**After fusion of epiphysis:** Causes excessive increase in width of bone called **acromegaly** in adults.

## LARON DWARFISM                              2 (2003)-IPU

This is a type of dwarfism in which plasma growth hormone concentration is normal or elevated but their growth hormone receptors are unresponsive as a result of loss of function due to mutations. This condition is also called **growth hormone insensitivity**. Plasma IGF-1 level is markedly reduced which is also growth hormone dependant.

## EXPLAIN WHY SOMATOMEDIN LEVELS ARE BETTER CORRELATED WITH GROWTH THAN PLASMA GROWTH HORMONE LEVELS                              1 (2003)

The effect of growth hormone on growth, cartilage and protein metabolism depends on interaction between growth hormone and somatomedins which are polypeptide growth factors secreted by the liver and other tissues. Hence somaotomedin levels are better correlated with growth than plasma GH levels. The somatomedins are part of a large family of growth factors that affect many tissues and organs. These include IGF-I and IGF-II.

## THYROID GLAND

## ENUMERATE THE PRINCIPAL ACTIONS OF THYROID HORMONES

**DESCRIBE THE REGULATION OF THEIR SECRETION. HOW WOULD YOU TEST FOR THYROID FUNCTIONS**      10 (1993)
**THYROID FUNCTION TESTS**                    2.5 (2003)-IPU
**THYROID HORMONES**                          2.5 (2011)
### Actions of Thyroid Hormones

I. **Metabolic effects**

   a. Thyroid hormones stimulate metabolism of various body tissues except brain, testes, lymph nodes and spleen. They increase their oxygen consumption. This is known as calorigenic effect of thyroid hormones.

b. **Carbohydrate metabolism:** Increases absorption of glucose from intestines. This action is not related to metabolic effect of the hormone. If hormones are present in excess, it can lead to hyperglycemia.

c. **Lipid metabolism:** They decrease blood cholesterol level by increasing the number of LDL receptors. In general, it stimulates lipid metabolism at all stages, i.e. synthesis, mobilization and degradation of lipids.

d. **Protein metabolism:** Thyroid hormones promote protein synthesis required for growth in the body.

e. **Vitamin metabolism:** They are necessary for conversion of β-carotene to vitamin A.

II. **Effects on growth and maturation**

They are essential for physical, nervous and mental growth.

1. They potentiate the effects of growth hormones by:
   a. Stimulating protein synthesis
   b. Promoting bone growth.
2. Growth of nervous tissue: Essential for development and maturation of the brain and for development of central synapses and myelination of nerves.
3. Ossification of cartilage
4. Development of teeth
5. Development of facial contours
6. Development of normal body proportions.

III. **Effect on other tissues**

a. **CVS**–can increase β-adrenergic activity when in excess.

b. **Reproductive system:** Important for maintaining normal reproductive cycle in females and spermatogenesis in males.

c. In small amount it is essential for normal erythropoiesis.

d. Stimulate appetite and GIT motility.

## Regulation of Thyroid Hormones

Thyroid hormones are regulated by following mechanisms (Fig. 8.2):

   i. Anterior pituitary control
  ii. Hypothalamic control
 iii. Autoregulation

i. **Anterior pituitary control**—anterior pituitary exerts control on thyroid hormones through thyroid stimulating hormone (TSH). TSH stimulates synthesis and release of thyroid hormones. These hormones in turn control TSH by their negative feedback effect.

ii. **Hypothalamic control**—hypothalamus by secreting thyrotropin releasing hormone (TRH) controls the release of TSH from the anterior pituitary and regulates secretion of thyroid hormones. Thyroid hormones also exert a negative feedback effect on the release of TRH.

Cold and stress also affect the TRH release from the hypothalamus. In general day-to-day level is maintained through feedback to TSH and hypothalamus comes into action under special circumstances like stress.

iii. **Autoregulation**—thyroid gland itself maintains a constant level of hormones in spite of wide variation in iodine intake. If excess of iodine is taken in the diet, excess hormone is not formed. Under this condition iodine trapping is less efficient, organification is also less and more of iodine is excreted.

If iodine intake is less, efficiency of gland increases. More hormones are formed and less of iodine is excreted.

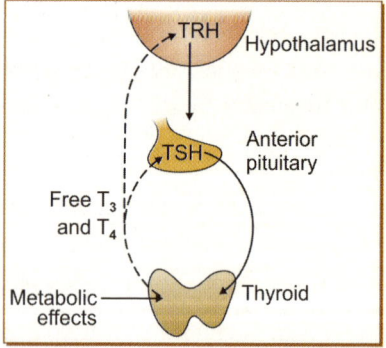

**Fig. 8.2:** Feedback control of thyroid secretion

## Mechanism of Autoregulation

Deficiency of iodine makes the gland more sensitive to TSH. If iodine is in excess, more of MIT is formed. MIT depresses iodine uptake by decreasing sensitivity of the gland to TSH.

## THYROID FUNCTION TESTS

I. Direct

II. Indirect

I. **Direct**

    a. Levels of $T_3$ and $T_4$ are determined by using radioimmunoassay.

    Levels are increased when the gland is hyperactive and decreases when the gland is hypofunctioning.

    *Normal values:*

    $T_4 = 80\ \mu gm/dL$

    $T_3 = 0.15\ \mu gm/dL$

    b. Radioactive iodine uptake by the gland: Uptake of radioactive iodine increases in hyperfunctioning of the gland and decreases in the hypoactive state.

II. **Indirect**

    a. **Protein bound iodine (PBI):** Level of PBI is directly related to the level of thyroid hormones. Normal level is 3.5–7.5 $\mu gm/dL$.

    PBI is increased if hormones increase in amount and decrease in the hypofunctioning of the gland.

    b. **Blood cholesterol:** Increases in a hypofunctioning gland and decreases in hyperfunctioning of the gland, as these hormones influence LDL receptors.

    c. **Basal metabolic rate:** Increases in hyperthyroidism and decreases in the hypofunctioning of the gland.

## COMPARE AND CONTRAST $T_3$ AND $T_4$ HORMONES    (2001)

| | $T_4$ | $T_3$ |
|---|---|---|
| 1. **Total plasma level** | More (3–8 $\mu gm/dL$) | 50 times less compared to $T_4$ (0.15 $\mu gm/dL$) |
| 2. **Secretion into plasma** | In large amount | In small amount |
| 3. **Distribution** | It is an extracellular hormone and acts as a prohormone | It penetrates tissue fluids and cells readily, therefore, it is an intracellular hormone |
| 4. **Protein binding** | 99.95% to 99.98%, mainly to TBG, | 99.98% mainly bound to TBG and albumin and |

*Contd.*

*Contd.*

| | $T_4$ | $T_3$ |
|---|---|---|
| | small amount to transthyretin and very little to albumin | very little to transthyretin |
| 5. **Free plasma level** | Less, therefore, more stable in the body | More, 4 times more free, therefore, comparatively less stable in the body |
| 6. **Duration of action** | Longer but onset of action on tissues is slow | Much shorter but more rapid onset of action on tissues. As free level is more and is more rapidly absorbed than $T_4$, therefore, it is more potent and active (approximately 3 to 5 times the biological activity of $T_4$) |

## GRAVES' DISEASE                                    5 (1986)

## EXPLAIN WHY THERE IS EXOPHTHALMOS IN GRAVES' DISEASE                                    1 (2005)

Grave's disease is a clinical condition arising due to hypersecretion of thyroxine and tri-iodothyronine. It is the commonest form of hyperthyroidism.

### Main Features of Graves' Disease

  i. Moderate diffuse enlargement of the thyroid gland

 ii. Signs of excessive thyroid secretion

iii. Exophthalmos

This condition is also known as **exophthalmic goitre** or **thyrotoxicosis**.

  i. Gland enlarges due to its marked stimulation

 ii. Signs of excessive hormone secretion are:

    a. Nervousness and irritability—due to increased responsiveness to catecholamines, stimulating the reticular activating system of the brain.

    b. Increase rate of metabolism and also raised resting metabolic rate.

    c.  Weight loss and hyperphagia—as a result of raised level of metabolism.

    d.  Heat intolerance—due to increased heat production.

    e.  Warm and moist skin—due to excessive sweating to promote heat loss.

    f.  Tachycardia and raised pulse pressure due to cardiac stimulation.

    g.  High sleeping pulse rate

    h.  Undue fatigability, muscle weakness and fine muscular tremors.

iii. Eye signs

Exophthalmos and lid retraction give the patient a staring look. It occurs due to the eyeball being pushed forward and happens due to the following reasons:

    1.  Increased muscle mass.

    2.  Increased fat content

    3.  Infiltration by lymphocytes

    4.  Increased water and mucopolysaccharide content in tissues behind the eyeball.

## Cause of Graves' Disease

It is an autoimmune condition. The condition occurs due to circulating antibodies against TSH receptors present in the thyroid gland. These antibodies are known as thyroid stimulating immunoglobulins (TSI). TSI mimics the actions of TSH and stimulates the gland causing hypersecretion of thyroid hormones. Consequently TSH levels are depressed. It is probably due to an autoimmune reaction, producing antibodies against muscle proteins. It is postulated that TSH receptor-stimulating antibodies (TSA) in the circulation cause release of cytokines that promote inflammation and oedema.

    The condition can be treated by antithyroid drugs like perchlorate and thiourea.

## EXPLAIN WHY NON-PITTING OEDEMA OCCURS IN HYPOTHYROIDISM    1 (2010)

Normally, skin contains a variety of proteins combined with mucopolysaccharides, hyaluronic acid and chondroitin sulphuric acid. In hypothyroidism because of decreased catabolism, these complexes deposit under the skin and subcutaneous tissues exerting an osmotic pressure causing retention of water and sodium chloride. Eventually this produces dry, coarse and puffy appearance of skin called 'myxoedema' which is a non-pitting oedema commonly seen around the eyes, hands and the supraocular fossa.

## EXPLAIN WHY IT IS NECESSARY TO EVALUATE THYROID STATUS IN NEWBORN     1 (2009)

$T_4$ is necessary for normal activity and development of the CNS. $T_4$ deficiency up to 2 years of age or in foetus causes the following features:

- Defective myelination in axons of cortical neurons
- Branching and development of dendrites decreases and synapses develop abnormally
- Marked reduction in the vascular bed of the brain.

All these changes result in an infantile brain. The most severely affected areas are the cerebral cortex, basal ganglia and cochlea. Critical period for this is up to 1 year of age. After one year even excessive administration of $T_4$ cannot restore the normal mental functions and irreversible mental retardation develops. Hence, it is essential to evaluate the thyroid status in a newborn.

## CALCIUM METABOLISM

### DEPOSITION AND REABSORPTION OF BONE     2 (2010)

The cells responsible for bone formation are the osteoblasts and the cells responsible for bone resorption are called osteoclasts. Osteoblasts are modified fibroblasts. Osteoclasts are members of the monocyte family.

Osteoclasts erode and absorb previously formed bone. They become attached to the bone via integrins in a membrane extension called the **'sealing zone'**. This creates an isolated area between the bone and a portion of the osteoclast. This sealed-off space formed by the osteoclasts resemble a large lysosome.

Throughout life, bone is constantly resorbed and new bone is formed. Bone remodelling is generally a local process carried out in a small areas by a population of cells called the bone-remodeling units. First osteclasts resorb the bone, and then osteoblasts lay down new bone in the same area. This cycle takes about 100 days.

In remodelling of cortical bone osteoclasts tunnel into the cortical bone followed by osteoblasts. In trabecular bone remodelling occurs on the surface of the trabeculae. The renewal rate for compact bone is 4% per year and is 20% per year for trabecular bone. The remodelling is related in part to the stresses and strains imposed on the skeleton by gravity.

Bone remodelling process is primarily controlled by hormones. Parathyroid hormone (PTH) accelerates bone resorption, whereas oestrogens slow-down resorption by inhibiting the production of bone eroding cytokines. A new finding is that intracerebroventricular but not intravenous leptin decreases bone formation.

## ROLE OF PARATHYROID GLAND IN REGULATING CALCIUM LEVEL IN THE BLOOD     2.5 (2004)

**Role of parathyroid hormone in regulating calcium level in the blood is as under:**

- PTH directly acts on the bone to increase bone resorption and mobilizes $Ca^{2+}$.
- In addition to increasing plasma levels of calcium, it increases phosphate excretion in the urine and depresses plasma phosphate levels (phosphaturic action).
- It increases reabsorption of calcium in the distal tubules in the kidney, but calcium excretion is increased in the urine in hyperparathyroidism because the increase in the load of filtered calcium overwhelms the effect on reabsorption.
- It increases the formation 1, 25-dihydroxycholecalciferol and this increases absorption of calcium from the intestine.
- On a long-term basis PTH stimulates the action of osteoblasts and osteoclasts.

## REGULATION OF SERUM CALCIUM     2 (2009)

|  | PTH | 1, 25-DHCC | Calcitonin |
| --- | --- | --- | --- |
| **On bone** | Increases bone resorption (osteolytic effect) | Mobilizes calcium and phosphate | Inhibits bone resorption |
| **On GIT** | Increases calcium and phosphate absorption | Increases calcium and phosphate absorption | Decreases calcium and phosphate absorption |

*Contd.*

*Contd.*

|  | **PTH** | **1, 25-DHCC** | **Calcitonin** |
|---|---|---|---|
| **On kidney** | Decreases phosphate absorption from PCT and increases excretion in DCT<br><br>Increases calcium reabsorption from DCT | Increases reabsorption of calcium from DCT and that of phosphate from PCT | Inhibits renal formation of 1, 25-DHCC<br>Increases excretion of calcium and phosphate |
| **Effect on serum calcium** | Increases | Increases | Decreases |

## CALCITONIN                     2.5 (1986, 1987, 1990)

Calcitonin is a calcium lowering hormone. It is produced mainly by the parafollicular or 'C cells' present in the thyroid gland, hence also known as thyrocalcitonin.

It is secreted whenever calcium level of blood rises above 9.5 mgm/dL and amount secreted is directly related to blood calcium level.

### Actions of Calcitonin

### On bones

1. It exerts its $Ca^{+2}$ lowering effects by inhibiting osteoclastic activity
2. It inhibits the $Ca^{+2}$ permeability of osteoclasts and osteoblasts
3. It decreases the number and activity of osteoclasts
4. Calcitonin activity is associated with an increase in alkaline phosphatases synthesis from the osteoblasts.

### On kidneys

1. Decreases renal formation of 1, 25-DHCC which in turn decreases serum $Ca^{2+}$ and $pO_4^{3-}$.

### On GIT

1. Increases intestinal secretion of water and electrolytes
2. Decreases gastric motility and acid secretion
3. Inhibits intestinal absorption of $Ca^{2+}$ and $pO_4^{3-}$.

## WHAT WILL HAPPEN AND WHY TO NEUROMUSCULAR EXCITABILITY IN PARATHYROID HORMONE DEFICIENCY 1 (2012)

## WHAT WILL HAPPEN AND WHY TO NEURONAL EXCITABILITY IN HYPOPARATHYROIDISM 1 (2006)

## EXPLAIN WHY HYPOCALCEMIA PRODUCES TETANY
1 (2005), 1 (2007)

There is an increase in neuromuscular excitability following hypocalcaemia produced due to parathyroid hormone deficiency leading to tetany. A decrease in the extracellular calcium concentration increases the excitability of nerve and muscle cells by decreasing the amount of depolarisation necessary to initiate changes in the $Na^+$ and $K^+$ conductance that produce the action potential. Conversely, an increase in the ECF calcium level can stabilize the membranes by decreasing their excitability.

## WHAT WILL HAPPEN AFTER PARATHYROIDECTOMY
2.5 (2003)-IPU

## WHAT WILL HAPPEN AND WHY IF PARATHYROID GLAND IS ACCIDENTALLY DAMAGED DURING THYROIDECTOMY
1 (2004)

Inadvertently parathyroidectomy occurs during the thyroid surgery in humans. This has serious consequences as PTH is considered essential for life. After parathyroidectomy plasma calcium level decreases leading to signs of hyperexcitability followed by full blown hypocalcemic tetany. Plasma phosphate level usually rises as the plasma calcium level falls. Symptoms usually develop 2–3 days postoperative but may appear after several weeks or more. The signs of tetany in humans include:

- **Chvostek's sign:** Quick contraction of ipsilateral facial muscles elicited by tapping over the facial nerve at the angle of the jaw.
- **Trousseau's sign:** Spasm of the muscles of the upper extremity that causes flexion of the wrist and thumb with extension of the fingers.
- **Neuromuscular hyperexcitability:** Numbness, tingling, stiffness with cramps in extremities due to extensive spasm of the skeletal muscles.
- **Laryngeal stridor** which is associated with airway obstruction producing asphyxia, convulsions and even death.

- **Visceral manifestations** include intestinal colic, bronchospasm and profuse sweating due to increased excitability of the autonomic ganglia.

- **ECG changes:** ST segment is prolonged with abnormal T wave.

- **Cataract** formation may occur due to excessive calcium accumulation in the lens.

- There are no clotting defects as the serum calcium level at which tetany occurs is above the level at which clotting defects would occur.

### Treatment

This centres around replacing the PTH. Injection of PTH can be given to correct the deficiency of the hormone along with injection of $Ca^{2+}$ salts to give temporary relief from the distressing symptoms.

**ADRENAL CORTEX**

## ENUMERATE GLUCOCORTICOID HORMONES. DISCUSS THEIR ROLE AS ANTI-INFLAMMATORY AND ANTI-STRESS HORMONE. ADD A NOTE ON CUSHING'S SYNDROME (2012)

**The glucocorticoid hormones include:** Cortisol or hydrocortisone and corticosterone.

### Anti-stress Action

Stress is defined as any change in the environment that changes or threatens to change an existing optimal steady state. Most type of the stress activate processes at the molecular, cellular or systemic levels that tend to restore the previous state, i.e. they are homeostatic reactions:

- Some but not all of the stresses stimulate ACTH secretion which is essential for survival.

- Most of the stressful stimuli that increase ACTH secretion also activate the sympathetic nervous system and part of the glucocorticoid (GC) function may be to maintain vascular reactivity to catecholamines.

- GC are also necessary for the catecholamines to mobilise free fatty acids which form an important emergency energy supply.

- Another theory holds that GC prevents other stress induced changes from becoming excessive.
- Stress causes release of GC to high pharmacological levels that in the short-run are life saving.
- Increase in ACTH which is beneficial on short-term basis becomes disruptive and harmful in the long run causing the **Cushing syndrome**.

## Anti-inflammatory Action

- GC inhibits the inflammatory response to tissue injury. They also suppress manifestations of allergic diseases that are due to the release of histamine from the tissues.
- Local injection of GC into an inflamed joint or near an irritated nerve produces a high local concentration of the steroid often without producing any side effects seen during systemic administration.
- GC decreases the circulating lymphocyte count and the size of the lymph nodes and thymus by inhibiting lymphocyte mitotic activity.
- They reduce secretion of cytokines by inhibiting the effect of NF-Kb on the nucleus. The reduced secretion of IL-2 leads to reduced proliferation of lymphocytes.
- GC inhibits inflammation by inhibiting phospholipase $A_2$. This reduces the release of arachidonic acid from tissue phospholipids and consequently reduce the formation of leukotrienes, thromboxanes, prostaglandins and prostacyclin.

## CUSHING SYNDROME                    2 (2002)

It is a clinical disorder which results from the exposure of the body tissues to sustained high blood levels of glucocorticoids. The causes are divided into two categories:

- **ACTH – independent**
  - Iatrogenic—prolonged treatment with high doses of GC
  - Adrenal cortex tumours
  - Adrenocortical cells with abnormally expressed receptors for ADH, GIP, IL-1 or GnRH
- **ACTH – dependent**
  - Ectopic ACTH production by non-pituitary tumours like cancers of the lungs

- Basophilic tumours of the pituitary
- CRH hypersecretion from tumours of non-endocrine tissue
- Iatrogenic—treatment with ACTH or its synthetic analogue.

## Characteristic Features
### Protein metabolism

1. Increase in protein catabolism that causes negative nitrogen balance and retarded growth.
2. Thinning of the skin and subcutaneous tissue
3. Muscles are wasted and poorly developed, called steroid myopathy. This along with hypokalemia produces marked muscular weakness.
4. Poor wound healing and minor injuries produce bruises and eccymoses.
5. Hair become thin and rough leading to loss of hair from the scalp.
6. Reduction in lymphoid tissue and dissolution of lymphocytes lead to increased uric acid secretion in the urine.

### Carbohydrate metabolism

GC excess produce hyperglycemia, glycosuria, increased resistance to insulin and increase in liver glycogen precipitating insulin resistant diabetes mellitus. This is associated with hyperlipidemia and ketosis.

### Fat metabolism

1. There is redistribution of body fat called 'centripetal distribution of fat'. The extremities are thin and there is deposition of fat in the abdominal wall leading to a 'pendular' abdomen.
2. The thin skin over the abdomen ruptures leading to the formation of purple striae.
3. Moon-like face is formed with narrow eye slits and fish-like mouth associated with $K^+$ depletion and weakness.
4. About 85% of the patients are hypertensive due to increased deoxycorticosterone secretion, increased angiotensinogen secretion or a direct glucocorticoid effect on blood vessels.
5. There is bone dissolution by decreasing bone formation and increased bone resorption. This leads to osteoporosis, a loss of bone mass that eventually leads to collapse of vertebral bodies and fractures.

6. CNS changes: GC in excess accelerate the basic EEG patterns and produce mental aberrations ranging from increased appetite, insomnia, euphoria to frank toxic psychosis.

7. Changes in blood: Eosinopenia, lymphopenia, basopenia, neutrophilia, polycythaemia, increase in platelet count and decrease in clotting time.

8. GIT: There is increased predisposition to peptic ulcers.

9. Increased susceptibility to infection.

10. Sexual changes:
    a. Increase in facial hair (hirsutism) and acne due to increased secretion of adrenal androgens.
    b. Impotency and hypogonadism in males and amenorrhoea in females.

## ENUMERATE HORMONES OF ADRENAL CORTEX AND DESCRIBE THE FUNCTIONS OF GLUCOCORTICOIDS  10 (1985)

### Hormones of Adrenal Cortex

Adrenal cortex is divided into 3 layers and each secrete a different type of hormone.

From outside inwards the 3 layers are:

1. Zona glomerulosa (outermost): Secretes mineralocorticoids, e.g. aldosterone and deoxycorticosterone.

2. Zona fasciculata (intermediate zone): Secretes glucocorticoids, e.g. cortisol, corticosterone.

3. Zona reticularis (innermost): Secretes sex steroids, e.g. dehydroepiandrosterone and androstenedione.

### FUNCTIONS OF GLUCOCORTICOIDS

i. **Antistress action**

   Glucocorticoids are secreted when a person is exposed to any kind of stress. They are found to be essential to cope up with stress. They are important for:
   i. Vascular reactivity of catecholamine
   ii. Mobilization of lipids as source of energy, during stress.

ii. **Action on intermediary metabolism**

   a. **Carbohydrate metabolism:** Increases blood glucose level and are physiologically important for maintaining blood glucose during starvation:

- By promoting gluconeogenesis
- Decreasing peripheral utilisation of glucose
- Anti-insulin action on peripheral tissues.

b. **Fat metabolism:** They are lipolytic and increase FFA levels causing ketosis.

c. **Protein metabolism:** Cause protein breakdown.

iii. **Permissive action**

  a. Play permissive role to catecholamines and glucagon in raising metabolic rate.

  b. Lipolytic action of catecholamines and glucagon.

  c. Pressor response of catecholamines.

  d. Bronchodilatation by catecholamines.

iv. **Maintenance of vascular reactivity**

Required for responsiveness of vascular smooth muscles to epinephrine and norepinephrine. In the absence of glucocorticoids, vessels do not constrict in response to these agents.

v. **Electrolyte and water balance**

Required for excretion of a water load so that excess water does not accumulate causing water intoxication. They influence the glomerular filtration rate.

vi. **Cellular elements of blood**

  a. They decrease eosinophils by causing their sequestration in spleen and lungs

  b. Decrease basophils

  c. Increase platelets, neutrophils and RBCs.

vii. **CNS effects**

  a. Have some influence on personality

  b. Maintain sensitivity to gustatory and olfactory stimuli.

viii. **Lung surfactant**: Essential for maturation of lung surfactant in foetus.

ix. In pharmacological doses, they have important anti-inflammatory and anti-allergic effects.

(*See* **previous questions for further details**)


## WHAT WILL HAPPEN AND WHY IF GLUCOCORTICOID THERAPY IS STOPPED ABRUPTLY
1 (2004)

When glucocorticoid therapy is stopped abruptly, not only is the adrenal atrophic and unresponsive after such treatment, but also even if its responsiveness is restored by injecting ACTH, the pituitary may be unable to secrete the normal amounts of ACTH for as long as a month. The cause is probably diminished synthesis of ACTH. Therefore, slowly ACTH increases to supranormal levels. This in turn stimulates the adrenal and glucocorticoid output which rises with feedback inhibition gradually reducing the elevated ACTH levels to normal. This complication of sudden cessation of steroid therapy can usually be avoided by slowly decreasing the steroid dose over a long period of time.

## EXPLAIN WHY GLUCOCORTICOIDS ARE GIVEN IN ORGAN TRANSPLANT                                          1 (2009)

Glucocorticoids are used in high doses in the treatment of inflammation and allergy. They prevent tissue damage, decrease local reaction, decrease fibroblastic activity and decrease the release of endogenous pyrogens. In late stages, they also decrease antibody formation by its destructive effect on fixed lymphoid tissues. Hence, glucocorticoids are used in the prevention or reduction of immune response of the recipient to an organ transplant.

## ADDISON'S DISEASE                                          2.5 (1993)

Addison's disease is a clinical condition arising due to insufficiency of adrenal corticoid hormones. Deficiency can occur due to an autoimmune process affecting the gland or due to a disease like tuberculosis. It is a chronic condition. Due to slow destruction of adrenal cortex, cortisol and aldosterone secretin is reduced.

Deficiency of hormones leads to decreased blood volume and hypotension. Patient often pulls along with life till some emergency arises which can precipitate a collapse called *Addisonian crisis.*

Clinical features are:

1. Muscle weakness

2. Hypotension

3. Mental confusion

4. Decreased ability to cope with stress

5. Hyperpigmentation due to raised ACTH levels.

## EXPLAIN WHY PIGMENTATION IS SEEN IN ADDISON'S DISEASE
1 (2006)

Primary adrenal insufficiency due to disease processes that destroy the adrenal cortex leads to Addison's disease. In this condition the circulating ACTH levels are elevated. The diffuse tanning of the skin and spotty pigmentation characteristic of chronic glucocorticoid deficiency are due to at least in part to melanocyte stimulating hormone (MSH) activity of ACTH when it is present in high levels in the blood. Pigmentation of skin creases of the hands and the gums is commonly seen.

## EXPLAIN WHY PATIENTS OF ADDISON'S DISEASE HAVE CRAVING FOR SALT
(2003)-IPU, 1 (2002)

Primary adrenal insufficiency due to disease processes that destroy the adrenal cortex is called Addison's disease. The normal function of aldosterone along with other mineralocorticoids is to increase the absorption of sodium from urine, sweat, saliva and the contents of the colon thus producing the retention of sodium in the ECF. Due to excess loss of salt in adrenal insufficiency this disease is accompanied by salt craving and severe hypotension and shock like condition which is called **Addisonian crisis.**

## DIFFERENTIATE BETWEEN PRIMARY AND SECONDARY HYPERALDOSTERONISM
2.5 (1987), 2 (2003)-IPU

**Primary hyperaldosteronism:** In this condition there is prolonged oversecretion of hormone aldosterone from adrenal cortex. The defect is in the gland itself usually a tumour of aldosterone producing cells of zona glomerulosa. It is characterised by:

1. Expansion of ECF volume due to increased $Na^+$ retention by the kidneys.
2. Hypertension due to raised ECF volume.
3. Hypokalemia due to excessive $K^+$ excretion.

**Secondary hyperaldosteronism:** Hypersecretion of aldosterone due to extra adrenal causes.

It is associated with clinical condition like congestive heart failure, nephrosis, cirrhosis of liver and toxaemia of pregnancy. In such patients level of renin and angiotensin II are raised in the circulation and is thought to be the reason for raised aldosterone secretion.

## ENUMERATE FUNCTIONS OF ALDOSTERONE
2.5 (1990), 2 (2004), 2.5 (2011)

**Aldosterone:** Aldosterone is the main mineralocorticoid secreted by the zona glomerulosa of adrenal cortex.

### Actions of aldosterone

1. It causes the retention of sodium in the body by acting on the DCT of the kidney.
2. Maintenance of ECF volume by retaining $Na^+$.
3. It promotes excretion of potassium ions and produces some diuresis.
4. It increases urinary acidity by causing secretion of $H^+$.
5. It also promotes sodium reabsorption from sweat, saliva and gastric juice to some extent.

## REGULATION OF ALDOSTERONE SECRETION        2.5 (2004)

The following factors are involved in the regulation of aldosterone secretion:

- **Renin-angiotensin system:** The secretion of aldosterone is influenced by changes in the circulating fluid volume which is sensed by the kidneys. The signals arising from the kidneys increase the aldosterone secretion when ECF volume is decreased and *vice versa*.

  Conditions that are associated with decreased ECF volume are:

  i. Sodium deprivation.

  ii. Haemorrhage.

  iii. Upright posture for several hours.

  iv. Acute diuresis.

- **Plasma potassium concentration:** There exists a potent negative feedback relationship between plasma potassium levels and aldosterone secretion.

- **Role of ACTH:** ACTH plays the following role in the secretion of aldosterone:

  - The direct stimulatory effect of ACTH is transient and mild
  - ACTH also stimulates the secretion of deoxycorticosterone from the zona fasciculata which has very mild mineralo-corticoid activity.

## ALDOSTERONE ESCAPE                    2 (2007)

A prominent feature of prolonged mineralocorticoid excess is potassium depletion due to prolonged $K^+$ diuresis. $H^+$ is also lost in the urine. $Na^+$ is retained initially but the plasma $Na^+$ is elevated only slightly because water is retained along with the sodium ions. When the ECF expansion rises beyond a certain point, sodium excretion is increased in spite of the continued action of mineralocorticoids on the renal tubules. This is called **aldosterone escape** and may be due to the release of ANP. Because of the increased excretion of sodium when the ECF volume is expanded, mineralocorticoids do not produce oedema in normal individuals and patients with hyperaldosteronism. However, this escape is not seen in certain diseases and in these situations continued expansion of ECF volume leads to oedema.

## EXPLAIN WHY OEDEMA IS NOT OBSERVED IN PROLONGED MINERALOCORTICOID EXCESS          1 (2009)

In patients with prolonged mineralocorticoid excess, the kidney escapes from its $Na^+$ retaining effects which is called **escape phenomenon**. Oversecretion of aldosterone produces hypernatremia with increase in extracellular fluid volume ( ECFV). When the ECFV expansion reaches a certain limit, sodium excretion is usually increased in spite of increased action of aldosterone on the DCT. This is probably due to the increased secretion of ANP. This phenomenon may not occur in patients with oedematous states like congestive heart failure, nephrosis, cirrhosis of the liver, etc. because of reduction in the amount of sodium reaching the DCT due to decreased renal blood flow.

## ADRENAL MEDULLA

## DIFFERENTIATING FEATURES OF EFFECTS OF EPINEPHRINE AND NOREPINEPHRINE          2.5 (1988)

| Effect | Epinephrine | Norepinephrine |
|---|---|---|
| Cardiac output | Increased | Decreased |
| Peripheral resistance | Decreased | Increased |
| Mean arterial pressure | May increase | Highly increase |
| Metabolic rate | Increased | Greater increase |

*Contd.*

*Contd.*

| Effect | Epinephrine | Norepinephrine |
|---|---|---|
| CNS stimulation | Present | Present |
| Blood glucose | Increase | Slight increase |
| FFA in blood | Increase | Greater increase |
| Bronchial dilatation | Marked | Slight |

## EXPLAIN WHY IV INFUSION OF NOREPINEPHRINE LEADS TO BRADYCARDIA RATHER THAN TACHYCARDIA  1 (2003)-IPU

When norepinephrine is infused slowly in humans or animals, the systolic and diastolic blood pressure rises. This hypertension stimulates the carotid and aortic baroreceptors producing reflex bradycardia that overrides the direct cardioacceleratory effect of norepinephrine.

## WHAT WILL HAPPEN AND WHY TO HEART RATE IF NOREPINEPHRINE IS INFUSED *IN VIVO*  (2001)

Norepinephrine by its direct action on the heart increases the heart rate via the $\beta_1$ receptors. But this increase in heart rate is overcome by the reflex stimulation of the aortic and carotid baroreceptors that ultimately leads to bradycardia.

## PANCREAS

## ENUMERATE THE HORMONES REGULATING BLOOD GLUCOSE LEVEL AND DESCRIBE THEIR ROLE IN ITS REGULATION
### 10 (1987)

### Hormones Regulating Blood Glucose Level

Normal blood glucose level varies between 60 and 90 mgm/dL. Following hormones interact to maintain this level:

1. Insulin
2. Glucagon
3. Glucocorticoids
4. Epinephrine
5. Growth hormone
6. Thyroid hormone
7. Somatostatin

1. **Insulin:** Insulin along with glucagon is the main hormone regulating the blood glucose level. It lowers the glucose level when it rises above normal.

**Actions of insulin:** It acts on almost all the body tissues except brain, kidney tubules and RBCs and promotes the entry of glucose in them. Its main actions are on the muscle, liver and fatty tissue. It lowers the blood sugar by the following mechanism:

i. Promoting entry of glucose in tissues and hence stimulates its peripheral utilization.

ii. Promotes glycogen synthesis in liver and muscle tissue.

iii. Inhibits gluconeogenesis in the liver.

iv. Decreases the release of amino acids for gluconeogenesis from muscle.

v. Decreases glucose output by the liver.

2. **Glucagon:** Its action is opposite to that of insulin. It increases blood glucose, whenever, hypoglycemia occurs. Hypoglycemia is a potent stimulus to release glucagon.

**Actions**

i. It promotes glycogenolysis in the liver and thus increases glucose output from the liver.

ii. It promotes gluconeogenesis in the liver from amino acids by stimulating various enzymes.

3. **Glucocorticoids:** They also have a hyperglycemic action and help to maintain blood glucose level, especially during fasting.

**Actions**

i. Glucocorticoids stimulate gluconeogenesis in the liver like glucagon. It mainly plays a permissive role to the action of glucagon.

ii. Decrease peripheral utilization of glucose by inhibiting glucose phosphorylation.

iii. Decrease affinity of insulin receptors.

4. **Epinephrine:** Epinephrine secretion is stimulated during hypoglycaemia. It is a glucose raising hormone.

**Actions of epinephrine**

It activates phosphorylase in the liver and promotes glycogen breakdown. As a result glucose output by the liver is increased and blood glucose level increases.

5. **Growth hormone:** It is a hyperglycemic hormone and has anti-insulin actions like:

i. Increases hepatic glucose output.

ii. Decreases peripheral utilisation of glucose by inhibiting glucose phosphorylation and inhibits futher entry of glucose.

iii. It may decrease the number of insulin receptors on cells.

6. **Thyroid hormones:** These hormones increase blood glucose by promoting its absorption in the intestine.

7. **Somatostatin:** Secreted in pancreas from islets of Langerhans which also secrete insulin and glucagon. It functions in a paracrine manner and inhibits the secretions of insulin and glucagon.

## ENUMERATE THE HORMONES SECRETED BY THE PANCREAS. DISCUSS THE FUNCTION OF ANY ONE OF THEM  10 (1988)

Islets of Langerhans of the pancreas have 4 types of cells secreting the following hormones:

1. α cells: Glucagon
2. β cells: Insulin
3. δ cells: Somatostatin
4. F cells: Pancreatic polypeptide

### Functions of Insulin

It is one of the major hormones regulating blood glucose level, maintaining it between 60 and 90 mgm/dL of blood. Besides blood glucose level, it plays an important role in the metabolism of fats and proteins also. For its action it combines with specialized insulin receptors present in the cell membrane of body tissues. Basically it is an anabolic hormone and causes the storage of carbohydrates, fats and proteins in the body.

I. **Action on carbohydrate metabolism**

1. Insulin facilitates entry of glucose in most body tissues except brain, kidney tubules and RBCs.

2. It produces major effects on muscle, liver and adipose tissue.

3. Main action is to lower blood glucose level, whenever it increases above normal, e.g. after intake of carbohydrate by the following actions:

   i. Facilitating entry of glucose in tissues and promoting peripheral utilisation of glucose.

   ii. Promotes glycogen synthesis from glucose in muscle and liver and hence stores carbohydrates by stimulating appropriate enzymes.

iii. Inhibits gluconeogenesis from amino acids in liver by inhibiting various enzymes needed for the purpose.

By actions (ii) and (iii), it decreases glucose output from the liver.

iv. Decreases release of glucogenic amino acids from muscle tissue and hence inhibits gluconeogenesis in the liver.

## II. Action on fat metabolism

1. Promotes fat deposition in adipose tissue by:
   a. Increased fatty acid synthesis
   b. Increased glycerol formation
   c. Promotes formation and deposition of triglycerides.
2. Prevents breakdown of neutral fats by inhibiting hormone sensitive lipase.
3. Increases uptake of ketone bodies by muscle.
4. Promotes lipid synthesis in liver.

## III. Action on protein metabolism

1. Promotes amino acid entry in muscle cells.
2. Increases protein synthesis in ribosomes.
3. Decreases protein breakdown in muscle.
4. Stimulates protein synthesis in the liver.

## IV. Effect on blood electrolytes

Insulin promotes the entry of potassium into cells thus lowers the plasma potassium levels.

At the same time insulin is known to increase the activity of $Na^+ - K^+$ pump in cell membrane, leading to hyper-polarisation. This probably increases negativity inside the cell which increases $K^+$ entry.

## DESCRIBE THE REGULATION OF SECRETION OF INSULIN

## ENUMERATE ITS MAJOR ACTIONS                    10 (1993)

## REGULATION OF SECRETION OF INSULIN           2 (2003)-IPU

Insulin secretion is regulated by following factors:

1. Substrate concentration
2. Hormonal control
3. Neural control

1. **Substrate concentration:** Glucose and amino acids in blood are the two substrates causing secretion of insulin. This is the major mechanism by which secretion of insulin is regulated. A rise in glucose level stimulates insulin secretion. It is believed that glucose molecules directly acts on β cells of islets of pancreas. Glucose molecules enter the β cells and its metabolites act in two ways.

   a. stimulate the release of insulin
   b. promote further synthesis of insulin.

   **Amino acids**

   Amino acids also stimulate β cells. A mixture of essential amino acids, particularly arginine and lysine, causes the release of insulin.

   A mixture of glucose and amino acids which are end-products of carbohydrate and protein digestion is a powerful stimulant for insulin release.

2. **Hormonal regulation**

   a. **Role of gastrointestinal hormones:** Hormones like gastrin, CCK-PZ, secretin and gastric inhibitory peptide stimulate insulin secretion. Except for GIP which is believed to have a physiologic role of the function of other hormones is not yet clear. It is known as physiologic GUT factor.

   b. **Pancreatic hormones:** Other pancreatic hormones like glucagon and somatostatin which are also secreted by islet cells, control the insulin secretion, by acting locally in a paracrine manner. Electron microscopy has revealed the presence of gap junctions between different types of islet cells.

   Glucagon stimulates insulin secretion and somatostatin inhibits it.

   c. **Other hormones:** Hormones which increase blood glucose level, e.g. cortisol and growth hormone, stimulate insulin secretion due to the hyperglycemia they produce. However, this is not an important regulatory mechanism.

3. **Neural regulation:** β cells are innervated by both vagal and sympathetic nerves.

Parasympathetic stimulation increases insulin secretion when blood glucose level is high.

## Sympathetic stimulation

Stimulation of β-adrenergic receptors stimulates insulin secretion, whereas stimulation of α-receptors causes inhibition.

## Actions of insulin

Insulin has actions on carbohydrate, fats and protein metabolism. Its main actions are on muscle, liver and adipose tissue. It is basically an anabolic hormone and promotes storage of carbohydrates, proteins and fats.

## Main actions (as discussed in previous question)

1. Reduces blood glucose by:
   a. Promoting peripheral utilization of glucose by tissues.
   b. Promotes glycogen synthesis in muscle and liver, by stimulating appropriate enzymes.
   c. Inhibits gluconeogenesis in liver by inhibiting various enzymes.
2. Promotes entry of amino acids and also protein synthesis in tissues.
3. Promotes fat deposition as neutral fats in adipose tissues.
4. Prevents lipolysis by inhibiting hormone sensitive lipase.

## INSULIN                                           2.5 (1991)

Insulin is a polypeptide hormone secreted by the β cells, present in islets of Langerhans of the pancreas. It is the principal hormone maintaining the blood glucose level at a normal value 60–90 mgm/dL.

It has action on various body tissues like muscle, liver and fat cells and promotes storage of carbohydrates, proteins and fats in the body. Hence it is an anabolic hormone.

**(Refer to previous questions for the main actions of insulin)**

## Actions of insulin

Amount of insulin secreted is directly related to the blood glucose level. Insulin combines with special insulin receptors present in the membrane of various body cells to produce its actions.

## ACTION OF GLUCAGON                2.5 (1991)

**Glucagon:** Glucagon is a polypeptide hormone secreted from α cells present in islets of Langerhans in pancreas. It is a hyperglycemic agent and plays an important role in regulation of blood glucose. It is secreted during hypoglycemia and raises blood glucose by acting on liver cells.

I. In the liver it causes:
   a. Glycogenolysis and increases glucose output by the liver.
   b. Promotes gluconeogenesis from amino acids.
   c. Increases ketone bodies formation in the liver.
II. It increases metabolic rate and hence calorigenic.
III. In large amount it increases myocardial contractility.
IV. Stimulates secretion of growth hormone, insulin and somatostatin.

Glucagon is glycogenolytic, gluconeogenic, lipolytic and ketogenic.

## DIFFERENTIATING FEATURES BETWEEN POLYURIA OF DIABETES MELLITUS AND DIABETES INSIPIDUS        2.5 (1986, 1988)
## COMPARE DIABETES MELLITUS AND DIABETES INSIPIDUS
                                                        2.5 (2006)

Polyuria of diabetes mellitus occurs due to the presence of excess glucose in the lumen of kidney tubules which cannot be reabsorbed, and is hence excreted. As the glucose is excreted through the kidney, large amount of water follows it producing osmotic diuresis and polyuria.

In diabetes insipidus reabsorption of water is defective in collecting ducts. Normally, water is reabsorbed in collecting ducts under the influence of ADH from the posterior pituitary. In diabetes insipidus, ADH secretion is absent or inadequate and large amount of water is excreted in the urine causing polyuria, but there is no glucose in the urine. Insipidus means tasteless in contrast to large amount of glucose in the urine of diabetes mellitus.

## CAUSE OF POLYURIA AND POLYPHAGIA IN DIABETES MELLITUS                2.5 (1989)

Hyperglycaemia, i.e. increase in blood glucose is the reason of ployuria and polyphagia. Hyperglycaemia causes hyperosmolarity of the blood. Large amount of glucose is filtered by the kidneys.

As the filtered amount exceeds the reabsorptive capacity, i.e. the transport maximum for glucose (TmG), large amount is excreted in the urine taking excess of water along with it called **osmotic diuresis** and polyuria occurs. As glucose is excreted, energy loss equivalent to 4.1 kcal per gram of glucose occurs from the body. This causes increased appetite and hunger causing polyphagia, i.e. excessive eating by the patient. Low glucose utilisation by glucostat cells of the ventromedial nucleus in the hypothalamus (satiety centre) results in no inhibition of lateral nucleus of the hypothalamus (feeding centre) which eventually produces increased hunger (polyphagia). Food intake causes hyperglycaemia leading to polyuria and a vicious cycle is set up.

## GLUCOSE TOLERANCE TEST IN DIABETIC AND NORMAL MAN                           2.5 (1991)

Glucose tolerance test is the response of the blood glucose to an oral test dose of glucose. Fasting blood glucose is measured and 75 gm of glucose in 300 ml of water ingested by the patient. Thereafter, plasma glucose level is determined every half an hour till two hours. A curve is plotted between the time and plasma glucose level (Fig. 8.3).

**Normal GTT:** When fasting venous plasma glucose level is < 115 mg/dL and after 2 hours of glucose administration value < 140 mgm/dL and no value is > 200 mgm/dL.

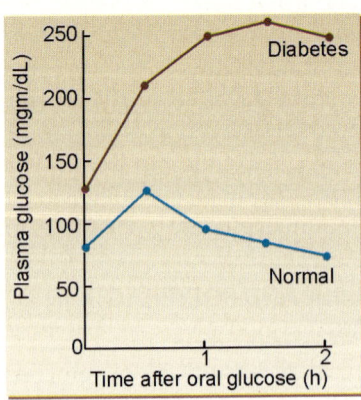

**Fig. 8.3:** Glucose tolerance test

**Diabetic GTT:** When fasting venous plasma glucose level is >115 mgm/dL and if the 2 hour postprandial (PP) value and one other PP value is > 200 mgm/dL.

**Impaired GTT:** When the fasting and PP values are above the upper limits of normal but below the values diagnostic of diabetic GTT.

## PATHOPHYSIOLOGY OF DIABETES MELLITUS     2 (2010)

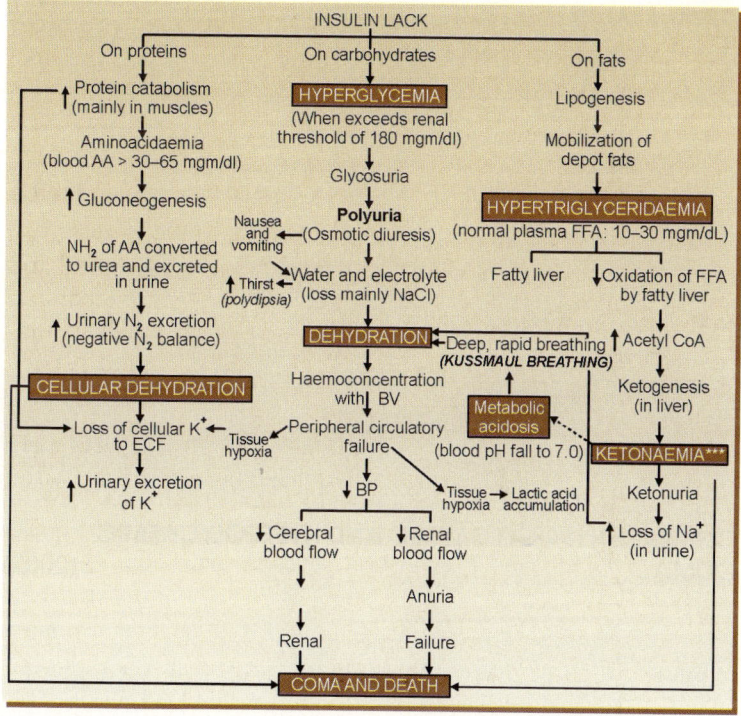

## COMPARE JUVENILE AND MATURITY ONSET DIABETES    2 (2005)

| Juvenile onset diabetes | Maturity onset diabetes |
|---|---|
| • It usually occurs before 14 years of age, patients are usually underweight | • This is the most common type of diabetes that usually occurs in patients over 40 years of age. Patients are normal or overweight |

*Contd.*

*Contd.*

| Juvenile onset diabetes | Maturity onset diabetes |
|---|---|
| • Family history is usually uncommon, however, a genetic factor may predispose to the development of antibodies against β cells of the pancreas | • Family history of diabetes is strongly positive |
| • Patient develops ketosis if left untreated | • Ketosis with infection is usually absent |
| • Patients are sensitive to insulin | • Initially insulin secretion is normal or increased but later it decreases. β cells are usually normal but main disturbance is (a) less active insulin production, (b) less cellular response to insulin due to deficiency of GLUT 4 in insulin sensitive cells, (c) presence of antibodies against insulin |
| • Insulin is the treatment of choice, hence it is also called **IDDM** (Insulin dependent diabetes mellitus) | • Insulin is needed only during infections, therefore, it is also called **NIDDM** (non-insulin dependent diabetes mellitus). Patient is usually treated using oral hypoglycemic agents |

## COMPARE HYPOGLYCAEMIC AND HYPERGLYCAEMIC COMA
**2 (2002)**

| | Hypoglycaemic coma | Hyperglycaemic coma |
|---|---|---|
| • **Cause** | It is usually due to fall in the blood glucose level < 40 mgm/dL and is generally considered to be a more serious medical emergency | It is usually due to increase in the blood glucose level more than 400 mgm/dL |
| • **Rate of onset** | Rapid, it develops within minutes | Invariably slow, it takes hours to days to develop |

*Contd.*

*Contd.*

|  | Hypoglycaemic coma | Hyperglycaemic coma |
|---|---|---|
| • Precipitating factors | Overdosage of insulin, missing meals and severe exercise | Insulin under dosage, infection and trauma |
| • Signs and symptoms |  |  |
| – Breathing | Laboured breathing | Deep and rapid (air hunger), also called Kussmaul breathing |
| – Sweating | Usually marked | Absent |
| – Hydration | Normal fairly hydrated | Marked dehydration |
| – CNS symptoms | Various, often bilateral extensor plantar response | Diminished reflexes |
| – Urine examination | No specific characteristic features seen | Marked glycosuria and ketonuria |

## WHY IS ESTIMATION OF GLYCOSYLATED Hb IS RECOMMENDED IN DIABETES                         1 (2004)

Glycosylated Hb has a glucose attached to the terminal valine in each β chain and is of special interest because its quantity in blood increases in poorly controlled diabetes mellitus. When plasma glucose level is episodically elevated over time, small amount of haemoglobin A are non-enzymatically glycated to form $HbA_{1C}$. Careful control of diabetes with insulin reduces the amount formed. Hence Hb $A_{1C}$ concentration is measured clinically as an integrated index of diabetic control for the 4 to 6 weeks period before its measurement.

## EXPLAIN WHY POLYPHAGIA IS COMMONLY ASSOCIATED WITH DIABETES MELLITUS ALTHOUGH BLOOD GLUCOSE IS HIGH                         1 (2004)

Low glucose utilization by the glucostat cells of the ventromedial nucleus of the hypothalamus (the satiety centre) in the deficiency or absence of insulin results in the lateral nucleus of the hypothalamus (feeding centre) being uninhibited which eventually leads to increased hunger called polyphagia in diabetic patients.

## EXPLAIN WHY INCREASED URINARY OUTPUT IS FOUND IN DIABETES INSIPIDUS
1 (2006)

Diabetes insipidus is produced either due to vasopressin deficiency **(central diabetes insipidus)** or when the kidneys fail to respond to the hormone **(nephrogenic diabetes insipidus)**.Vasopressin is also called anti-diuretic hormone **(ADH)** since it increases water reabsorption in the collecting ducts by increasing the permeability of their epithelium to water. As a result water enters the hypertonic interstitium of the renal pyramids hence the urinary concentration increases and its volume decreases. So if this hormone is deficient, water is not reabsorbed in the collecting ducts and a large volume of dilute urine is passed by the patient.

## EXPLAIN WHY HIGH BLOOD SUGAR CAUSES PERIPHERAL NEUROPATHY
1 (2003)-IPU

Long standing high blood glucose level is accompanied by micro-angiopathy, a vascular lesion in which the capillary basement membrane is thicker than normal. This hyperglycemia is ultimately responsible for neuropathy, i.e degeneration of sensory and motor nerves in the lower part of the body along with **retinopathy** (scarring of the retina) and **nephropathy** (renal diseases leading to renal failure).

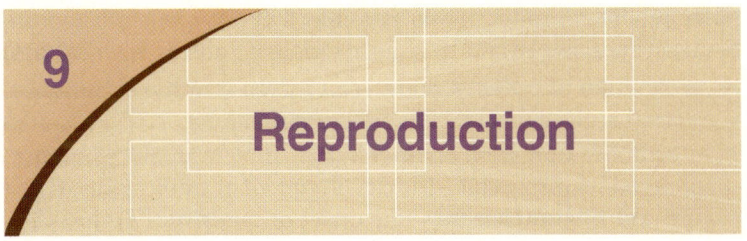

# Reproduction

# 9

## PHYSIOLOGY OF REPRODUCTION

**PSEUDOHERMAPHRODITE**        **2 (2004)**

**COMPARE TRUE AND PSEUDOHERMAPHRODITE**      **2 (2007)**

**Pseudohermaphrodites** are individuals in whom normal gonadal development occurs according with their chromosomal sex but later development of heterosexual characteristics takes place. They are divided into the following two categories:

- **Female pseudohermaphrodite:** An individual with female internal genitalia and masculine external genitalia. The chromosomal sex is female. It occurs due to congenital virilising adrenal hyperplasia.

- **Male pseudohermaphrodite:** An individual having male chromosomal sex with defective testes and has female internal and/or external genitalia. It may be due to the following causes:
  - Defective embryonic testes leading to deficiency of MRF
  - Androgen resistance: Male hormone cannot exert their full effects due to mutation in the androgen receptor gene or loss of receptor function. This results in androgen resistance syndrome.
  - Deficiency of adrenal androgen due to congenital deficiency of 17α-hydroxylase
  - Congenital deficiency of 5α-reductase that converts testosterone to DHT in the target organs.

## CHANGES DURING PUBERTY        **2 (2005)**

Puberty is defined as the period when the endocrine and gametogenic functions of the gonads have first developed to the point where reproduction is possible. Puberty generally occurs between the ages of 8 and 13 years in girls and 9 and 14 years in boys.

- At the time of puberty there is an increase in the secretion of adrenal androgens which is called **adrenarche**.
- In girls the first event is **thelarche**—development of breasts followed by **pubarche**—the development of pubic and axillary hair and then **menarche**—the onset of menstrual period. The initial menstrual cycles are generally anovulatory, with regular ovulation occurring about a year later.

| Stage of puberty | In boys | In girls |
|---|---|---|
| **1.** *Stage 1* (up to 7.5 years) | Preadolescent stage or stage of childhood. | Preadolescent stage. |
| **2.** *Stage 2* (12 years boys and 10.5 years girls) | Genital development begins by enlargement of the testes | Appearance of 'breast bud' (*thelarche*) **Note:** Regular ovulation (page 82) usually appears about a year later |
| **3.** *Stage 3* (14 years boys and 11.5 years girls) | Pubic and axillary hair begins, penis enlarges. | Pubic and axillary hair begin (*pubarche*), elevation and enlargement of the breasts, gain in height (*height spurt*) |
| **4.** *Stage 4* (15.5 years boys and 13 years girls) | Further growth of external and internal genitalia occurs with peak gain in height (*height spurt*) | Projection of areolas, appearance of the menses (*menarche*) |
| **5.** *Stage 5* (16.5 years boys and 14 years girls) | Adult genitalia with secondary sexual characteristics which include: | Adult genitalia with secondary sexual characteristics which include: |
| i. Body configuration | Broad shoulders, more muscular body | Narrow shoulders, broad hips, thighs that converge and arms that diverge (*wide carrying angle*), female distribution of |

*Contd.*

*Contd.*

| Stage of puberty | In boys | In girls |
|---|---|---|
| | | fat in the breast and hips giving the characteristic curves to the body |
| ii. Hair growth | Hair appears all over body, in axilla, over the pubis, face and chest; hairline on scalp recedes anterolaterally; male pattern of pubic hair (triangle with apex up) | Appearance of hair in the axilla and pubis; less body hair and more scalp hair; hair in pubic region concave upwards (female *flat-topped* pattern of distribution of hair caused by local conversion of weak androgens from the ovary and adrenal cortex to testosterone |
| iii. Voice | Larynx enlarges, vocal cords increase in length and thickness, therefore, voice becomes deep and breaks | Larynx does not enlarge to that extent as in males, therefore, voice becomes high pitch |
| iv. External genitalia | Penis increases in length and width, scrotal skin thickens, becomes pigmented and rugose. | Clitoris increases in length and width, labia majora and minora enlarge |
| v. Internal genitalia | Seminal vesicles, prostate and bulbourethral glands enlarge and secrete | Ovaries, uterus and vaginal growth increases and their activity increases |
| vi. Skin changes due to | Acne (pimples) appears increased secretion from sebaceous glands by the action of androgens | Acne and formation of comedones (*black heads*) is less as oestrogen antagonizes the action of androgen on sebaceous glands |
| vii. Psychological changes | Aggressive active attitude, interest in opposite sex develops. | Changes in mental and emotional behaviour; shyness; interest in opposite sex develops |

## MALE REPRODUCTIVE SYSTEM

### EXPLAIN WHAT WILL HAPPEN AND WHY IF FOETAL TESTES ARE REMOVED IN THE EIGHTH WEEK OF INTRAUTERINE LIFE
1 (2003), 1 (2004)

The development of male phenotype and genitalia occurs only in the presence of a functional testes. Thus removal of the testes at an early stage like 8th week of intrauterine life (castration) prevents the formation of male genitalia and results in completely female genitalia.

### EXPLAIN WHY TESTES ARE LOCATED IN THE SCROTUM OUTSIDE THE ABDOMINAL CAVITY
1 (2003)-IPU

Spermatogenesis requires a temperature considerably lower than the interior of the body. The testes are normally maintained at a temperature of 32°C in the scrotum. They are kept cool by the air circulating around the scrotum and probably by heat exchange in a countercurrent fashion between the spermatic arteries and veins.

### WHAT WILL HAPPEN AND WHY IF FAILURE OF TESTICULAR DESCENT OCCURS IN THE SCROTUM
1 (2011), 1 (2002)

### WHAT WILL HAPPEN AND WHY IF TESTES REMAIN INTRA-ABDOMINAL DURING PUBERTY
1 (2006)

The testes develop in the abdominal cavity and normally migrate to the scrotum during foetal development under the influence of MRF. Incomplete descent of the testes on one or both sides in newborn is called **cryptorchidism**. In this condition seminiferous tubules remain infantile due to higher temperature to which the gland is exposed in the abdomen compared to the scrotum, therefore, spermatogenesis fails to occur resulting in sterility. Since the Leydig cells are normal and continue to secrete testosterone, therefore, normal male secondary sexual characters develop.

### WHAT WILL HAPPEN AND WHY IF BLOOD-TESTES BARRIER WILL FAIL TO DEVELOP
2 (2002)

Blood-testes barrier helps to maintain the composition of fluid in the lumen of the seminiferous tubule which is quite different from that of the plasma containing very little protein and glucose but is rich in androgens, oestrogens, $K^+$, inositol, glutamic and aspartic acid.

The blood testes barrier protects the germ cells from blood-borne noxious agents. It prevents antigenic products of cell division and maturation from entering the circulation and generating an autoimmune response against the germ cells and thus protects them.

It may also help in establishing an osmotic gradient that facilitates movement of fluid into the tubular lumen.

## COMPARE AND CONTRAST SPERMATOGENESIS AND SPERMIOGENESIS     2 (2003)

The process of formation of sperms (spermatozoa) is called **spermatogenesis**.

**Spermiogenesis** is a part of spermatogenesis and is the process of conversion of spermatids to sperms (spermatozoa). This takes place within the cytoplasm of the Sertoli cells and depends on the presence of androgens locally.

## LEYDIG CELLS     3 (1986)

Leydig cells are present in the testes between the seminiferous tubules as nests of cells, containing lipid granules. They are responsible for secreting male sex hormone testosterone and are present in close proximity of blood vessels. These are internally secreting cells which are functional in foetal testes also.

### Functions of Leydig Cells

i. In the foetus testosterone is secreted by the Leydig cells which is essential for the development of internal reproductive organs, i.e. epididymis and vas deferens and also male external genitalia.

ii. After puberty, testosterone secreted by them is essential for the process of spermatogenesis by helping to maintain a high constant levels of testosterone locally, essential for normal spermatogenesis.

iii. It is also required for development and maintenance of secondary sexual characters in males.

## DESCRIBE BRIEFLY THE SECRETION OF TESTOSTERONE     5 (1992)

Testosterone is the male sex hormone produced by the testes. It is secreted by the specialised Leydig cells present in the interstitial tissue, present outside the seminiferous tubules of testis. It is synthesized from cholesterol and poured into the circulation via the small vessels present in close proximity of these cells.

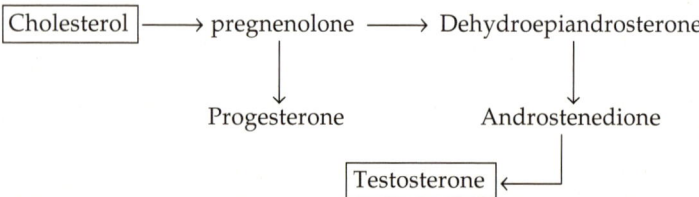

Testosterone secretion is under the control of luteinizing hormone (LH) secreted from the anterior pituitary. It acts on specific receptors present on Leydig cells, causing the formation of cAMP.

cAMP has the following functions:

1. It stimulates the formation of cholesterol from cholesteryl esters.
2. Conversion of cholesterol to pregnenolone via activation of protein kinase.

## REGULATION OF TESTICULAR FUNCTIONS        2 (2011)

Testes perform the following functions:

i. Spermatogenesis, i.e. formation of mature sperms capable of fertilising the ovum.

ii. Secretion of hormone testosterone

These functions are controlled by pituitary gonadotropins, i.e. FSH and LH.

**LH:** Regulates the secretion of testosterone from Leydig cells.

**FSH:** Regulates spermatogenesis along with testosterone. It is also trophic to Sertoli cells present in the seminiferous tubules which in turn secrete androgen binding protein (ABP).

**ABP:** Binds testosterone and maintains a high local level of it, essential for spermatogenesis.

Testes migrate outside the abdomen to the scrotum in foetal life. In the scrotum temperature is lower which is essential for normal spermatogenesis. If they do not descend due to some reason, it leads to testicular damage due to high abdominal temperature. The process of spermatogenesis is defective that can lead to male infertility.

## SPERMATOGENESIS                           5 (1987)

Spermatogenesis is the process of formation of new spermatozoa in seminiferous tubules of testis.

Sperms develop in the tubules of germinal epithelium lining seminiferous tubules, through successive stages and pass into the lumen of the tubules. Spermatozoa develop from primitive germ cells called spermatogonia which are located immediately adjacent to the basement membrane.

In between the developing sperms lie tall cells which extend from basement membrane to the lumen of the tubule called the supporting cells or **Sertoli cells**.

Process of spermatogenesis starts at puberty under the influence of pituitary gonadotropins and it continues throughout life.

## STAGES OF SPERMATOGENESIS

1. Primitive spermatogonia divide and form slightly more differentiated spermatogonia-B.
2. Spermatogonia-B undergo several more mitotic divisions giving rise to a large number of primary spermatocytes which are sperm precursors and have 23 pairs of chromosomes.
3. Primary spermatocytes undergo a reduction division and each give rise to 4 secondary spermatocytes containing 23 chromosomes. Secondary spermatocytes form spermatids.
4. Conversion of spermatids to spermatozoa: This transformation is also called **spermiogenesis**. In sperm the epitheloid character of the spermatids is lost and it elongates acquiring a head and a tail. Spermiogenesis occurs in close association with Sertoli cells (Fig. 9.1). Entire process of spermatogenesis is completed in 74 days.

## SERTOLI CELLS                    2 (2004), 2.5 (2004)-IPU

### Role of Sertoli Cells in Spermatogenesis

1. Contain glycogen and provide nourishment to growing sperms.
2. Converts spermatids to spermatozoa, probably by secreting certain digestive enzymes.
3. Secrete androgen binding protein and help to maintain a local high level of testosterone by binding it and releasing it slowly.
4. Secrete inhibin responsible for feedback control of FSH.

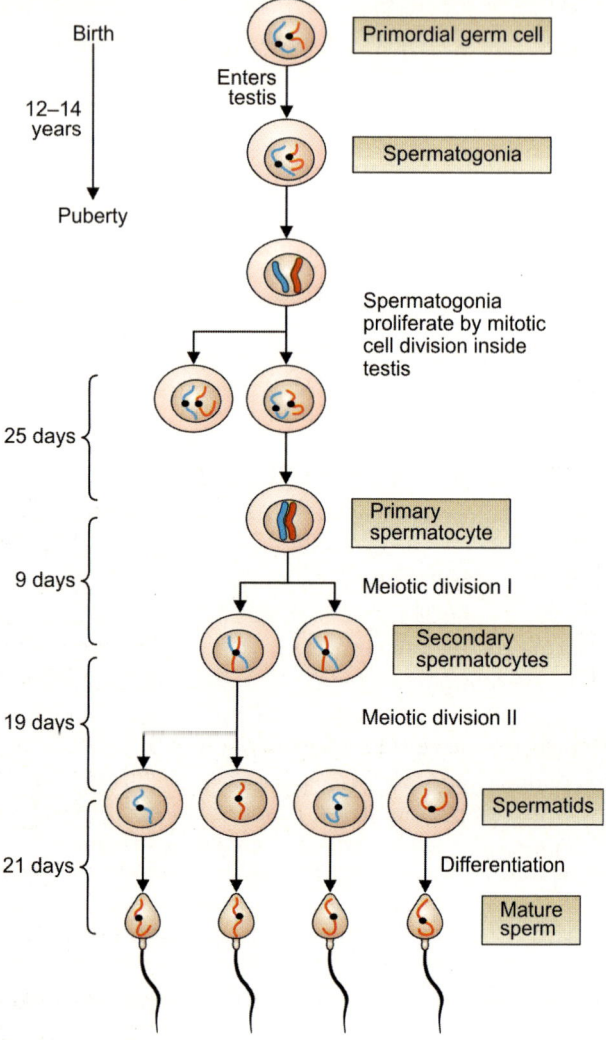

**Fig. 9.1:** Stages of spermatogenesis

5. Secrete MRF in foetal testes and control the development of male internal reproductive organs.
6. Provide blood-testis barrier and protect developing sperms against blood toxins.

## REGULATION OF SPERMATOGENESIS        2.5 (1988, 2001)

Factors controlling spermatogenesis:

1. Hormonal control
2. Temperature control

*Hormonal control:* A number of hormones control spermatogenesis:

   a. Testosterone: Secreted by Leydig cells under influence of LH from anterior pituitary, a high local level of testosterone is essential around developing sperms.
   b. LH: Stimulates testosterone formation by Leydig cells.
   c. FSH: Stimulates Sertoli cells and helps in conversion of spermatids to spermatozoa.
   d. Growth hormone: Promotes general metabolic growth. It specifically promotes early division of spermatogonia.

*Temperature control:* Spermatogenesis occurs at a temperature of about 32°C, i.e. lower than core body temperature. This is achieved by the descent of testis to scrotum which has lower temperature. Testes are kept cool in the scrotum by:

   a. Air circulating around scrotum
   b. Heat exchange by countercurrent mechanism between spermatic arteries and veins.

## FEMALE REPRODUCTIVE SYSTEM

### DESCRIBE THE ENDOMETRIAL, OVARIAN AND HORMONAL CHANGES DURING MENSTRUAL CYCLE        10 (1985)

### DESCRIBE HORMONAL CONTROL OF MENSTRUAL CYCLE        10 (1990)

### DESCRIBE BRIEFLY THE REGULATION OF MENSTRUAL CYCLE        5 (1992)

### COMPARE AND CONTRAST PROLIFERATIVE AND SECRETORY PHASE OF MENSTRUAL CYCLE        2 (2003)-IPU

### OVARIAN CYCLE        2.5 (2004)

### CHANGES AND CONTROL OF MENSTRUAL CYCLE

Menstrual cycle includes the cyclical changes occurring in reproductive organs in women of reproductive age group, under the influence of female hormones. Average duration of the menstrual cycle is 28 days (range: 25–35 days) and it is divided into three phases, namely:

1. Proliferative phase
2. Secretory phase
3. Menstruation

**1. Proliferative phase:** It follows the menstrual phase during which the endometrium of the uterus is shed off. This period lasts till the 14th day of the menstrual cycle. During proliferative phase following changes take place in the uterus, ovary and hormone levels.

## Uterine Changes

- Growth of endometrium takes place
- Uterine glands increase in length
- Epithelial cells proliferative
- Blood vessels grow (angiogenesis).
- Increase in stroma

This is also known as **preovulatory** or **follicular phase.**

## Ovarian Changes

Several primordial follicles grow in the beginning of the cycle. At around 6th day, one of the follicles starts growing faster than others called dominant follicle. It continues to grow into a mature graafian follicle. Theca interna cells of graafian follicle secrete oestrogen.

## Hormonal Control (Fig. 9.2)

- At beginning of proliferative phase oestrogen level is low because the follicle is not fully grown and not secreting in large amounts. FSH level is substantial and is responsible for the growth of ovarian follicle into graafian follicle.
- Amount of oestrogen is gradually rising and is responsible for proliferative changes in the endometrium.
- As oestrogen level rises there is feedback inhibition of FSH and by this time graafian follicle has matured.
- Oestrogen peak occurs around 14th day of the cycle and is maintained for some time.
- A high maintained level of oestrogen has a positive feedback effect on LH. So the LH is secreted in large amount called **LH**

**surge**. LH surge is responsible for ovulation with discharge of ovum from the follicle. The follicle is then transformed into corpus luteum.

Corpus luteum secretes large quantities of progesterone and also oestrogen. The secretory phase then starts under the effect of progesterone.

**2. Secretory phase:** Lasts till the 28th day of the cycle.

## Uterine Changes

Endometrium starts secreting a fluid hence the name secretory phase. Endometrial glands become tortuous and get filled with secretions. Arteries get coiled called spiral arteries. Glycogen content of epithelial cells increases.

## Ovarian Changes

Corpus luteum grows and secretes progesterone and oestrogens from luteal cells.

If fertilization of ovum does not take place, corpus luteum starts regressing around 24th day of the cycle and eventually is replaced by scar tissue called **corpus albicans**.

## Hormonal Changes

Levels of progesterone and oestrogen are rising, both showing a peak in this phase and decline after the peak, because corpus luteum starts regressing by then as abovementioned hormones are increasing, levels of FSH and LH decline.

**3. Menstrual phase:** Duration is 3–5 days. Day 1 of this phase is the 1st day of the menstrual cycle. It occurs as a result of regression of the corpus luteum and consequent fall in oestrogen and progesterone levels.

## Uterine Changes

As the corpus luteum regresses, hormonal support of endometrium is absent, therefore, arteries go into spasm. As a result of the spasm parts of endometrium undergo necrosis and are sloughed off and bleeding occurs, forming the menstrual blood flow.

In menstrual flow superficial 2/3rd of the endometrium called **stratum functional** is denuded and deeper 1/3rd called **stratum basale** remains. In proliferative phase new endometrium is formed from the stratum basale.

## Ovarian Changes

Ovaries contain corpus albicans of previously formed graafian follicles.

## Hormonal Levels

Oestrogen and progesterone are very low along with FSH and LH. After the menstrual phase FSH begins to rise as oestrogen is low. Under the effect of FSH further primordial follicles begin to grow and a new cycle starts.

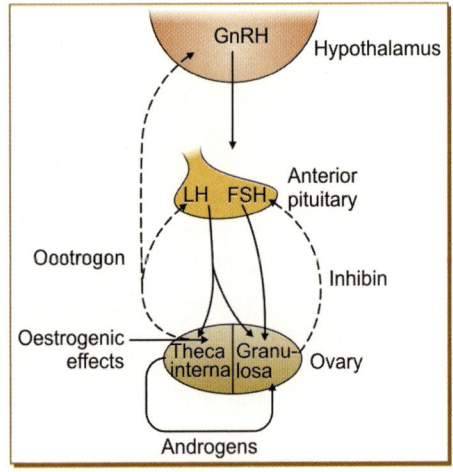

**Fig. 9.2:** Feedback regulation of ovarian function

## WHAT ARE GONADAL HORMONES? DESCRIBE SYNTHESIS AND FUNCTIONS OF ANY ONE OF THEM          10 (1989)

Gonadal hormones are produced by the ovary in females and testes in males.

## Ovarian Hormones

1. **Oestrogens:** Secreted in the proliferative and secretory phases of menstrual cycle.

2. **Progesterone:** Secreted mainly during the secretory phase.
3. **Relaxin:** Produced in small amounts by the corpus luteum during the secretory phase.

## Testicular Hormones

1. **Testosterone:** Main male hormone
2. **Oestrogen:** Produced in very small quantities.

## Oestrogen

This is the female hormone secreted by the ovary from:

i. Theca interna cells
ii. Granulosa cells
iii. Corpus luteum.

**During pregnancy it is secreted by**

1. Corpus luteum (till 3 months)
2. Placenta

**Synthesis of oestrogen:** It is synthesised from cholesterol. Biosynthetic pathway is as follows:

$$
\begin{array}{c}
\text{Cholesterol} \\
\downarrow \\
\text{Pregnenolone} \\
\downarrow \\
\text{Hydroxyprogesterone} \\
\downarrow \\
\text{Androstenedione} \\
\downarrow \text{Aromatisation} \\
\text{Oestradiol}
\end{array}
$$

## Actions of Oestrogens

Secretion of oestrogens starts at puberty and has the following actions.

I. **In non-pregnant female**
   1. Development of breast and reproductive organs and other secondary sexual characters at puberty, e.g. body configuration and hair distribution.
   2. Responsible for proliferative changes in the endometrium after menstruation in the female reproductive cycle.

3. Cyclical changes in cervix and vagina. Produces ramification of vaginal epithelial cells, which help to make the vaginal pH acidic and protect it against infections.
4. Responsible for female sexual behaviour.

II. **Actions during pregnancy**
1. Causes the growth of uterine muscles. It produces hypertrophy of muscle fibres and also increases contractile proteins in fibres.
2. Increases excitability of myometrium and increases the responsiveness of the myometrium to oxytocin, especially towards the end of pregnancy.
3. Causes breast development in preparation for lactation by promoting the growth of ducts.

III. **Other actions**
1. Causes salt and water retention in the body.
2. Makes the sebaceous secretions thin thus preventing acne.
3. Lowers plasma cholesterol and helps to prevent atherosclerosis.
4. Feedback control of FSH and LH.

## PROGESTERONE                                    2.5 (1991)

Progesterone is one of female sex steroids. It is secreted by the corpus luteum in non-pregnant female in the luteal phase of the menstrual cycle. During pregnancy it is also secreted by the placenta in large amounts. Small amounts are also secreted by the graafian follicle.

## Actions of Progesterone

1. Responsible for the secretory phase of uterine cycle.
2. Produces cyclic changes in cervix and vagina.
3. It is thermogenic.
4. During pregnancy it decreases the excitability of myometrium and hence maintains pregnancy.
5. Development of alveolar tissue of breast during pregnancy in preparation for lactation later on.
6. Has stimulatory effect on respiration.
7. In large doses it produces natriuresis by blocking the action of aldosterone on the kidneys.

## EXPLAIN WHY RISE IN BBT OCCURS DURING AN OVULATORY CYCLE      1 (2004), 1 (2005)

## EXPLAIN WHY RISE IN BBT IS AN INDICATOR OF OVULATION      1 (2010)

There is an increase in the basal body temperature at the time of ovulation by 0.3°C to 0.5°C due to the thermogenic action of progesterone at the level of the hypothalamus.

## INDICATORS OF OVULATION      3 (1987)

These are clinical and laboratory tests by which one can know if ovulation has occurred or not. These tests are based on the fact that if ovulation takes place progesterone is secreted in large amount from the ovary and has the following effects on the body:

1. **BBT charting:** Basal body temperature is recorded every morning before the woman gets up from the bed. A special BBT thermometre with wide graduations is used. If ovulation occurs, there is an abrupt rise in BBT by at least 0.5°C and persists for the rest of the cycle. It is probably due to progesterone secretion which is a thermogenic hormone.

2. **Pre-menstrual endometrial biopsy (EB):** Presence of functioning corpus luteum indicates that ovulation has occurred, which can be determined by doing a premenstrual endometrial biopsy which will show a secretory pattern.

3. **Examination of cervical mucus:** Cervical mucus shows a **fern-like pattern** in the oestrogen phase. The mucus is thinnest at the time of ovulation. In the presence of progesterone its elasticity increases, so that a drop can be stretched into a thread 8–12 cm long (*spinnbarkeit*).

4. **Levels of progesterone** in blood and its metabolites can be estimated. These tests are useful clinically in cases of sterility.

5. **Ultrasound scanning** can record the process of ovulation.

## LH SURGE      3 (2004)

At 36–48 hours before ovulation in the menstrual cycle, the oestrogen feedback effect becomes positive and this initiates the burst of LH secretion **(LH surge)** that produces ovulation. This is called the LH surge and ovulation occurs about 9 hours after this surge.

At a moderate constant level of circulation, oestrogen exerts a negative feedback on LH secretion, whereas during this period in the cycle, an elevated oestrogen level exerts a positive feedback effect and stimulates LH secretion.

## FUNCTIONS OF FSH IN MALES AND FEMALES    2 (2002)

### Role of FSH in Males

Role of FSH in males is uncertain, however, less androgen is required if FSH is present for spermatogenesis.

- It appears to facilitate the last stage of spermatid maturation via an action on Sertoli cells.
- It promotes the production of androgen binding protein (ABP), thereby stabilizing the high supply of androgen to the developing germ cells in the seminiferous tubule lumen.

### Role of FSH in Females

- It promotes the development of the ovarian follicle.
- Increases the secretion of oestradiol (oestrogen) from the theca interna cells which leads to the proliferative changes in the endometrium.
- The rise in FSH concentration increases the serum concentration of oestradiol to reach a peak at 12–13 days called **oestrogen surge**.

## RELAXIN    2.5 (2004)

Relaxin is a polypeptide hormone that is produced in the corpus luteum, uterus, placenta and mammary glands in women and the prostrate gland in men.

### Functions in Females

- Facilitates delivery by:
  1. Relaxation of the symphysis pubis and other pelvic joints
  2. Softening and dilation of cervix
  3. May play a role in development of breasts.

### Function in Males

In men it is found in the semen where it helps to maintain sperm motility and aids in penetration of the ovum by the sperm.

## COMPARE OVULATORY AND ANOVULATORY CYCLE   2 (2009)

In some cases ovulation fails to occur during the menstrual cycle known as an anovulatory cycle. Such cycles occur for the first

12–18 months after menarche and again before the onset of menopause. When ovulation does not occur, no corpus luteum is formed and the effects of progesterone on the endometrium are absent. Oestrogen continues to cause growth, however, and the proliferative endometrium becomes thick enough to breakdown and slough off. The time taken for menstruation to occur is variable, but it usually occurs in less than 28 days from the last menstrual period. The flow is variable and ranges from scanty to relatively profuse.

## WHAT WILL HAPPEN AND WHY TO GONADOTROPIN LEVELS AFTER MENOPAUSE       1 (2012)

The human ovaries become unresponsive to gonadotropins with advancing age and their function declines. This is associated with and probably caused by a decline in the number of primordial follicles. They no longer secrete progesterone and 17β-estradiol in appreciable quantities and oestrogen is formed only in small amount. As the negative feedback of oestrogen and progesterone is reduced, FSH secretion is increased along with LH levels.

In women a period called perimenopause, which precedes menopause and can last for up to 10 years. During this time FSH levels increase before an increase in LH is observed due to a decrease in oestrogen, progesterone and inhibins and the menses become irregular. This occurs between 45 and 55 years of age.

## EXPLAIN WHY BONE DENSITY IS REDUCED AFTER MENOPAUSE       1 (2011)

Bone density is reduced after menopause due to the deficiency of oestrogen. Oestrogen inhibits the secretion of cytokines such as IL-1, IL-6 and TNF-α and these cytokines foster the development of osteoclasts. Oestrogen also stimulates the production of TGF-β which increases apoptosis of osteoclasts.

## CONTRACEPTIVE MEASURES

### SAFE PERIOD       2.5 (1985)

### DESCRIBE THE BASIS OF RHYTHM METHOD OF CONTRACEPTION       2.5 (1991)

**Safe period:** It is time period during the reproductive cycle of a female when the chances of conception are minimal.

It is decided on the basis that in an average cycle of 28 days:

1. Ovulation occurs on 14th–15th day of the cycle.
2. Discharged ovum is probably fertilizable for 36 hrs.
3. Sperms can survive in female genital tract for about 48 hrs.

So the fertile period during a cycle is very short but could be extended between 10th and 17th day of the cycle. The period outside the fertile period is called the **'safe period'**. This fact is applied in the rhythm method of contraception. As the time of ovulation is variable even in women with regular cycles, this method is not considered reliable for the prevention of conception.

## DESCRIBE THE PRINCIPLES UNDERLYING METHODS OF CONTRACEPTION IN THE FEMALE. EXPLAIN THE MECHANISM OF ACTION OF ORAL CONTRACEPTIVES     10 (1992)

## MECHANISM OF ORAL CONTRACEPTIVES   2.5 (1991), 2 (2004)

## MECHANISM OF ACTION OF INTRAUTERINE CONTRACEPTIVE DEVICES     2.5 (1989), 2 (2002)

## PHYSIOLOGICAL BASIS OF ORAL CONTRACEPTIVES
    2.5 (1988), 4 (2004)-IPU, 2.5 (2006)

## ORAL CONTRACEPTIVES     2.5 (2010)

Contraceptives are the measures taken to prevent conception. It may be used as a temporary measure to prevent pregnancy for a desired period or as a permanent measure. Contraception can be achieved by the following methods:

### A. Temporary Methods

  **I. Preventing union of sperm and ovum:**

    a. **Rhythm method:** The physiological basis of this method is:

      1. In a normal cycle ovulation occurs around 14th day.
      2. Ovum is fertilizable till 48 hrs after ovulation.
      3. Sperm can survive in the female genital tract for 48–72 hrs.

      Based on the above facts fertile period is between 10 and 17 days of the cycle and the rest of the cycle is 'safe period' where there are minimal chances of fertilisation of ovum. At the same time it is based on the assumption that reproductive cycle of female is regular.

    b. **Mechanical barriers:** A mechanical barrier is created so that sperms cannot get access to ovum, e.g. diaphragm inserted in vagina and cervical cap fitted on the cervix.

c. **Spermicidal jellys and creams:** These are placed in the vagina and they kill the sperms.

II. **Prevention of ovulation by interfering with normal reproductive cycle.** Oral contraceptives if used properly are considered 100% successful in the prevention of conception. They are of the following types:

1. **Classical or combined pill:** These pills contain high doses of oestrogen and progestins as a 'combined' pill. It is administered for 21 days and then withdrawn for 5–7 days to allow menstrual bleeding. Physiological basis is that high doses of oestrogen probably depresses FSH and prevent the normal LH surge that occurs prior to ovulation and thus ovulation is prevented. Progesterone thickens the cervical mucus and hinders sperm migration.

2. **Sequential pill:** It involves administration of high doses of oestrogen for 15 days followed by 5 days of oestrogen and progesterone. This inhibits ovulation by suppressing the release of FSH and LH.

3. **Administration of large doses of oestrogen:** This decreases FSH levels with multiple irregular peaks of LH secretion rather than a single mid-cycle peak, thereby producing anovulatory cycle.

4. **Mini pill or micropill:** It involves the administration of low doses of progesterone through the entire period of menstrual cycle. This prevents fertility without inhibiting ovulation. It may act on the cervical mucus, endometrium or decrease the motility of the fallopian tube.

5. **Post-coital pill or morning after pill:** It is recommended within 48 hours of unprotected intercourse. A double dose of combined pill is given followed by another 2 pills 12 hours later.

6. **Progesterone antagonists:** Mifepristone is helpful in producing abortions after conception. It acts by inhibiting the progestational effects on the uterus.

   Disadvantages of contraceptive pills are:
   - Increase risk of thromboembolic phenomenon
   - Precipitate diabetes mellitus
   - Increase systemic arterial blood pressure by their salt retaining properties.

III. **Prevention of implantation:** Intrauterine contraceptive devices (IUDs) are used for the prevention of implantation. They are divided into the following types:
  - Non-medicated IUD, e.g. Lippe's loop
  - **Copper IUD, e.g Copper T:** It acts by altering the composition of the cervical mucus and also decreases sperm motility
  - **Hormone releasing IUD:** It is filled with progesterone and acts by increasing the viscosity of cervical mucus. It makes the endometrium unfavourable for implantation of the fertilized ovum
    **Mechanism of action of IUDs**
    - It speeds the passage of the fertilized ovum preventing its implantation in the endometrium
    - It disturbs the orderly sequential changes taking place in the endometrium during the normal menstrual cycle

IV. **Suppression of normal menstrual cycle:** Long acting progestins are used to suppress menstrual cycle, e.g. once a month pill and subcutaneous implants of progestins. Progesterone is released slowly and normal cycles do not occur.

## B. Permanent Methods

**Tubectomy:** Fallopian tubes are cut and tied so that the ovum released after ovulation cannot enter the tube and so cannot be fertilized. These days tubectomy is not a major surgery and can be performed through a laproscope.

## Termination of Pregnancy

Even if conception has occurred, pregnancy can be terminated known as medical termination of pregnancy (MTP). The cervix is dilated and products of conception are taken out. It is safe if done within 12 week of conception.

## PHYSIOLOGY OF PREGNANCY

### HORMONES OF PLACENTA                    2.5 (2003)

The following hormones are secreted by the placenta:
- Human chorionic gonadotropin (HCG)
- Human chorionic somatomammotropin (HCS)
- Oestrogen
- Progesterone

- Relaxin
- GnRH
- Human chorionic thyrotropin
- Leptin
- Inhibin

## Human Chorionic Gonadotropin (HCG)

- This is a glycoprotein formed by the syncytiotrophoblastic cells of the placenta immediately after implantation of the fertilised ovum.
- It is a primarily a luteinizing and luteotrophic hormone and also has some FSH activity.
- It helps to maintain the corpus luteum of pregnancy which continues to secrete oestrogen and progesterone till 3 months of pregnancy.
- It can be detected in the serum after 10 days and as early as 14 days after conception in the urine. Its detection in the urine forms the basis of pregnancy diagnosis test. If foetal death occurs in early pregnancy, HCG disappears from the serum and urine.

## Human Chorionic Somatomammotropin (HCS)

- It is synthesised by placental syncytiotrophoblastic cells.
- It is lactogenic and has small amount of growth stimulating activity. It is called the maternal growth hormone of pregnancy. It brings about nitrogen, potassium and calcium retention and decreases glucose utilisation.
- It promotes the growth and development of the breasts during pregnancy. If foetal death occurs in late pregnancy, HCS secretion falls.
- Its serum concentration rises steadily from 70 days of conception till term. The amount of HCS secreted is directly proportional to the size of the placenta, therefore, low HCS level is a sign of placental insufficiency.

## Oestrogen and Progesterone

- Both these hormones are required for the initiation and maintenance of pregnancy.
- Both these hormones are produced mainly by the corpus luteum during the first 6 to 8 weeks of pregnancy. After this the fetoplacental unit takes over the formation of oestrogen and progesterone.

## FUNCTIONS OF PLACENTA                         2 (2010)

Placenta serves mainly three functions:

1. Hormonal secretion
2. Transport of substances between mother and foetus
3. Protection of the foetus

   I. **Hormonal secretion:** The syncytiotrophoblastic cells of the placenta serves as an endocrine gland and secretes the following hormones:
   - Human chorionic gonadotropin
   - Human chorionic somatomammotropins
   - Human chorionic thyrotropin
   - Placental oestrogens
   - Placental progesterone
   - Relaxin

   (For details refer to question on hormones secreted by the placenta).

   II. **Transport of substances between the mother and foetus**
   - **Transport of nutrients:** The major function of the placenta is to transport nutrients between the mother and foetus.
   - Excretion of waste products through the placenta.
   - **Diffusion of respiratory gases:** Transport of oxygen and carbon dioxide.
   - **Transport of antibodies:** Maternal antibodies are transported to the foetus and are responsible for innate immunity.
   - **Transport of harmful substances:** Certain viruses and many drugs (mainly nicotine and barbiturates) can easily cross the placental barrier and may produce harmful effects on the foetus.

   III. **Protection of the foetus:** Placenta protects the foetus in many ways:
   - It acts as a barrier against many harmful substances
   - It provides nutrition to the foetus
   - Its hormonal secretion is required for proper foetal growth
   - Placental progesterone decreases uterine contractions and thus protects the foetus from being expelled before the full term.

## PHYSIOLOGICAL BASIS OF PREGNANCY TEST    2.5 (1991)
## PREGNANCY DIAGNOSTIC TESTS    4 (1986, 1988, 1989)

Pregnancy diagnosing tests are based on the presence of chorionic gonadotropin hormone secreted by the placenta called human chorionic gonadotropins (HCG). It can be detected as early as 7 days after conception in blood by radioimmunoassay. HCG appears in the urine of pregnant females also and can be detected as early as 14 days after conception.

Clinically urine of females is tested for the presence of HCG.

### HCG has Following Properties

  i. It has luteinising action like LH

  ii. It is basically a glycoprotein and antibodies can be generated against it. This property is used in biological test done on laboratory animals.

Urine of the female is injected in animals and occurrence of ovulation in animal indicates that conception has taken place.

This fact is also utilised in immunological test to diagnose pregnancy.

These days biological tests have become obsolete and have been replaced by immunological tests which are easier to perform and results are available after a short time.

### Principle of Immunological Pregnancy Diagnosis Test

Human chorionic gonadotropins (HCG) are secreted in large amount by the placenta during pregnancy. It is a glycoprotein and hence antibodies can be raised against it.

### Test

1. Antibodies against HCG are raised and antisera obtained.
2. Sheep red cells or latex particles are coated with HCG
3. Antisera is first added to the urine. If urine contains HCG these will be neutralised by the antisera.
4. Coated RBCs are then added and the presence (or absence) of agglutination is observed.

    • If agglutination of RBCs takes place, it indicates absence of pregnancy. This is because as there is no HCG in urine, antibodies in the antisera are not consumed and when RBCs coated with HCG are added, antibodies react with them and cause their agglutination.

- **No agglutination:** Indicates that conception has taken place or the pregnancy test is +ve as explained above.

## HORMONAL CONTROL OF LACTATION 5 (1989)
## HORMONES RESPONSIBLE FOR BREAST DEVELOPMENT
4 (1987)
## DESCRIBE THE ACTIONS OF OESTROGEN AND PROGESTERONE ON THE BREAST 2.5 (1990)
## DESCRIBE THE INITIATION OF LACTATION 10 (1986)
## PHYSIOLOGY OF LACTATION 2 (2009), 3 (2012), 2.5 (2003)

Lactation is the process of milk secretion by the mammary gland after the baby is born.

A number of hormones interact in the process. It involves the following stages:

i. Breast development
ii. Secretion of milk
iii. Initiation and maintenance of secretion
iv. Milk ejection

**Breast development:** An increase in the growth of breasts occurs during pregnancy specially during the first half under the influence of following hormones:

1. Oestrogen
2. Progesterone
3. Prolactin
4. Growth hormone
5. Insulin
6. Adernal corticoids
7. Chorionic somatomammotropin

Oestrogen and progesterone secreted from the placenta are primarily responsible for the growth of the mammary gland.

- **Oestrogen:** Causes proliferation of ducts and their branching.
- **Progesterone:** Causes the growth of alveolar tissue and increases their number.
- **Prolactin:** Has synergistic effect with oestrogen for development but oestrogen inhibits the milk secretion by

prolactin. It acts directly on the mammary epithelial cells to produce localized alveolar hyperplasia. This action is increased by growth hormone, corticosteroids and thyroxine.

- **Role of placenta:** During pregnancy in addition to oestrogen and progesterone, the placenta also produces a prolactin growth hormone like factor called placental lactogen.

## Milk Secretion

It is the process of synthesis of milk by the alveolar epithelium and its passage into the lumen of alveoli.

### Milk secretion can be divided into two phases

1. **Initiation of secretion or lactogenesis:** It is under the hormonal control of prolactin. Though some milk secretion occurs in the later half of pregnancy, under the effect of increasing level of prolactin, it is kept in check by the high circulating level of oestrogen.

   After delivery, with expulsion of placenta oestrogen levels decline and activity of prolactin is unopposed, so secretion of milk droplets occurs which are poured into the ducts.

2. **Maintenance of secretion or galactopoiesis:** Hormone prolactin is important for the continued milk secretion. It also involves neural reflexes. Suckling by the baby through a neuroendocrinal reflex causes the further secretion of prolactin.

   Hence prolactin is essential for the initiation of milk secretion as well as its continuation.

**Milk ejection:** It is process of discharge of milk from the mammary gland through nipples. It is controlled by the hormone oxytocin secreted from the posterior pituitary. Oxytocin produces contraction of myoepithelial cells present in the duct lining. With their contraction milk is ejected through the nipple.

Oxytocin release is also reflexly controlled. Suckling by the newborn stimulates certain receptors present in the nipple and areola and a neuroendocrinal reflex is initiated. Impulses are carried to the supraoptic and paraventricular nuclei of the hypothalamus and then to posterior pituitary causing the release of oxytocin. So the process of milk secretion and its ejection is maintained as the baby suckles the breast and continues as long as breastfeeding is continued.

Oxytocin is used clinically to cause ejection of milk from engorged breast when child is not breast fed due to some reason. Hormone oestrogen is some time injected to suppress lactation, e.g. after a still birth.

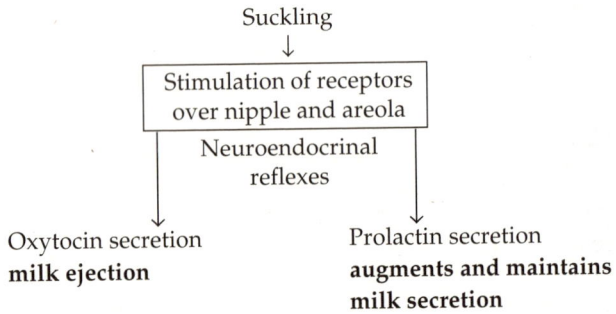

LACTATION AMENORRHOEA **3 (2004)-IPU**

WHY LACTATION IS A NATURAL CONTRACEPTIVE **1 (2004)**

WHY AMENORRHOEA IS OBSERVED DURING LACTATION **1 (2006)**

Lactation is associated with amenorrhoea and temporary sterility, probably due to the inhibitory action of prolactin on the secretion of gonadotropins FSH and LH by inhibiting GnRH. Ovulation is inhibited and the ovaries are inactive, so oestrogen and progesterone output falls to low levels. This period is variable from 6 weeks (in women who do not nurse their infants) to 25–30 weeks in women who nurse regularly.

CONTROL OF PARTURITION **5 (1993)**

PHYSIOLOGY OF PARTURITION **2.5 (2004)**

Parturition is the process of delivery or birth of the newborn. The uterine contractions that are painless and of mild intensity during the first trimester gradually increase after the 30th week of pregnancy until labour to become stronger, more frequent and painful.

Normal delivery occurs after 270 days of fertilization or 284 days after the 1st day of the menstrual period preceding the conception. What exactly initiates the process is not known but maternal and foetal factors are involved. Process of parturition is under the control of hormone oxytocin.

## Oxytocin Produces

i. Softening and dilatation of the cervix.

ii. Intermittent uterine contractions which push the baby downwards along the birth canal.

## Control of Oxytocin (Fig. 9.3)

Increase in myometrial oxytocin receptors occurs in pregnancy under the influence of oestrogen and it reaches to the maximum at the end of pregnancy.

- At the onset of parturition, oxytocin action is increased due to increase in the number of receptors though concentration of oxytocin does not increase, the cause is not understood.

- Once the uterine contraction are initiated further, secretion of oxytocin occurs by positive feedback effect as follows.

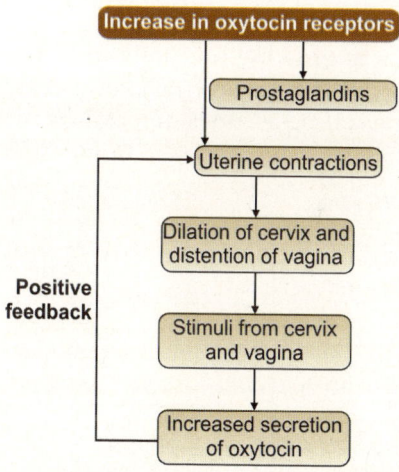

**Fig. 9.3:** Role of oxytocin in parturition

This positive feedback mechanism is repeated till delivery is completed.

In addition parturition is aided by **spinal reflexes** arising in cervix and unknown stimuli from the foetus itself. Exact foetal mechanism involved is not completely understood as yet.

## PHYSIOLOGY OF FOETUS AND NEWBORN

### FOETOPLACENTAL UNIT                    2.5 (1991)

Large amount of oestrogen which is essential for pregnancy is secreted by the placenta.

Placenta alone cannot synthesize this hormone as some of the enzymes required for the synthesis are not present in the placenta. However, enzymes so needed are present in foetal adrenal cortex. Some intermediaries in oestrogen synthesis are formed in foetus. So, both placenta and foetal adrenal gland function as a unit to form oestrogen and is known as foetoplacental unit (Fig 9.4).

### Steps in Synthesis of Oestrogens

1. Cholesterol → Pregnenolone

2. Pregnenolone → Progesterone

3. Progesterone → Dehydroepiandrosterone

4. Dehydroepiandrosterone → Oestradiol

Unless foetus is growing normally, oestrogen synthesis in pregnancy will not increase. Hence, an estimation of urinary oestriol excretion is used as index of foetal growth.

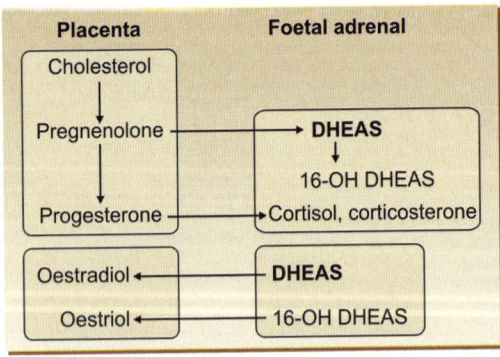

**Fig. 9.4:** Interaction between the placenta and foetal adrenal cortex in the synthesis of steroids

# 10

# Central Nervous System

**EXPLAIN THE MECHANISM OF SYNAPTIC TRANSMISSION. NAME ANY TWO INHIBITORY TRANSMITTERS** 10

Impulse transmission across a synapse occurs by the following mechanisms:

a. Release of a chemical, known as neurotransmitter as is seen in **chemical synapses**.

b. Electrical changes in **electrical synapse**.

**Mechanism of transmission across chemical synapse**

A transmitter is released into the synaptic cleft from the presynaptic nerve terminals which is responsible for bringing about an electrical change in postsynaptic membrane. Electrical change so produced in the postsynaptic membrane may excite or inhibit the postsynaptic neuron depending upon the nature of the transmitter released from the presynaptic neuron.

1. **Mechanism of excitation of postsynaptic neuron**

   • As the action potential passes along the axon of presynaptic neuron, it opens voltage-gated $Ca^{2+}$ channels in the synaptic knobs. Entry of $Ca^{2+}$ causes the release of an excitatory neurotransmitter, e.g. ACh from vesicles at synaptic knobs.

   • Neurotransmitter travels across the synaptic cleft and binds with certain specialised receptors in postsynaptic membrane.

   • Binding with these receptors triggers the opening of voltage-gated $Na^+$ channels causing the entry of $Na^+$ across the membrane along concentration and electrical gradient.

   • Entry of $Na^+$ causes a transient depolarisation of the postsynaptic membrane, which makes the membrane more excitable and hence known as **excitatory postsynaptic**

**potential,** i.e. EPSP. EPSP is a local non-propagated electrical response but they can be summated.

- A spatial or temporal summation of EPSPs produces an action potential which is propagated and postsynaptic neuron is thus excited and impulse is passed on to it. Some excitatory neurotransmitters act by closing $K^+$ channels in the postsynaptic membrane, thus preventing $K^+$ efflux, making the membrane less negative inside and hence more excitable.

2. **Mechanism of inhibition of postsynaptic neuron:**

At certain synapses the neurotransmitter released is such that it makes the postsynaptic membrane more negative by producing transient non-propagating inhibitory potentials in the postsynaptic membrane known as inhibitory postsynaptic potentials. IPSPs like EPSP are a local potentials but they hyperpolarise the postsynaptic membrane and inhibit the postsynoptic neuron. This type of inhibition is called **direct inhibition.** At these synapses neurotransmitters act by opening $Cl^-$ channels or $K^+$ channels or even by closing $Na^+$ or $Ca^{2+}$ channels in the postsynaptic membrane.

**Mechanism of action at electrical synapses**
At electrical synapses impulse reaching the presynaptic membrane generates EPSPs in the postsynaptic membrane by promoting passage of ions through gap junctions between the two membranes. EPSPs at electrical synapses have shorter latency than at chemical synapses, e.g. some neurons in the lateral vestibular nucleus.

**Inhibitory neurotransmitters**
1. GABA
2. Glycine

**MECHANISM OF PRESYNAPTIC INHIBITION**      2.5 (1989)

**SYNAPTIC INHIBITION**      2.5 (2004)

**COMPARE AND CONTRAST PRESYNAPTIC INHIBITION AND POSTSYNAPTIC INHIBITION**      2 (2004)-IPU

Presynaptic inhibition in CNS is mediated by neurons that end on excitatory endings forming axo-axonal type of synapses. These neurons inhibit presynaptic endings so that the amount of neurotransmitter released by them is less and in turn degree of excitation of postsynaptic neuron is less. Possible mechanisms of presynaptic inhibition are:

1. Increase Cl⁻ conductance at presynaptic ending so that size of the action potential reaching them is smaller and the transmitter released is less.
2. Decrease $Ca^{2+}$ entry and hence reduction in amount of neurotransmitter which is released.
3. Opening of voltage-gated $K^+$ channels and increased $K^+$ efflux.
4. Inhibition of transmitter release independent of $Ca^{2+}$ GABA is a known transmitter producing presynaptic inhibition, e.g. presynaptic inhibition of afferents carrying pain sensation at the level of spinal cord producing analgesia (Fig. 10.1).

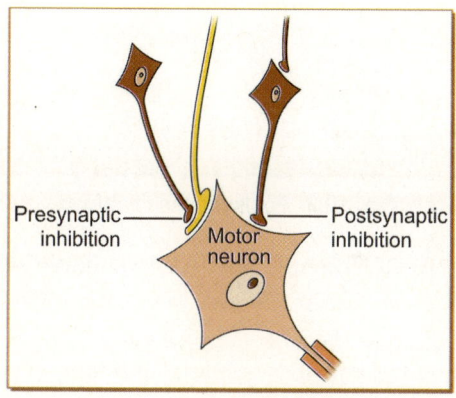

**Fig. 10.1:** Presynaptic inhibition

## MECHANISM OF POSTSYNAPTIC INHIBITION 2.5 (1991)

Postsynaptic inhibition also known as direct inhibition occurs, due to generation of inhibitory postsynaptic potentials, i.e. IPSPs in postsynaptic neurons.

IPSP occurs due to the nature of the neurotransmitter released at presynaptic nerve terminals. It increases the permeability of postsynaptic membrane for chloride ions, which moves in with the concentration gradient and increases negativity inside.

This takes the membrane potential away from the firing level thus inhibiting the postsynaptic neuron.

This type of inhibition occurs in the spinal cord. As a group of neurons supplying agonist muscle are excited, collateral branches through interneurons, end on neurons supplying the antagonistic group of muscles producing IPSPs and inhibit them. Here the inhibitory neurotransmitter is glycine (Fig. 10.2).

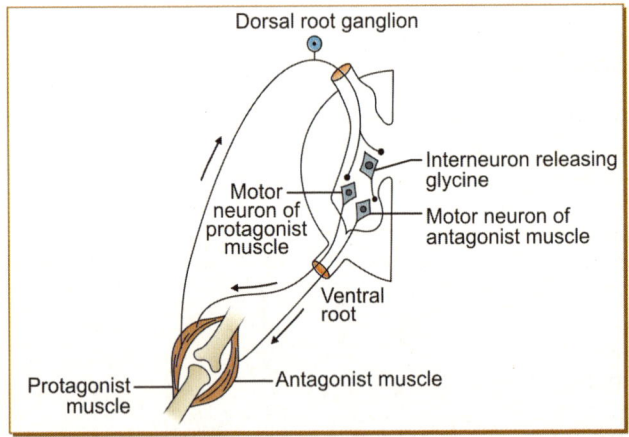

**Fig, 10.2:** Postsynaptic inhibition

## COMPARE AND CONTRAST: SPATIAL AND TEMPORAL SUMMATION 2 (2003)-IPU

The EPSP is a graded response. It does not follow all-or-none law like action potential and shows spatial and temporal summation.

**Temporal summation:** This occurs when repeated stimuli are applied at very short intervals, i.e. before the previous EPSPs have decayed.

**Spatial summation** occurs when postsynaptic membrane receives impulses from a large number of presynaptic terminals simultaneously. The effect of all the impulses is added up and enough transmitter substance is released to cause a greater response.

Both types occur simultaneously in the neuronal pool. When temporal or spatial summation bring the membrane potential of the cell to the firing level, an action potential is generated and is propagated in the postsynaptic neuron.

## COMPARE AND CONTRAST: OCCLUSIONAL AND SUBLIMINAL FRINGE IN NEURONS
**2 (2003)-IPU**

**Occlusion:** This is the decrease in response due to the presynaptic fibres sharing postsynaptic neurons. Thus occlusion is due to afferent fibres overlapping in their central distribution.

**Subliminal fringe:** Neurons are said to be in subliminal fringe if they are not discharged by an afferent volley but do have their excitability increased. The neurons that have few knobs ending on them are in subliminal fringe and those with many are in the discharge zone.

## COMPARE EPSPs AND IPSPs
**(2000)**

| EPSPs | IPSPs |
|---|---|
| 1. It is the initial depolarising response produced by a single stimulus to a sensory nerve | 1. IPSP is produced by stimulation of certain presynaptic fibres which regularly initiate a hyperpolarising response in spinal motor neurons |
| 2. It begins 0.5 msec after the impulse enters the spinal cord reaching its peak in 1.0–1.5 msec and then declines slowly over the next 4 msec | 2. It begins 1–1.5 msec after the entry of the afferent impulse into the spinal cord and rises to a peak in 1.5–2 msec after its onset. It declines exponentially with a time constant of 3 msec |
| 3. **Neurotransmitters:** Glutamate | 3. **Neurotransmitter:** GABA and glycine |
| 4. **Ionic basis:** The EPSPs are produced when the excitatory transmitter opens $Na^+$ or $Ca^{2+}$ channels in the postsynaptic membrane, producing inward current | 4. **Ionic basis:** They are produced by movement of chloride ions into the cell or opening of $K^+$ channels with movement of potassium out of the postsynaptic cell, or by closure of $Na^+$ or $Ca^{2+}$ channels |
| 5. Summation produces action potential | 5. Summation cannot lead to an action potential |

## DIFFERENCE BETWEEN EPSPs AND ACTION POTENTIAL
**2.5**

| EPSPs | Action potential |
|---|---|
| • Transient partial depolarization at postsynaptic | • Potential change when a nerve or a muscle is stimulated |

*Contd.*

*Contd.*

| EPSPs | Action potential |
|---|---|
| membrane in a synapse in response to a single stimulus | with threshold stimulus |
| • Local response that is not propagated | • Action potential is propagated along the nerve or muscle |
| • EPSP show both spatial and temporal summation for reaching the firing level | • Obeys all-or-none law. Summation of action potential is never possible |
| • Excitability of the synapse is increased during EPSPs | • Tissue is refractory to another stimulus during action potential |

## RECEPTORS

### PACINIAN CORPUSCLE                    2.5 (1985, 1986)

Pacinian corpuscle is a type of mechanoreceptor present in the skin and deep fibrous tissue.

It is the most widely studied receptor, due to its relatively larger size and accessibility in the mesentery of experimental animals. It consists of straight unmyelinated terminal surrounded by concentric lamellas of connective tissue, giving it an appearance of so-called 'cocktail onion'. Myelin sheath of sensory nerve commences inside the connective tissue capsule and the 1st node of Ranvier is also inside it.

Experiments have proved that unmyelinated portion of nerve is the site of generation of receptor potentials. Further once the receptor potential reaches firing level, action potential is produced in the first node of Ranvier and propagated through the sensory nerve.

Pacinian corpuscle is a fast adapting touch receptor and is specially adapted to respond to vibrations.

### ENUMERATE THE PROPERTIES OF RECEPTORS       2.5 (1991)

#### Properties of Receptors

1. **Specificity of response**, i.e. responds to a particular type of stimulus called **adequate stimulus**.
2. Sensation evoked by impulse generated in a receptor depends on the particular part of sensory cortex stimulated.

3. Whenever a sensory pathway is stimulated anywhere along its way to the cortex, the sensation evoked is that for which the receptor is specialised known as **Muller's doctrine of specific nerve energies**.

4. No matter where a sensory pathway is stimulated along its course, the conscious sensation perceived is referred to the site of receptor called **law of projection**.

5. **Adaptation**—receptors adapt to a variable degree. Some are fast adapting, e.g. touch receptors while some are slow like muscle spindle. Temperature receptors are considered intermediate.

6. **Intensity discrimination:** Magnitude of sensation felt is proportional to intensity of stimulation, known as '**Weber-Fechner law**'.

## RECEPTOR POTENTIAL                                  2.5 (1995)

Receptor potential is the electric response in the form of depolarisation of a sensory receptor when it is stimulated. It is a type of generator potential. This property of sensory receptor has been widely studied in pacinian corpuscles.

- Site of the receptor potential is the non-myelinated nerve terminal of the receptor.
- It is a graded response proportional to the intensity of stimulus pressure in case of a pacinian corpuscle till the firing level of 10 mV of depolarisation, when an action potential is generated.
- The receptor potential is responsible for initiating depolarisation in sensory nerve fibres.
- Mechanism of generation is opening of $Na^+$ channels, thereby increasing sodium permeability of the membrane and depolarisation of the membrane.

## WHAT ARE PROPRIOCEPTORS ? WRITE IN BRIEF THE FUNCTION OF ANY ONE OF THEM                              2.5 (1991)

Proprioceptors are a type of exteroceptors which give information regarding the position of the body in relation to its external environment and passive movement of body parts. These include:

- Muscle spindle
- Golgi tendon organ
- Joint receptors
- Vestibular apparatus

## Function of muscle spindle

It is a stretch receptor present in the skeletal muscle. It is stimulated when the muscle is stretched which causes reflex contraction of the muscle thus maintaining the muscle, length in a feedback manner.

### SENSORY SYSTEM

### ENKEPHALINS                                        2.5 (1992)

Enkephalins are peptide inhibitory neurotransmitters secreted from certain neurons in GIT and central nervous system like:

1. Dorsal horns of spinal cord
2. Spinal trigeminal nucleus
3. Periaqueductal grey matter
4. Raphe nuclei

In the brain these peptides along with endorphins bind to opiate receptors and hence are known as opioid peptides. They play a role in relieving pain by:

  i. Activating descending inhibitory pathway from the mid-brain ending in lateral funiculus of the spinal cord.
 ii. Inhibit nociceptive neurons in substantia gelatinosa of spinal cord. They also decrease intestinal motility. They are one of the natural ligands for opiate receptors, present in the CNS.

### COMPARE VISCERAL AND SOMATIC PAIN
                                           2 (2004), 2 (2004)-IPU

| Visceral pain | Somatic pain |
|---|---|
| • This involves muscles and hollow viscera | • It involves the skin and subcutaneous tissue |
| • It is dull and poorly localised because receptors are relatively few and also due to the relative deficiency of Aα nerve fibres | • It is sharp in character and well localised which is based on the richness of the skin innervation with receptors |
| • It produces faintness, nausea, vomiting, sweating, brady-cardia and fall in blood pressure | • It leads to reflex withdrawl movements, increase in heart rate, blood pressure and respiration |
| • It is both local and radiates to distant sites | • It usually does not radiate |

## WHAT WILL HAPPEN AND WHY WHEN PAIN FIBRES IN THE STUMP OF AN AMPUTATED LIMB GET STIMULATED  **2 (2012)**
## EXPLAIN WHY PAIN IS SEEN IN PHANTOM LIMB  **1 (2007)**

Around 50 to 80% of amputees experience phantom sensation usually pain in the region of the amputated limb called **phantom limb pain**. The current theory is that the brain can reorganise if the sensory input is cut off. The ventral posterior thalamus nucleus is one example where this change can occur. Thalamic region that received input from the foot and leg now respond to stimulation of the stump. Others have demonstrated remapping of the somatosensory cortex producing this effect.

## THALAMIC SYNDROME  **(2001)**

Damage to the thalamus experimentally or following vascular blockage may be associated with a peculiar reaction to painful stimuli known as **thalamic syndrome**. In this condition even minor stimuli lead to prolonged, severe and very unpleasant pain. Such sudden attacks of pain may occur spontaneously.

## REFERRED PAIN  **2.5 (2005), 2.5 (2007)**
## THEORIES OF REFERRED PAIN  **2 (2010)**

When the sensation of pain is experienced at a site other than the injured or diseased part, it is called referred pain. Examples of referred pain are:

- Referral of cardiac pain to the inner aspect of the left arm
- Pain in the tip of the shoulder caused by irritation of the central part of the diaphragm
- Pain in the testicle due to stone in the ureter.

Pain is usually referred to a structure that developed from the same embryonic segment or dermatome as the structure in which the pain originates from, e.g. the heart and arm have the same segmental origin and the testicle migrated with its nerve supply from the primitive urogenital ridge from which the kidney and ureter also developed. This is called '**dermatomal rule'**.

### Theories of referred pain

- **Convergence theory:** The basis of referred pain may be convergence of somatic and visceral pain fibres on the same second-order neurons in the dorsal horn that project to the thalamus and then to the somatosensory cortex. This is called the **convergence–projection theory**. Somatic and visceral neurons converge in the ipsilateral dorsal horn. The somatic nociceptive fibres normally do not activate the second-order neurons but when the visceral stimulus is prolonged, facilitation of the somatic fibre endings occur. They now stimulate the second-order neurons and of course the brain cannot determine whether the stimulus comes from the viscera or from the area of referral.

- **Facilitation theory:** The afferent impulses from the visceral structures produce subliminal fringe effects that lower the excitability threshold of spinothalamic neurons that receive afferent fibres from the somatic areas. Therefore, any slight activity in the pathways transmitting pain impulses from the somatic regions and which normally would die out within the spinal cord is facilitated, thus reaching conscious levels.

## GATE CONTROL THEORY OF PAIN                              2 (2005)

Transmission in nociceptive pathways can be interrupted by actions within the dorsal horn of the spinal cord at the site of sensory afferent termination. The relief from pain by shaking or rubbing an injured area may be due to simultaneous activation of innocuous cutaneous mechanoreceptors whose afferents emit collaterals that terminate in the dorsal horn. The activity in these cutaneous mechanoreceptors may reduce the responsiveness of the dorsal horn neurons to their input from nociceptive afferent terminals. This is called **gate control theory of pain** modulation and it serves the rationale behind **TENS** (transcutaneous electrical nerve stimulation) for pain relief.

## CENTRAL INHIBITION OF PAIN                               2 (2002)

Descending inhibitory pathways from the brainstem to rexed lamina I, IV and V in the spinal cord can produce analgesia. One such pathway is mesencephalic pain inhibitory system. This system arises from the midbrain and descends to the dorsal horn cells in the spinal cord. It contains opiate receptors and is stimulated by the following structures:

- Structures immediately surrounding the IIIrd ventricle
- Periaqueductal grey (PAG) matter in the midbrain

- Substantia nigra in midbrain
- Raphe magnus nucleus in the medulla.

An injection of opiods into the PAG induces analgesia. PAG is part of a descending pathway that modulates pain transmission by inhibition of primary afferent transmission in the dorsal horn. These PAG neurons project directly to and activate two groups of neurons in the brainstem:

1. Serotonergic neurons in the raphe magnus nucleus
2. Catecholaminergic neurons in the rostral ventromedial medulla.

Neurons in both these regions project to the spinal cord where the released serotonin and norepinephrine inhibit the activity of the dorsal horn cell that receives input from nociceptive afferent pathways. There is also a group of catecholaminergic neurons in the locus coeruleus that are elements of this descending pain modulating pathway. These pontine fibres also exert their analgesic effect by the release of norepinephrine in the dorsal horn.

## EXPLAIN WHY COUNTER-IRRITANTS WHEN APPLIED CAUSE LOCAL PAIN RELIEF                    1 (2011)

Transmission in the nociceptive pathway can be interrupted by actions within the dorsal horn of the spinal cord at the sensory afferent termination. Counter-irritants when applied to the skin reduce the pain due to injury. This relief may be due to simultaneous activation of innocuous cutaneous mechanoreceptors whose afferents emit collaterals that terminate in the dorsal horn. The activity of these afferents may reduce the responsiveness of the dorsal horn neurons to their input from nociceptive afferent terminals. This is called the **gate control theory of pain.**

## EFFECTS OF LESION OF PRIMARY SENSORY CORTEX    2.5 (1992)

In a lesion of primary sensory cortex there is loss of fine sense of discrimination on the opposite side of the body.

1. One cannot appreciate small differences in:
   i. Intensity of touch
   ii. Temperature
2. Loss of tactile localisation
3. Loss of two point discrimination

4. Astereognosis, i.e. loss of recognition of size, shape and form of objects with eyes closed.

Experimental data shows that lesion in the sensory cortex do not abolish sensations, but they are affected to a variable extent.

Proprioception and fine touch are most affected and pain is affected only slightly.

## REFLEXES

### ROLE OF MUSCLE SPINDLE IN REGULATION OF MUSCLE TONE                                   4 (1993), 2 (2006)

**Muscle tone:** Skeletal muscles are in a state of partial tension in the body known as muscle tone. Muscles offer resistance to stretch. Tone in the muscle is due to a state of partial contraction and muscle contract sub-tetanically to produce tension or tone. Muscle spindle is the receptor present in skeletal muscle which is sensitive to stretch. However, as the muscle is stretched, muscle spindle is also stretched and is hence stimulated causing reflex contraction of the muscle, called **stretch reflex**.

### Pathway of Stretch Reflex

Muscle stretch → spindle stretch → afferent impulses from distorted ending of spindle are set up → spinal centre → efferent impulses from motor neurons go to muscle fibres → contraction of muscle fibre.

As the muscle contracts and shortens, spindle is no more stimulated as the stretch on the spindle is removed, hence the stretch reflex is terminated and muscle relaxes.

To produce tone or tension in the muscle it should contract continuously which is achieved through the stimulation of muscle spindle through γ-efferent discharge from higher centres. Stimulation through γ-efferents shortens the contractile ends of the intrafusal fibres of muscle spindle, producing deformity and setting up afferent impulses from muscle spindle, thus causing reflex contraction of the muscle. There is a continuous discharge to γ-efferent from higher centres. There is evidence that there is a simultaneous discharge to α and γ motor neurons from higher centre. Because of this **α-γ linkage**, the muscle spindle also shortens as the muscle shortens. Thus muscle spindle is stimulated continuously and muscle contraction is sustained hence the muscle tone is maintained. Thus the muscle spindle functions to produce and maintain tone in skeletal muscles (Fig. 10.3).

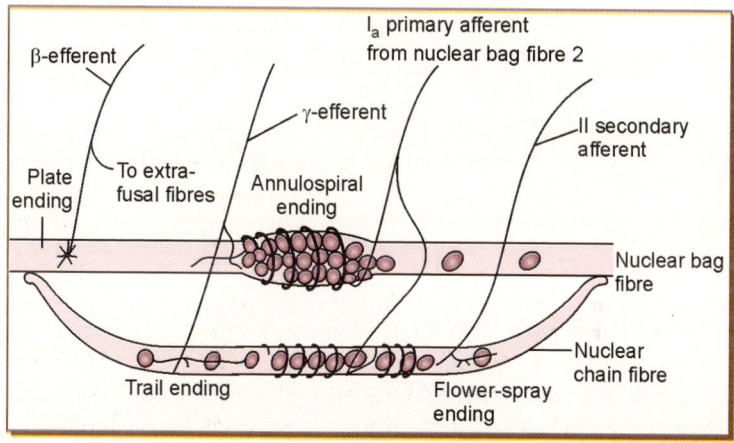

**Fig. 10.3:** Muscle spindle

## ESSENTIAL COMPONENTS OF REFLEX ARC            2.5 (1985)

A reflex arc is constituted by the following components:

1. Receptor
2. Afferent neuron
3. Synapse is integrating centre which may be in spinal cord or higher up in various parts of brain. Centre integrates the signal brought by the afferents and the message sent by the efferents.
4. Efferent neuron
5. Effector organ

Stretch reflex is the simplest reflex that is integrated in the spinal cord. In a stretch reflex:

- **Receptor** is the muscle spindle
- **Afferent** via type I fibres enter the spinal cord and synapse which forms the integrating centre
- **Efferents** via motor nerve supply
- **Effector organs,** i.e. extrafusal muscle fibres and cause their contraction (Fig. 10.4).

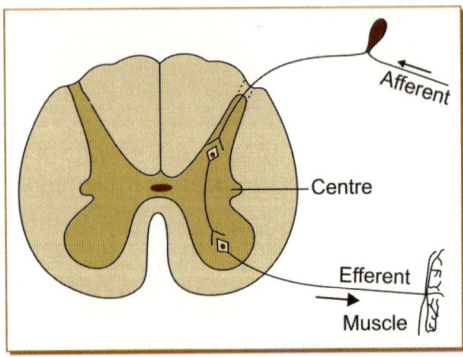

**Fig. 10.4:** Reflex arc

## STRETCH REFLEX, NEURAL PATHWAY OF STRETCH REFLEX
2.5 (1988, 1991, 2000)

When a muscle is stimulated by stretch, it responds by contracting called the stretch reflex. It is a monosynaptic reflex.

**Pathway of stretch reflex**

When a muscle is stretched, stretch receptor, i.e. muscle spindle is stimulated. Afferent impulses are conducted by fast conducting fibres to motor neurons in the spinal cord which innervate the same muscle. Efferent impulses after integration in the spinal cord, cause contraction of the muscle. In this reflex neurotransmitter released at the synapse in the spinal cord is glutamate (Fig. 10.4).

## MUSCLE SPINDLE AND GOLGI TENDON ORGANS 2 (2003)-IPU

| Muscle spindle | Golgi tendon organ |
|---|---|
| • This is the receptor for the stretch reflex. This is a small encapsulated spindle like or fusiform shaped structure located within the fleshy part of the muscle | • This forms the receptor for the inverse stretch reflex. It consists of a netlike collection of knobby nerve endings among the fascicles of a tendon |
| • They are innervated by $I_a$ fibres | • They are innervated by $I_b$ fibres |
| • **Physiological significance:** When a muscle is stretched passively the spindles are | • **Physiological significance:** It acts as a protective reflex to prevent tearing of the muscle. |

*Contd.*

*Contd.*

| Muscle spindle | Golgi tendon organ |
|---|---|
| also stretched which sets up action potentials in the sensory fibres whose frequency is proportionate to the degree of stretch and produces muscle contraction | A strong and potentially damaging muscle force reflexly inhibits the contraction of the muscle producing relaxation instead of trying to maintain the force and risking damage |

**(Refer to question on comparison between stretch and inverse stretch reflex also)**

## COMPARE FLEXOR AND STRETCH REFLEX
**2 (2004)-IPU**

| Flexor reflex | Stretch reflex |
|---|---|
| • This is a type of polysynaptic reflex | • This is a monosynaptic reflex |
| • This occurs in response to painful or noxious stimuli that cause contraction of flexor group of muscles and inhibition of extensor muscles, therefore, the limb stimulated is flexed and withdrawn from the stimulus | • When a skeletal muscle with an intact nerve supply is stretched, it contracts. This response is called the stretch reflex or myotactic reflex |
| • This shows after-discharge and irradiation of the impulse | • They do not show after-discharge or irradiation of the impulse |
| • This has a longer latent period due to slow conducting fibres in the polysynaptic pathway | • This has a shorter latent period because of rapidly conducting afferent fibres |

## COMPARE STRETCH REFLEX AND INVERSE STRETCH REFLEX
**2 (2006, 2009, 2011)**

| Stretch reflex | Inverse stretch reflex |
|---|---|
| • When a skeletal muscle with an intact nerve supply is stretched, it contracts. This response is called the stretch reflex or myotactic reflex | • The relaxation in response to strong stretch is called the inverse stretch reflex |
| • This is a monosynaptic reflex | • This is a bisynaptic reflex |

*Contd.*

*Contd.*

| Stretch reflex | Inverse stretch reflex |
|---|---|
| • The receptor for this reflex is the muscle spindle | • Golgi tendon organ forms the receptor for this reflex |
| • $I_a$ fibres form the afferents for this reflex | • $I_b$ fibres form the afferents for this reflex |
| • This is the fundamental reflex which plays an important role in the control of body postures. It is particularly well developed in posture maintaining muscles, i.e. the back muscles, extensors of the legs and flexors of the arm | • It acts as a protective reflex to prevent tearing of the muscle It also plays an important role in regulating tension during normal muscle activity, i.e. when a muscle contracts, the force developed within the muscle acts as a stimulus for its own relaxation. This is called autogenic inhibition |

## LENGTHENING REACTION                    3 (2004)-IPU

Lengthening reaction or clasp knife effect is response of the spastic muscle to lengthening due to operation of stretch reflex and inverse stretch reflex.

When muscles are hypertonic, moderate stretch produces reflex contraction of the muscle (due to stretch reflex) while strong stretch produces relaxation (due to inverse stretch reflex).

Clinically this sequence of resistance to flexion followed by relaxation when a limb is moved passively is known as **clasp knife effect** (because of its resemblance to the closing of a pocket knife). The physiological name for it is the lengthening reaction because it is the response of a spastic muscle to lengthening.

## MOTOR SYSTEM

### WHAT IS A MOTOR UNIT ? WHAT ARE THE FEATURES OF LOWER MOTOR NEURON LESION?                    2.5 (1990)

A motor unit is constituted by a single motor nerve fibre, i.e. an axon and all the muscle fibres innervated by its terminal branches. All muscle fibres in a motor unit contract together on excitation of the axon. Number of muscle fibres in a unit is variable, but all fibres in a motor unit are of the same type. Motor units may be fast or slow depending upon the type of muscle fibres they have.

Features of lower motor neuron (LMN) lesion:

1. Voluntary muscle contraction and muscle power is lost causing paralysis.
2. Muscle tone is lost producing flaccid paralysis.
3. Marked wasting of muscles occurs (disuse atrophy)
4. Deep tendon reflexes are absent.
5. Plantar reflex is present unless neurons supplying the concerned muscles are affected.
6. Superficial abdominal reflexes are generally retained.
7. Clonus is absent

## WHAT WILL HAPPEN AND WHY IF THERE IS LESION OF PYRAMID IN THE MEDULLA                                        1 (2003)

Lesion of pyramids in the medulla leads to **upper motor neuron (UMN)** type of disorder. Affected muscles become hypertonic producing spastic paralysis due to two causes:

• **Release phenomenon:** Loss of higher inhibitory control
• **Denervation sensitivity** of centres below the transection.

## UPPER MOTOR NEURONS AND THEIR LESION                    2.5 (1993)

Upper motor neurons are neurons present in the brain and brainstem which modulates the activity of α-motor neurons of the spinal cord. From these neurons fibres descend as:

a. Pyramidal
b. Extrapyramidal fibres (EP) and end on α-neurons, directly or indirectly through γ-motor neurons and regulate their activity.

## FEATURES OF UMN LESION

1. Loss of voluntary muscle activity, i.e. paralysis.
2. Increased tone of muscles producing rigidity or spasticity due to lesion in EP pathways.
3. Deep tendon reflexes are exaggerated due to lesion in EP pathways.

4. Babinski sign present due to lesion in pyramidal pathways.
5. Clonus present.
6. Muscle atrophy is not severe.

## FUNCTIONS OF EXTRAPYRAMIDAL SYSTEM　　4 (1985)

- Extrapyramidal (EP) system is composed of descending brainstem and spinal motor pathways which do not pass through medullary pyramids. It is a part of upper motor neurons (UMNs). These fibres descend in anterolateral columns of the spinal cord and relay in motor neurons (mainly the γ-motor neurons) and modulate their activity.
- Anatomically recognisable tracts in this system are:
  1. Vestibulospinal arising from lateral vestibular nucleus in medulla
  2. Rubrospinal from red nucleus located in the midbrain
  3. Tectospinal from superior colliculus
  4. Olivospinal from inferior olivary nucleus
  5. Reticulospinal originating in the reticular formation in the pons and medulla

Through these tracts reticular formation influences the activity of spinal motor neurons. Activity in these tracts is influenced by extrapyramidal fibres arising from the cerebral cortex. Extrapyramidal system has inhibitory as well as facilitatory influence on spinal motor neurons through reticular formation and thus modulate their discharge to skeletal muscles. These tracts discharge to motor neurons innervating postural muscles all the time, and hence produce certain amount of tone in them.

Depending upon the degree of tone or tension in different muscles the posture of the body is adjusted and regulated.

Tone and a balanced posture of the body is essential for performing voluntary motor activity. Extrapyramidal system thus by modulating the γ-efferent discharge maintains the tone in muscles and a stable body posture, thus providing a background for voluntary motor activity.

## EXPLAIN WHY UMN LESIONS PRODUCE SPASTICITY　　1 (2007)

Upper motor neuron lesions are produced due to lesions of the upper motor neurons, i.e neurons in the brain and spinal cord that influence the activity of lower motor neurons. Affected muscles become hypertonic **(spastic paralysis)** due to release phenomenon, i.e. loss of higher inhibitory control over LMNs and denervation hypersensitivity of centres below the transection.

## COMPARE UMN AND LMN LESION 2 (2005)
## BABINSKI'S SIGN                    2.5 (1985, 1986, 1987)

| Lower motor neuron lesion | Upper motor neuron lesion |
|---|---|
| 1. This is due to the lesion of lower motor neurons, i.e the spinal and cranial motor neurons that directly innervate the muscles | 1. It is due to lesion of upper motor neurons, i.e. the neurons in the brain and spinal cord that can influence the activity of the lower motor neurons |
| 2. Single or individual muscle is affected | 2. It involves a group of muscles |
| 3. Muscle becomes completely paralysed (flaccid paralysis) | 3. Affected muscles become hypertonic (spastic paralysis) |
| 4. Disuse atrophy of the muscle occurs | 4. The muscle atrophy is not severe |
| 5. All reflexes (superficial and deep) are completely lost | 5. Deep reflexes are hyperactive due to increased γ-motor discharge. Amongst superficial reflexes only abdominal, cremastric and anal reflexes are lost |
| 6. Babinski sign is not elicited | 6. Babinski sign is elicited |

## EXPLAIN WHAT WILL HAPPEN TO PLANTAR REFLEX IF THE PYRAMIDS ARE DAMAGED                    1 (2004)

The Babinski's sign will become positive if the pyramids are damaged. Babinski's sign is a neurological sign of clinical importance. It is elicited by stretching the skin of the lateral aspect of sole of the foot. This sign is said to be present when the abovementioned stimulation results in dorsiflexion of the big toe and fanning of other toes. It is only present when there is a neurological lesion affecting the pyramidal tracts in upper motor neuron lesion.

In a normal person it is seen as plantar flexion, i.e. stimulation of lateral aspect of foot produces plantar flexion of toes. The Babinski's sign is believed to be a withdrawl reflex normally held in check by the pyramidal tracts.

It is normally present in infants (a child less than 1 year of age) as the pyramidal tracts are not fully developed till the age of 1 year. It is of value in localizing a lesion of the nervous system.

## EXPLAIN WHY LESIONS OF THE INTERNAL CAPSULE PRODUCE CONTRALATERAL SPASTIC HEMIPLEGIA    1 (2003)-IPU

In the lower part of the medulla 80 to 85% of the fibres of the descending pyramidal tract cross to the opposite side, enter the lateral white column and descend down as lateral corticospinal tract or indirect pyramidal tract. Because of this crossing of the fibres lesions of the internal capsule through which pyramidal tract fibres pass produces contralateral spastic hemiplegia.

## DIFFERENCE BETWEEN PYRAMIDAL AND EXTRAPYRAMIDAL SYSTEM    2.5 (1989)

## COMPARE MEDIAL AND LATERAL DESCENDING MOTOR SYSTEMS    2 (2004)-IPU

| Pyramidal tracts lateral | Extrapyramidal tracts medial |
| --- | --- |
| 1. Origin: 30% of fibres arise from the motor cortex, area 4 in the precentral gyrus, 30% from the premotor cortex and remaining 40% from the somatosensory areas I and II and adjacent parietal lobe association cortex | 1. This is made up of those areas in the CNS that are concerned with muscular movements and posture. Its fibres have many synapse in their descending path with cells of nuclear masses on the way which include: Nuclei of the cerebral cortex, basal ganglia, hypothalamus and nuclei of the reticular formation in the brainstem. |
| 2. Its axons pass without relay to the spinal segmental levels where they form synapses with either interneurons in the dorsal horn or directly with motor neurons themselves | 2. They have many synapses in their descending path with cells of nuclei of the striatum (caudate and putamen), the globus pallidus, the hypothalamus and the nuclei of the reticular formation |
| 3. They have greater influence over motor neurons that | 3. They are more involved with coordination of the large muscle |

*Contd.*

*Contd.*

| Pyramidal tracts lateral | Extrapyramidal tracts medial |
|---|---|
| control muscles involved in fine movements particularly of fingers and hands | groups used in maintenance of upright posture, in locomotion, and in head and body movements when turning towards a specific stimulus |
| 4. Lesion of this tract produces spasticity | 4. Its lesion produces rigidity |

## DIFFERENTIATE BETWEEN SPASTICITY AND RIGIDITY
**2.5 (1986), 2 (2000)**

Spasticity and rigidity both are clinical signs due to hypertonia of skeletal muscles.

The term spasticity is used to describe hypertonia due to lesions of pyramidal tract. The hypertonia is of clasp-knife type and is seen when the limb is passively flexed or extended. Hence it is said to be stretch sensitive. Spasticity due to cerebral or brainstem lesion has a characteristic distribution. The upper limb flexors and lower limb extensors are mainly involved.

Rigidity is hypertonia seen due to lesion of basal ganglia. It is of two types:

   i. **Cog-wheel:** Where resistance to passive stretch is variable
  ii. **Lead pipe type:** Resistance to passive stretch is uniform, throughout the passive movement.

## SPINAL CORD

## EFFECTS OF THE DORSAL NERVE ROOTS SECTION    2.5 (1985)

Dorsal nerve roots carry afferent impulses to the spinal cord. Section of dorsal nerve roots brings about the following effects in corresponding body segments.

1. **Sensory loss:** All sensation, i.e. pain, touch and temperature sensation from the skin is lost
2. Loss of visceral sensibility
3. Loss of muscle tone
4. Absence of superficial and deep reflexes
5. Postural disturbances and defective gait may occur due to loss of input to higher centres from proprioceptors regarding the position and movement of joints.

## TABES DORSALIS                              2 (2002)
## WHAT WILL HAPPEN AND WHY TO SENSATIONS IN TABES DORSALIS                                      1 (2007)

In tabes dorsalis degeneration of the dorsal (sensory) roots occur affecting specially fibres in the dorsal columns and fibres that convey pain. This disease is usually caused by syphilis.

### Characteristic Features

- **Lightening pain** of varying intensity which comes in attacks with pain free intervals in between. This is due to stimulation of pain fibres in the dorsal nerve roots.
- Loss or decrease in **pain sensibility** produces:
  - Trophic disturbances such as perforating ulcers at pressure points.
  - Anaesthesia around the anus, legs, upper chest and inner border of the hands due to involvement of the dorsal nerve roots in the lumbosacral and cervicothoracic regions of the spinal cord.
  - Anaesthesia of the central part of the face due to involvement of the Vth cranial nerve.
  - Charcot joints occur due to repeated trauma to the joints
- **Loss of deep sensibility:** Loss of position sense, passive movements and vibration sense.
- **Reflexes.** Deep tendon reflexes that depend on intactness of the reflex arc are lost like knee jerk, ankle, biceps and triceps jerk
- Marked disturbance of voluntary movement.

## SPINAL SHOCK              2.5 (1993), 2 (2006), 3 (2012)
## EXPLAIN WHY COMPLETE TRANSECTION OF THE SPINAL CORD PRODUCES SPINAL SHOCK                       1 (2003)-IPU

Spinal shock occurs when there is complete transection of the spinal cord. It is the period immediately following transection. During which there is no sensory and motor activity below the site of the lesion.

### Clinical Features

1. Patient feels he is cut into two portions, the upper portion (higher centres and the mind) are clear but the entire body below the level of the lesion is completely deprived of all activity.

2. Muscles are completely paralysed **(flaccid paralysis)**. There is complete loss of muscle tone.
3. All reflexes (superficial and deep) are markedly decreased or lost.
4. All the sensations below the lesion are lost.
5. The urinary bladder and rectum are generally paralysed, however, the sphincter vesicae recovers very rapidly resulting in retention of urine.
6. All the sympathetic vasoconstrictor fibres leave the spinal cord between $T_1$ and $L_2$ spinal segments, therefore:
   a. A transection below $L_2$ produces no effect or very little fall of blood pressure
   b. A transection at $T_1$ level cuts off all thoracolumbar sympathetic neurons from the medullary cardiovascular centre producing a marked fall in MBP from a resting value of 100 mm Hg to 40 mm Hg
   c. Fall in blood pressure is less marked as the section shifts more distally towards $L_2$.
7. If lesion is at the level of $T_6$, all impulses coming from the abdominal viscera are cut off from the brain.

Duration of spinal shock is a direct function of the degree of encephalisation of motor functions, i.e. level of development of motor functions. It lasts for about 3 weeks in man.

## Cause of Spinal Shock

Cessation of tonic bombardment of spinal neurons by excitatory impulses in descending pathways plays a role in the development of spinal shock. In addition spinal inhibitory interneurons that normally are inhibited themselves may be released from this descending inhibition to become disinhibited.

## DIFFERENCES BETWEEN COMPLETE AND INCOMPLETE TRANSECTION OF SPINAL CORD   **2.5 (1987)**

| Complete transection | Incomplete transection |
|---|---|
| 1. Spinal cord is completely cut into two and is an acute condition | 1. Lesion may be acute or slow in onset. Some fibres particularly those of the extrapyramidal tract escape injury |

*Contd.*

*Contd.*

| Complete transection | Incomplete transection |
|---|---|
| 2. Stage of spinal shock is always present with loss of sensory and motor activity | 2. If the destruction of the cord is gradual, stage of spinal shock is missing |
| 3. During recovery phase reflex activity first appears in the flexor muscles, later in the extensors producing paraplegia in flexion | 3. Reflex tone returns in the extensor group of muscles first, producing paraplegia in extension |
| 4. Cross extensor reflex is feeble | 4. Marked crossed extensor response is seen |
| 5. Deep reflexes are feeble | 5. Deep reflexes are exaggerated |
| 6. All sensations below the level of lesion are permanently abolished | 6. Some ascending tracts have escaped injury, hence some sensations may be present |

## BROWN SEQUARD SYNDROME

**2 (2003)-IPU, 2, 2.5 (2003), 2 (2007)**

A hemisection of the spinal cord causes a characteristic and easily recognisable clinical picture that reflects damage to ascending sensory (dorsal column pathway, ventrolateral spinothalamic tract) and descending motor (corticospinal tract) pathways, which is called **Brown Sequard syndrome**.

**Changes below the lesion of hemisection (on the opposite side)**

### Sensory Changes

- Complete loss of pain, temperature and crude touch due to damage to the spinothalamic fibres which come from the opposite side.
- Kinaesthetic sensations, fine touch, etc. will persist because the posterior column of the opposite side are not damaged.

### Motor Changes

Either no paralysis or paralysis of few muscles occurs of the upper motor neuron type. This is due to the possible involvement of some fibres of direct pyramidal tracts of the same side when these fibres cross.

Therefore, below the level of lesion on the same side there is extensive motor loss but little sensory loss, while on the opposite side, there is extensive sensory loss but little motor loss. This phenomenon is called **Brown Sequard syndrome**.

Although a pure hemisection is rare the syndrome is fairly common because it can be caused by spinal cord tumour, spinal cord trauma, degenerative disc diseases and ischaemia.

## Treatment

Drug treatment depends on etiology and time since onset of the syndrome. High doses of corticosteroids are of value particularly if administered after the onset of such a spinal cord injury. Steroids decreases the inflammation by suppressing polymorphonuclear leukocytes and reverse the increase in capillary permeability.

## WHAT IS SYRINGOMYELIA? MENTION ITS CHARACTERISTIC FEATURES                                        2.5 (1991)

## EXPLAIN WHY DISSOCIATED ANAESTHESIA IS PRESENT IN PATIENTS SUFFERING FROM SYRINGOMYELIA       1 (2003)-IPU

## WHAT WILL HAPPEN AND WHY IF CAVITATION OCCURS AROUND CENTRE OF CANAL IN SPINAL CORD       1 (2004)

Syringomyelia is a clinical condition in which an excess outgrowth of neuroglia in grey matter around central canal of spinal cord occurs. Cavity formation may also be there.

The lesion though rare mostly involves the cervical region of the cord, thus affecting arms and hands. Ascending sensory tract carrying sensation of crude touch, pain and temperature to opposite side are affected but dorsal column afferents are spared.

## Clinical Sign

1. Loss of pain and temperature sense due to damage to fibres carrying these sensations which cross in the anterior white commisure.
2. Touch is retained as it has a dual pathway, fibres that cross in the grey column get damaged while the fibres which descend in the dorsal column escape.

   (1) and (2), thus producing dissociated anaesthesia, i.e. loss of temperature and pain sensation while sense of touch is retained.

3. At the level of lesion initially the cavitation and gliosis spreads and involves the anterior horn cells producing flaccid paralysis of the muscles (usually of the hands).

In later stages involvement of the pyramidal and extra-pyramidal tracts leads to progressive spastic paraplegia, i.e. spastic paralysis of the legs.

## CONTROL OF BODY MOVEMENTS AND POSTURE

### COMPARE DECORTICATE AND DECEREBRATE RIGIDITY   **2** (2010)

| Decorticate rigidity | Decerebrate rigidity |
|---|---|
| 1. Here the whole cerebral cortex is removed but the basal ganglia and the brainstem are intact | 1. This is produced by transection of the brainstem at the superior border of the pons in animals between the two colliculi. |
| 2. **Postural findings:** Moderate rigidity is present due to loss of cortical area that inhibits spinal γ motor neuron discharge via the reticular formation: | 2. **Postural findings:** There is a marked increase in tone of the extensor group of muscles |
| i. The legs are fully extended, arms lie across the chest, semi-flexed at the elbow, forearm slightly pronated and the wrists and fingers flexed | i. The limbs are hyperextended, the tail and head are dorsiflexed and the back is concave due to extreme hyperextension of the spine |
| ii. It is seen only when the animal is at rest | ii. The animal stays in the position in which it is placed since there are no righting reflexes |
| 3. **Postural reflexes:** The typical neck reflexes and righting reflexes can be obtained Hopping and placing reactions are seriously disrupted by decortications | 3. **Postural reflexes:** Tonic neck and tonic labyrinthine reflexes are present |
| 4. **Significance in man:** It is seen commonly on the hemiplegic side after haemorrhage or thrombosis in the internal capsule | 4. **Significance in man:** In true decerebrate rigidity there is extension of all 4 limbs. Although the defect that is produced is incompatible with life but it helps in supporting the body against gravity |

## DIFFERENCE BETWEEN MIDCOLLICULAR AND ISCHAEMIC DECEREBRATION      2.5 (1987, 1993)

## COMPARE CLASSIC AND ISCHAEMIC DECEREBRATION
### 2 (2003)-IPU

| Classic decerebration | Ischaemic decerebration |
|---|---|
| 1. It involves transection of brainstem between two colliculi called Sherrington (or classical) decerebration | 1. It is produced by tying both the carotid arteries and the basilar arteries at the junction of the pons and medulla |
| 2. It is usually a fatal traumatic procedure | 2. It is relatively a safe procedure |
| 3. It leads to decerebrate rigidity of the Sherringtonian type that is particularly evident in the extensor antigravity muscles | 3. It produces a marked increase in the muscle tone that resembles decerebrate rigidity |
| 4. Mechanism of development: It is due to a release phenomenon which increases γ-motor neuron activity called **γ-rigidity** | 4. It is due to excessive discharge of the α motor neurons from vestibulospinal tracts, therefore, also called **α-rigidity** |
| 5. Effect of deafferentation: Hypertonia is abolished indicating that it is reflex in nature | 5. Hypertonia in no way is reduced indicating that hypertonia is induced indirectly |
| 6. It gets abolished by administration of chlorpromazine or local anesthetic procaine which abolishes γ-motor neuron activity | 6. It remains unaffected by administration of such drugs |
| 7. Removal of the anterior lobe of the cerebellum increases the rigidity | 7. It is not affected by removal of the anterior lobe of the cerebellum |

## EFFECT OF LESION OF MIDBRAIN      2.5 (1992)

In the midbrain long ascending and descending nerve tracts and nuclei of third and fourth cranial nerves are packed in a small area. Lesion of midbrain hence produces:

1. Hemiplegia and loss of sensations on opposite half of the body excluding the head region.
2. Movements of eyeball are affected on the same side of the body.
3. Light reflex is absent on the same side and the pupil is dilated.
4. Ptosis on the affected side may occur.

## HOW IS NORMAL POSTURE OF BODY MAINTAINED    10
## CONTROL OF POSTURE    2.5 (2011)

Normal posture of the body is maintained due to tone in postural muscles. Tone in postural muscle is essential for the following:

1. Support body weight
2. To maintain upright balanced position of the body.
3. Produces a stable background posture by adjusting tone in certain muscles during performance of voluntary motor activity.

Tone in muscles is a state of tension due to subtetanic contraction of muscles. Muscles of neck, trunk and lower limbs are main postural muscles and in a normal person certain amount of tone is always present in them.

Muscles are in contracted state due to the presence of stretch reflex. Stretch reflex is a basic reflex integrated in the spinal cord causing muscle contraction, but to maintain tone, the contraction of muscles has to be sustained. So, there is supraspinal control on stretch reflex through γ-motor neurons to sustain muscle contraction and consequently the muscle tone. Various extrapyramidal motor pathways influence the activity of γ-motor neurons through brainstem reticular formation. Through the influence on γ-motor neurons tone in postural muscles is reflexly maintained. These reflexes are known as postural reflexes (Fig. 10.5).

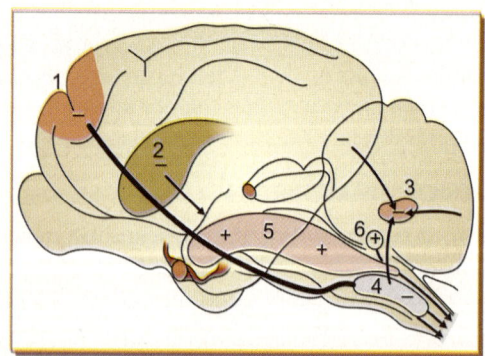

**Fig. 10.5:** Areas in the cat brain where stimulation produces facilitation or inhibition of stretch reflexes, (1) motor cortex, (2) basal ganglia, (3) cerebellum, (4) reticular inhibitory area, (5) reticular facilitatory area, (6) vestibular nuclei

**Postural reflexes:** Various postural reflexes are initiated from sensory receptors in the skin, muscles, joints and vestibular apparatus and are integrated at different levels of CNS. Postural reflexes operate to adjust tone in neck, trunk and limb muscle to produce and maintain errect and balanced body posture. Postural reflexes are:

1. **Static:** Causing sustained contraction of muscles at rest.

2. **Dynamic:** Causing momentary contraction of muscles to support body during movements.

   I. **Spinal reflexes:** To support the body weight

     a. **Stretch reflex:** Basic reflex

     b. **Positive supporting reaction:** Increases tone in limb extensors and limbs act like pillars to support body weight. This reflex is initiated as the sole touches the ground.

  II. **Tonic labyrinthine reflexes:** As the position of the head in space is altered receptors in vestibular apparatus are stimulated. Reflexes with centre in the medulla is initiated and tone in extensors is altered to maintain balanced posture.

 III. **Tonick neck reflexes:** As the position of head is changed in relation to the body, afferents from proprioceptors in neck are stimulated and tone is increased in limb muscles accordingly to maintain a balanced posture.

 IV. **Righting reflexes:** If the stable attitude of body is disturbed, righting reflexes are initiated from vestibular apparatus and tone reflexly increases in neck and trunk muscles and the posture is maintained. These reflexes are integrated in the midbrain. There are neck and body righting reflexes. Righting reflexes are also initiated from visual cues and integrated in the cerebral cortex to correct body posture.

## DECEREBRATE RIGIDITY      3 (2004)-IPU, 2.5 (2007)

Transection of the brainstem at the superior border of the pons in animals between the two colliculi is called **decerebrate preparation**. There is a marked increase in tone of extensors, i.e. antigravity muscles occurring immediately after decerebration. This is called **decerebrate rigidity**.

**Table 13.1:** Principal postural reflexes

| Reflex | Stimulus | Response | Receptor | Integrated in |
|---|---|---|---|---|
| Stretch reflexes | Stretch | Contraction of muscle | Muscle spindles | Spinal cord, medulla |
| Positive supporting (magnet) reaction | Contact with sole or palm | Foot extended to support body | Proprioceptors in distal flexors | Spinal cord |
| Negative supporting reaction | Stretch | Release of positive supporting reaction | Proprioceptors in extensors | Spinal cord |
| Tonic labyrinthine reflexes | Gravity | Contraction of limb extensor muscles | Otolithic organs | Medulla |
| Tonic neck reflexes | Head turned: | Change in pattern of extensor contractions | Neck proprioceptors | Medulla |
| | 1. To side | 1. Extension of limbs on side to which head is turned | | |
| | 2. Up | 2. Hind legs flex | | |
| | 3. Down | 3. Forelegs flex | | |
| Labyrinthine righting reflexes | Gravity | Head kept level | Otolithic organs | Midbrain |
| Neck righting reflexes | Stretch of neck | Righting of thorax and shoulders, then pelvis | Muscle spindles | Midbrain |
| Body on head righting reflexes | Pressure on side of body | Righting of head | Exteroceptors | Midbrain |
| Body on body righting reflexes | Pressure on side of body | Righting of body even when head held sideways | Exteroceptors | Midbrain |
| Optical righting reflexes | Visual cues | Righting of head | Eyes | Cerebral cortex |

## Characteristic Features

- Hyperextension of all four limbs
- Dorsiflexion of tail and head
- Extreme hyperextension of the spine (opisthotonos) produces concave configuration of the back
- The animal can be made to stand on all four limbs but is easily toppled by a slight push
- Righting reflexes are absent, the animal stays in the position in which it is placed.

**Postural reflexes** present in decerebrate animal are those which have their integration centre in the spinal cord or medulla or pons. These include:

- Stretch reflex
- Positive supporting reaction
- Negative supporting reaction
- Crossed extensor reflex
- Tonic neck and tonic labyrinthine

Decerebrate rigidity is a **release phenomenon**. It is a state of release in which hyperactive proprioceptive reflexes are responsible for a state of increased muscle tone. The hyperactivity of muscle reflexes is due to:

- Release of γ-motor neurons from an inhibitory extrapyramidal discharge, which increases muscle spindle sensitivity to stretch.
- A residual facilitatory discharge from descending facilitatory reticular projection to γ-motor neurons contributes to the state of functional increase of the stretch reflexes.

### Significance of decerebrate rigidity in man

The extensor muscles of the lower limb, the muscles of the back and flexor muscles of the upper limb are the antigravity muscles. Contraction of these muscles helps to maintain a comfortable balanced posture in the upright position.

In man true decerebrate rigidity causes extension of all the four limbs. Although the defect that is produced is incompatible with life but helps in providing support against gravity.

## EXPLAIN WHY RIGIDITY DISAPPEARS IN A DECEREBRATE ANIMALS AFTER DEAFFERENTATION      1 (2004)

Decerebrate rigidity is a release phenomenon. It is a state of release in which hyperactive proprioceptive reflexes are responsible for a state of increased muscle tone. The hyperactivity of muscle reflexes is due to:

- Release of γ-motor neurons from an inhibitory extrapyramidal discharge.
- A residual facilitatory discharge from descending facilitatory reticular projection to γ-motor neurons contributes to the state of functional increase of the stretch reflexes. Rigidity disappears after deafferentation as the stretch reflex is abolished.

## RETICULAR FORMATION

### FUNCTIONS OF RETICULAR FORMATION OF BRAINSTEM
### 4.5 (1993)

Situated in the core of the brainstem, i.e. medulla, pons and mesencephalon are areas of diffused neurons known as *reticular formation* (RF). The lower end of RF is continuous with the interneurons of spinal cord.

Various ascending and descending fibre tracts between spinal cord and brain give collaterals to reticular neurons. Reticular neurons are both motor and sensory and it also contains various centres for regulating autonomic activity. It also has certain specific nuclei like vestibular, raphe, etc.

Input signals to RF are from:

1. Spinothalamic tract
2. Spinoreticular tract
3. Vestibular nuclei
4. Cerebellum
5. Basal ganglion
6. Sensory and motor tracts
7. Hypothalamus

Output pathways from the reticular formation:

1. Medial and lateral vestibulospinal tracts from vestibular nuclei.
2. Reticulospinal tracts from pontine and medullary nuclei.

3. To higher centres—A diffuse output to various areas of the cerebral cortex.

Autonomic centres situated in the RF are:

1. Cardiac and vasomotor centres
2. Centres controlling respiration
3. Vomiting centre
4. Deglutition centre

Functions of reticular formation:

1. The RAS and related reticular components are concerned with conscious alert state of mind that makes perception possible.
2. There is a major input from the anterolateral systems into the midbrain reticular formation which activates the RAS, which in turn maintains the cortex in the alert state.
3. The descending fibres in it:
   - Inhibit transmission in sensory pathways in the spinal cord
   - They are concerned with spasticity and adjustment of stretch reflexes that control body movement and posture.
4. It contains many of the areas concerned with regulation of heart rate, BP and respiration.
5. It contains cell bodies and fibres of many of the serotonergic, cholinergic, noradrenergic and adrenergic systems.

## CEREBELLUM

### FUNCTIONAL DIVISION OF CEREBELLUM          2.5 (2003)-IPU

Functionally, the cerebellum is divided into different parts depending upon the connections they make with other parts of the motor control system:

- The flocculonodular lobe is functionally related to the vestibular apparatus and therefore also called **vestibulo-cerebellum**. It is concerned with control of body posture, equilibrium and the vestibulo-ocular reflex.
- The anterior lobe and parts of the posterior lobe that receive information from parts of the spinal cord constitute the **spinocerebellum**. It occupies the median portion of the cerebellar cortex and receive proprioceptive input from the body.

It is concerned with control of axial and limb muscles and postural reflexes.

• The remaining part of the posterior lobe receives information from the cerebral cortex and pons, thus called the **neocerebellum**. It occupies the lateral portions of the cerebellar cortex. It is concerned with skilled voluntary movements.

**NEURONAL CIRCUIT OF CEREBELLUM**     **3 (2004)-IPU**

**CONNECTIONS AND FUNCTIONS OF CEREBELLUM**

       **5 (2004)-IPU**

**FUNCTIONS OF CEREBELLUM**     **2.5 (2004)**

**CEREBELLAR FUNCTION TESTS**     **2.5 (2002)**

**ROLE OF CEREBELLUM IN MOTOR CONTROL**    **4 (2003)-IPU**

**CEREBELLAR CIRCUITRY**     **(2001)**

**DESCRIBE THE IMPORTANT AFFERENT AND EFFERENT CONNECTIONS OF CEREBELLUM. DESCRIBE SOME OF THE SYMPTOMS OF CEREBELLAR DISEASE**     **10 (1987)**

**FUNCTIONS OF CEREBELLUM**     **4 (1993)**

**ENUMERATE CONNECTIONS OF CEREBELLUM. DESCRIBE THE FUNCTIONS OF CEREBELLUM. WHAT IS DYSDIADOCHO-KINESIA?**     **10 (1994)**

### Connections of Cerebellum

**Afferent pathways**

I. **From central nervous system**

   a. Corticopontocerebellar pathway: Originates from motor and some sensory areas of cerebral cortex → pontine nuclei → opposite cerebellum.

   b. Olivocerebellar pathway: From inferior olivary nucleus to all parts of cerebellum. This pathway is excited by fibres from motor cortex, basal ganglia, reticular formation and spinal cord.

   c. Vestibulocerebellar: From vestibular apparatus → vestibular nuclei → flocculonodular lobe.

   d. Reticulocerebellar: Originates in various portions of reticular formation and terminates mainly in the vermis.

   e. Tectocerebellar: From superior and inferior colliculi carrying auditory and visual impulses to the cerebellum.

II. **From periphery**

    a. Dorsal and ventral spinocerebellar tracts: Bringing proprioceptive sensations from all parts of the body except head and neck.

    b. Cuneocerebellar: Carries proprioceptive impulse from head and neck and joins dorsospinocerebellar tracts.

    c. Spinoreticular pathway: Originate in dorsolateral part of the spinal cord to reticular formation and then to cerebellum.

    d. Spino-olivary pathway: From spinal cord → olivary nucleus → cerebellum.

## Efferent Pathways

I. From lateral hemisphere to ventrolateral and ventrobasal nuclei of thalamus.

II. From vermis through fastigial nucleus to reticular formation.

III. From intermediate zone to:

    a. Basal ganglia

    b. Thalamus

    c. Reticular formation of brainstem

IV. Flocculonodular lobe to vestibular nuclei

**(Note: If the connection are to be enumerated, just name the pathways)**

## Functions of Cerebellum

Functionally, cerebellum is divided into three parts (Fig. 10.6).

I. Vermis and adjacent medial part of hemisphere also known as spinocerebellum.

II. Lateral parts of hemisphere or neocerebellum.

III. Flocculonodular lobe or vestibulocerebellum.

**I. Function of spinocerebellum**

    1. Spinocerebellum functions to bring about **coordinated, smooth motor activity** by controlling rate, range and direction of movement by breaking and damping the motor activity at the appropriate moment. Cerebellum receives information from the peripheral parts of body through sensory receptors continuously. It also receives information on the desired program of muscle contraction from cerebral motor control areas. It compares

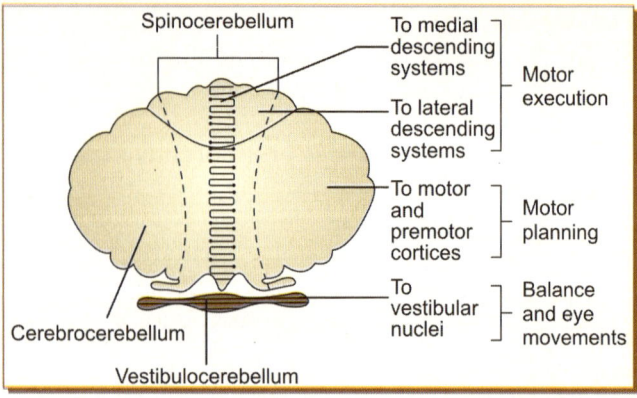

**Fig. 10.6:** Functional division of the cerebellum

the instantaneous state of body as depicted by peripheral information with the status initiated by motor cortex and transmits required corrective signals if needed to motor cortex to vary the level of activation thus making the movements smooth and orderly.

2. **Control of muscle tone and posture:** Through its connection with reticular formation and other structures in the brainstem it influences the stretch reflex and hence muscle tone and postural reflexes. In humans it facilitates the stretch reflex.

3. **Control of fast ballistic movements**

4. **Extramotor predictive functions:** It functions to predict the rate of progression of visual and auditory stimuli in space.

II. **Functions of neocerebellum:** This part has connections with association areas of the neocortex and helps in planning and programming of motor activity along with the basal ganglia. Information in turn is transmitted to the motor and premotor areas of the cerebral cortex.

III. **Functions of flocculonodular lobe:** This part functions to maintain body equilibrium. It has connections with vestibular nuclei of the brainstem and helps to maintain reflex tone in certain neck and trunk muscles to maintain erect balanced body posture.

## Symptoms of Cerebellar Disease

I. **Disturbance in posture**

a. **Atonia or hypotonia:** The muscle tone is either completely lost or reduced on the affected side due to loss of facilitatory effect of the neocerebellum.

- **Nystagmus:** It is defined as a tremor of the eyeball which occurs when the subject tries to fix his eyes at an object.
- **Deep reflexes:** Deep reflexes become weak and pendular. This is due to hypotonia of the quadriceps muscles.

II. **Disturbance of voluntary movements**

- **Asthenia:** Feebleness of movement
- **Ataxia:** Incoordination of movement
- **Decomposition of movement:** The movement seems to occur in stages
- **Asynergia:** Lack of coordination between protagonists, antagonists and synergists
- **Dysmetria:** The movement is poorly carried out in direction, range and force, therefore, the movement overshoots the intended mark called past-pointing **(hypermetria)** or falls short of it **(hypometria)**. It results in the loss of the neural circuit required to control the strength and duration of movement.
- **Intentional tremors:** patients cannot perform activity smoothly. If they reach for an object their movements are jerky and accompanied by oscillating to and fro tremors that become more marked as the hand approaches the object. The tremors are course and occur at the rate of 4–6 times/second and can be clearly seen when that part is used in voluntary movement. They occur because an entire movement cannot be directed by a single motor command.
- **Gait:** Drunken gait.
- **Speech:** It is slow and slurring due to the imperfect use of movements of the laryngeal muscles and tongue.

## Cerebellar Function Tests

i. **Finger-nose test:** The patient is asked to place the index finger of his extended arm over his nose with his eyes closed.

ii. **Rebound phenomenon:** If the patient is asked to flex his forearm against resistance, then the resistance is suddenly released, the patient cannot break the movement and the released forearm flies backward and strikes his face.

iii. **Adiadochokinesia:** The patient is unable to carry out rapidly alternate and opposite movements like rapid supination and pronation of the forearm.

iv. **Heel-knee test:** The patient lies in the lying down movement. He is asked to touch his knee by the opposite heel, then moving the heel along the tibia downwards. This test detects decomposition of movement.

## COMPARE FUNCTIONS OF NEOCEREBELLUM AND SPINOCEREBELLUM                                   2 (2007)

**Spinocerebellum** is the region of the cerebellum that receives proprioceptive input from the body as well as a copy of the 'motor plan' from the motor cortex. By comparing plan with performance, it smoothes and coordinates ongoing movements.

It is also concerned with movement of the trunk and limb muscles as well as the postural reflexes.

**Neocerebellum (cerebrocerebellum)** is phylogenetically the newest part of the cerebellum that reach their maximum development in humans. It interacts with the motor cortex in the planning and programming of movements along with basal ganglion.

## EXPLAIN WHY IN CEREBELLAR LESIONS SYMPTOMS ARE SEEN ON THE SAME SIDE          1 (2004)

Each cerebellar hemisphere influences the opposite cerebral cortex. The motor cortex in turn via the corticospinal tracts, controls the movements of the opposite side of the body. Because of this double decussation, each cerebellar hemisphere controls voluntary movement on its own side of the body. Hence, cerebellar lesions lead to symptoms on the same side of the body.

## THALAMUS

## FUNCTIONS OF THALAMUS                                              2.5 (1988)

Thalamus is a subcortical mass of grey matter and a part of diencephalon. It lies on each side of the IIIrd ventricle and form posteromedial boundary of internal capsule.

Through its extensive input and output fibres, it performs various functions like:

1. Dorsoventral nuclei of thalamus are important **relay station** for specific ascending sensory pathways except sense of smell.

2. Ventrolateral nuclei are relay station for **cerebellocerebral projections**. This pathway between cerebellum and motor cortex is essential for smooth and coordinated motor activity. It also receives input from the basal ganglia for motor control.

3. Non-specific ascending reticular activating system (RAS) relays in the intralaminar nuclei and then to various diffuse areas of the cerebral cortex and produces an alert wakeful, conscious state of mind.

4. Through its connections (involving anterior nuclei) with hypothalamus and cerebral cortex, thalamus plays an important role in **emotions and personality**.

5. **Role in memory:** Plays a role in **memory process** through its connections with the hypothalamus.

## EEG AND SLEEP

### PHYSIOLOGICAL BASIS OF EEG                    3 (2004)

The activity recorded in the EEG is that of rhythmically discharging cell bodies in the most superficial layers of the cortical grey matter. The EEG is due to graded potentials which are summated postsynaptic potentials in the brain neurons.

The EEG recorded from the scalp is a measure of the summation of dendritic postsynaptic potentials rather than action potentials. The dendrites of the cortical neurons are a forest of similarly oriented densely packed units in the superficial layers of the cerebral cortex. Propagated potentials can be generated in the dendrites. In addition recurrent axon collaterals end on dendrites in the superficial layers. As excitatory and inhibitory endings on the dendrites of each cell become active, current flows into and out of these current sinks and sources from rest of the dendritic processes and the cell body. The cell body–dendritic relationship is therefore of a constantly shifting dipole. Current flow in this dipole produces wave-like potential fluctuations in a volume conductor. When the sum of the dendritic activity is negative relative to the cell body, the neuron is depolarised and hyperexcitable, when it is positive the neuron is hyperpolarised and less excitable.

## ALPHA RHYTHM OF EEG                         2.5 (1985, 1989)

Alpha rhythm of EEG is one of the fundamental rhythms seen in adult EEG in relaxed state of mind with eyes closed. Usual frequency of alpha rhythm varies between 8 and 13 cycle/sec and have average amplitude of 50 μV.

It is a predominant rhythm when EEG is recorded over parietal and occipital areas of the scalp.

It is believed to arise primarily from diencephalon via non-specific thalamocortical projections.

It appears as a result of synchronized activity of neurons and disappears if eyes are opened or an external stimulus is given or if one concentrates or the person is engaged in some mental activity. This disappearance of alpha activity is known as **alpha-block**, when alpha waves are replaced by fast and irregular waveform due desynchronised activity of neurons (Fig. 10.7).

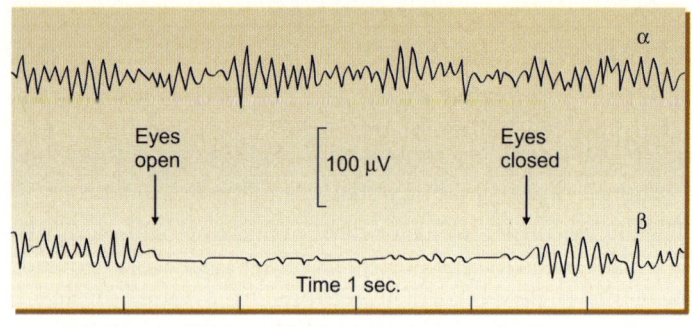

**Fig. 10.7:** Normal human electroencephalogram (EEG)

## REM SLEEP              2.5 (1992), 3 (2004)-IPU, 4 (2003)-IPU

Sleep is the period of decreased cortical activity which appears to be essential for proper functioning of the brain.

There are two different kinds of sleep:

1. REM sleep
2. Non-REM sleep

## REM Sleep

Also known as '**paradoxical sleep**' because it is characterized by rapid, irregular and low-voltage activity in the EEG which is characteristic of an alert mind though the person is asleep. It has the following features:

1. During this phase the sleep is associated with dreams.

2. Threshold of arousal by external stimuli is elevated.

3. There are rapid and roving movements of eyeball, hence the name rapid eye movement, i.e. REM sleep.

4. Large phasic potentials originating from the pons and pass rapidly to the lateral geniculate bodies and finally to the occipital cortex called pontogeniculo-occipital or PGO spikes can be observed during REM sleep.

5. There is decreased tone in skeletal muscle due to activation of an area in the reticular formation of the medulla which functions to decrease muscle tone by inhibiting the stretch-reflex.

## REM AND NON-REM SLEEP                          2.5 (1988)
## COMPARE SLOW WAVE AND REM SLEEP        2 (2002, 2003)

REM and non-REM are the two types of sleep, but they are different from each other.

| REM sleep | Non-REM sleep |
|---|---|
| 1. It is also called paradoxical sleep | 1. It is also called slow wave sleep |
| 2. EEG shows rapid, irregular and low-voltage activity | 2. EEG shows slow- and high-voltage activity called sleep spindles |
| 3. Muscle tone is reduced | 3. Tone not reduced |
| 4. There are rapid and roving movements of the eye | 4. No such movements occur |
| 5. PGO spikes can be recorded during REM sleep | 5. PGO spikes are not observed. Synchronizing activity from the thalamus is seen |
| 6. Associated with dreaming | 6. Dreaming does not occur usually |

## BASAL GANGLIA

**Basal ganglia:** Include a group of distinct subcortical nuclei of forebrain, namely:

1. Caudate nucleus
2. Putamen
3. Globus pallidus

Caudate nucleus and putamen are together known as **corpus striatum** or **neostriatum**.

Putamen and globus pallidus together constitute **lenticular nucleus**. The globus pallidus is divided into an external and internal lyments.

**Closely associated with these nuclei are:**

a. Substantia nigra of midbrain
b. Subthalamic nucleus

Functionally basal ganglia are closely related to:

I. Thalamus
II. Reticular formation

**Connections of basal ganglia**

## Afferent From (input is to neostriatum)

1. Motor areas of the cerebral cortex
2. Association areas of cerebral cortex called corticostriatal projection.
3. Substantia nigra of midbrain, called **nigrostriatal pathway**.
4. Thalamus from centromedian nuclei of thalamus.

## Efferent (Through globus pallidus)

1. To venteroanterior and ventromedial nuclei of thalamus.
2. From neostriatum to substantia nigra.
3. From globus pallidus to substantia nigra down to reticular formation of brainstem.
4. Short pathways from striatum to globus pallidus
5. Caudate nucleus to thalamus
6. Caudate nucleus to hypothalamus (Fig. 10.8).

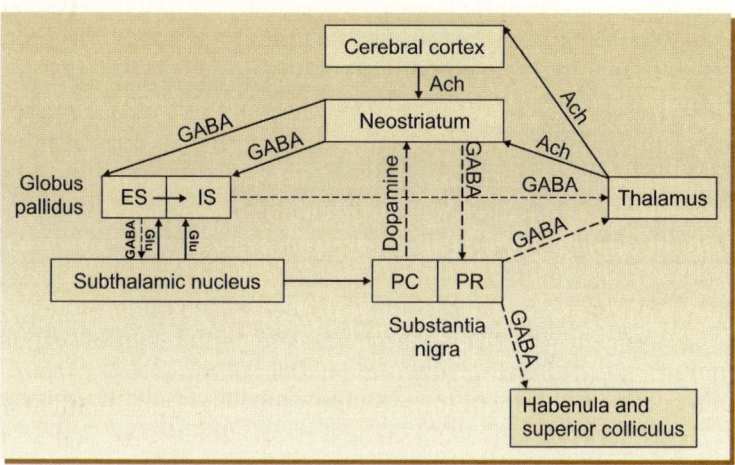

**Fig. 10.8:** Connections of the basal ganglia

Feedback closed loop connection between basal ganglia and cerebral cortex.

There is a feedback circuit between the cerebral cortex and basal ganglia. The neostriatum receives extensive inputs from the cerebral cortex and thalamus, via the internuclear connections, the neostriatum sends most of its output to the globus pallidus and to the reticular nucleus of the substantia nigra. This in turn projects to the thalamus. The information received by the thalamus is conveyed back to the cortex thus completing the feedback circuit.

This feedback circuit is integrated in the ventrolateral nucleus of the thalamus with another circuit, i.e. cortico-ponto-dentato-thalamocortical circuit and inhibits excessive activity of the motor cortex, areas 4 and 6.

**Functions of basal ganglia:** Play an important role in motor functions:

1. **Planning and programming of voluntary motor activity:** Cerebellar hemisphere function along with basal ganglia in planning motor activity. Electric activity in neurons of basal ganglia is observed before any voluntary motor activity occurs. For this purpose they function in close association with the cerebral cortex.

   Experimental evidence suggests that ideas or thoughts are generated in neocortical areas of the cerebrum and transmitted to basal ganglia where the abstract thoughts are converted into a definite programmed patterns of muscle activity and relayed to motor cortex through thalamus. From motor cortex via corticospinal tracts impulses are sent to appropriate motor neurons supplying the skeletal muscles.

2. **Maintenance of muscle tone and body posture:** Through its connection with extrapyramidal tracts, it helps to maintain tone in skeletal muscle and thus the erect and balanced body posture is produced.

   Extrapyramidal fibres originating from motor cortex relay in the basal ganglia pass onto substantia nigra and then relay in the reticular formation of the brainstem and finally to γ-motor neurons via the reticulospinal pathways and influence muscle tone.

   Fibers from basal ganglia to reticular formation are generally inhibitory and influence the activity of γ-motor neurons. Through their influence on the tone of axial and girdle muscle, basal ganglia helps to provide a stable background posture for performing voluntary actions.

3. Basal ganglia **prevent involuntary static tremors**: The exact neuronal circuits involved are not known.

4. Probably plays a role in **cognitive functions** through connection of caudate nucleus to pre-frontal cortex.

**Parkinsonisms:** *Paralysis Agitans* (originally described by James Parkinson).

It is the commonest of clinical disorders due to lesions in the basal ganglia. There is damage to dopamine secreting neurons of nigrostriatal pathways. As a result dopamine content of neostriatum is decreased, causing an imbalance between dopamine and acetylcholine content of striatum, thus causing derangement of motor activity.

Causes:

- Primary or idiopathic
- Cerebral arteriosclerosis
- Complications of encephalitis
- Complication of drugs such as phenothiazine which blocks the $D_2$ dopamine receptors.

Dopaminergic neurons and dopamine receptors are steadily lost with aging in basal ganglia in normal individuals. However, symptoms appear when the loss exceeds 60–80%.

## Clinical Features

1. **Rigidity**
   - This effects only large proximal muscles of the limbs, involving both protagonists and antagonists.
   - The commonly affected muscles are biceps, knee flexors and sternocleidomastoids.
   - Posture is that of a flexion attitude. In advanced cases as a result of marked rigidity, statue like state is produced and voluntary and involuntary movements become progressively difficult.

2. **Tremor**
   
   It consists of regular, rhythmic alternate contraction of antagonists and agonists muscles at the rate of 6–8 times/second. Its frequent presence can be seen as pill-rolling movements. Commonest sites are fingers, hands, lips and tongue. These tremors are present at rest and disappear on activity, therefore, they are called static (resting) tremors.

3. **Akinesia and hypokinesia:** In early stages the weakness and poverty of movements leads to:
   - Difficulty in initiating voluntary movement
   - Slow and monotonous speech

- Mask like facial expressions
- Loss of normal subconscious movements like swinging of the arms while walking
- Festinant gait (shuffling gait)
- The tendon jerks become progressively difficult to elicit as the rigidity increases.

## EXPLAIN WHY LEVODOPA IS PRESCRIBED IN PARKINSON'S DISEASE                          1 (2011)

Parkinson's disease is produced due to degeneration of dopaminergic nigrostriatal tract. Therefore, concentration of dopamine in this region, i.e. nigrostriatal system is reduced. Administration of levodopa (L-dopa) a precursor of dopamine decreases the rigidity and tremors. Dopamine cannot cross the blood-brain barrier but L-dopa can. Hence, this is prescribed instead of dopamine in patients of Parkinson's disease.

## COMPARE AND CONTRAST CEREBELLAR AND PARKINSON'S TREMORS               2 (2004)-IPU, 2 (2004, 2006)

## TREMOR OF CEREBELLAR DISEASE AND PARKINSONISM
2.5 (1986)

### Corobollar Tromor

- Patients cannot perform activity smoothly. If they reach for an object, their movements are jerky and accompanied by oscillating to and fro tremors that become more marked as the hand approaches the object (intentional tremors).
- The tremors are course and occur at the rate of 4–6 times/ second. They can be clearly seen when that part is used in voluntary movement.
- They occur because an entire movement cannot be directed by a single motor command.
- Clinically, these tremors are demonstrated by the following tests:
  - Finger-nose test
  - Rebound phenomenon
  - Adiadochokinesia
  - Heel-knee test

## Tremors of Parkinsonism

1. It consists of regular, rhythmic alternate contraction of antagonistic and agonist muscles at the rate of 6–8 seconds. Its frequent presence can be seen as pill-rolling movements, i.e. rhythmic contraction of thumb over first two fingers.
2. **Common site:** Fingers, hands, lips, tongue and it often causes movement of pronation and supination.
3. It is present at rest but disappears on activity, therefore, popularly called resting (static) tremors.
   **Mechanism:** During voluntary movements impulses from the motor cortex pass down the descending pathways and stimulate both α- and γ-motor neurons. The γ-efferents stimulate the stretch reflex to stop the involuntary movements. This is called damping effect.
4. It increases in emotional states, excitement or anxiety due to the increase secretion of epinephrine from the adrenal medulla which in turn excites the RAS. However, the tremors disappear during sleep due to decreased activity of RAS.
5. **Cause of tremors:** It may be due to associated degenerative lesion in the reticular formation and its ascending connections.

## HYPOTHALAMUS

### EXPLAIN WHY HYPOTHALAMUS IS CALLED THE HEAD GANGLION OF THE NERVOUS SYSTEM    1 (2011)

Sherrington called the hypothalamus the 'head ganglion of the nervous system' since stimulation of the hypothalamus produces autonomic responses but does not seem to be concerned with visceral function per se. The autonomic responses triggered in the hypothalamus are part of a more complex phenomenon such as eating, emotions and rage. Stimulation of various parts of the hypothalamus particularly the lateral areas produce diffuse sympathetic discharge and increases medullary adrenal secretion in response to stress called the flight or fight reaction.

### WHAT WILL HAPPEN AND WHY IN LESIONS OF THE VENTROMEDIAL NUCLEUS OF THE HYPOTHALAMUS    1 (2009)

Lesions of the ventromedial nucleus cause hyperphagia (excessive eating) and the animal becomes grossly obese called **hypothalamic obesity**.

The ventromedial nucleus of the hypothalamus acts as the satiety centre which is the primary centre that controls the food intake. It functions by inhibiting the feeding centre which is chronically active. Therefore, lesion of the satiety centre leads to uninhibited action of the feeding centre.

## COMPARE GLUCOSTATIC AND LIPOSTATIC THEORY OF FOOD INTAKE                                    2 (2010)

### Glucostatic Theory

The cells of the ventromedial nucleus of the hypothalamus act as a satiety centre due their functioning as glucoreceptors, also called glucostats. They sense the glucose level of the blood. The activity of the satiety centre is thus governed by the level of glucose utilisation of cells within this centre. This is called as **glucostatic theory**.

If the glucoreceptors are inadequately supplied with glucose, their activity is decreased. As a result the activity of the feeding centre is unchecked, their activity increases and the individual is hungry. The reverse phenomenon is seen if the glucoreceptors are supplied with adequate glucose.

### Lipostatic Theory

Neurons in the hypothalamic feeding centre also respond to changes in the level of fatty acids and amino acids. The size of the body fats initiate either neural or hormonal signals that are relayed to the hypothalamus, thus controlling food intake (Fig. 10.9).

Leptin is a circulating protein hormone produced mainly in the adipose cells that act on the hypothalamus to decrease the

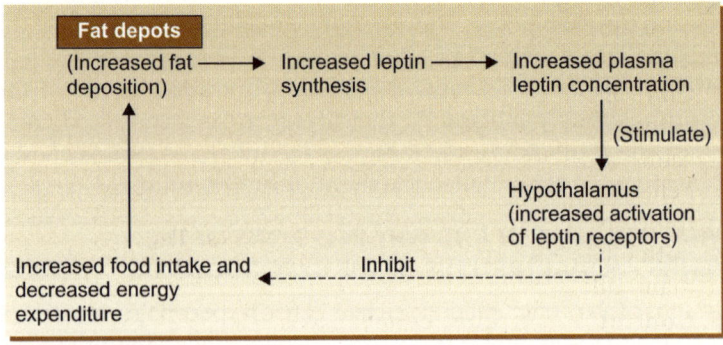

**Fig. 10.9:** Feedback control, i.e. control of fat depots by leptin

release of neuropeptide Y and produces decreased food intake and increased energy expenditure.

## ROLE OF HYPOTHALAMUS IN REGULATION OF FOOD INTAKE                                    8 (2003)-IPU
## ROLE OF HYPOTHALAMUS IN FOOD AND WATER INTAKE
                                                      5 (2004)-IPU
## ROLE OF HYPOTHALAMUS IN THIRST MECHANISM    2.5 (2004)
## TEMPERATURE REGULATING MECHANISMS
                                        2.5 (2010), 2.5 (2009)

## ENUMERATE THE FUNCTIONS OF HYPOTHALAMUS. DESCRIBE ANY ONE OF THEM IN DETAIL. ADD A NOTE ON LEPTIN   (2012)

### Functions of Hypothalamus

1. **Regulation of body temperature:** Hypothalamus is the centre for various reflexes to maintain constant body temperature. In response to heat anterior hypothalamus initiates mechanisms to lower temperature and posterior hypothalamus responds to cold.

2. **Control of autonomic activity:** Stimulation of posterior and lateral hypothalamus activates sympathetic activity. Stimulation of preoptic area has parasympathetic effects.

3. **Control of pituitary activity**
   a. Hypothalamus through releasing factors controls the release of hormones of anterior pituitary and thus influences growth, metabolism and reproduction.
   b. It is the site of formation of posterior pituitary hormones, i.e. oxytocin and ADH are secreted by the supraoptic and paraventricular nuclei of the hypothalamus.

4. **Control of feeding behaviour:** Lateral hypothalamus when stimulated induces feeding and hence acts as the feeding centre. Dorsomedial nucleus when active inhibits feeding and hence is the satiety centre. It is believed that feeding centre is tonically active and is inhibited by the satiety centre intermittently for short periods. Feeding reflexes are initiated from mammillary body.

5. **Control of drinking behaviour:** Osmoreceptor that sense osmolarity of plasma and accordingly modify drinking is located in the lateral preoptic area.

6. Control of **sexual behavior and mating:** Anteroventral hypothalamus regulate this behaviour.
7. Control of **emotions** in association with limbic system-hypothalamus is responsible for exteriorisation of emotions like rage and anger.
8. Control of **biological rhythms:** It is the function of suprachiasmatic nuclei and it controls circadian rhythm of ACTH secretion.

### Role of Hypothalamus in Regulation of Food Intake

The body weight of an individual is maintained relatively constant over a long time. It is determined by the balance between caloric intake and energy expenditure. There are many inputs that control food intake and hypothalamus integrates all these afferent inputs. There are two hypothalamic centres that are concerned with the regulation of food intake:

• Ventromedial nucleus acts as the satiety centre
• Lateral hypothalamus that acts as the feeding centre.

### Mechanism

I. The satiety centre is the primary centre that controls food intake. It functions by inhibiting the feeding centre.

II. The feeding centre is chronically active and its activity is inhibited by the satiety centre following ingestion of food.

III. There are four main theories that are concerned with the regulation of food intake:

1. **Glucostatic theory:** The cells of the ventromedial nucleus of the hypothalamus acts as a satiety centre due to their functioning as glucoreceptors, also called glucostats. They sense the glucose level of the blood. The activity of the satiety centre is thus governed by the level of glucose utilisation of cells within this centre. This is called **glucostatic theory**.

   If the glucoreceptors are inadequately supplied with glucose, their activity is decreased. As a result the activity of the feeding centre is unchecked, their activity increases and the individual is hungry. The reverse phenomenon is seen if the glucoreceptors are supplied with adequate glucose.

2. **Lipostatic theory:** Neurons in the hypothalamic feeding centre also responds to changes in the level of fatty acids

and amino acids. The size of the body fats initiate either neural or hormonal signals that are relayed to the hypothalamus, thus controlling food intake.

Leptin is a circulating protein hormone produced mainly in the adipose cells that act on the hypothalamus to decrease the release of neuropeptide Y and produces decreased food intake and increased energy expenditure.

3. **Gut-peptide theory:** Food in the GIT causes release of peptide/hormones which act on the hypothalamus to inhibit food intake. Circulating CCK seems to play an important role. It acts via both CCK-A (peripheral/visceral) and CCK-B receptors (central/hypothalamic).

4. **Thermostatic theory:** A fall in the core body temperature stimulates the food intake, whereas a rise inhibits it.

## Role of Hypothalamic Peptides

Principal hypothalamic peptides concentration increases during feeding and decreases during satiety. Thus they seem to play an important role in the regulation of food intake:

- **Food intake is increased by** neuropeptide Y, orexin A, orexin B, ghrelin
- **Food intake is decreased by** α-MSH, CART, CRH, malonyl-CoA.

## Leptin

This is a circulating protein hormone produced mainly in the adipose cells. It acts on the hypothalamus to decrease the release of neuropeptide Y and produces decrease in food intake and increased energy expenditure.

Leptin receptors are found in various body tissues as well as in brown adipose tissues and are abundant in brain microvessels. Leptin thus acts to control the size of body's fat depots. Therefore, any defect in the leptin receptor gene results in obesity.

## Role of Hypothalamus in Thirst Mechanism (Fig. 10.10)

The hypothalamus is involved in regulating the fluid balance by participating in the control of water intake as well as in the water loss by the body.

### Role in control of water intake—thirst

- The osmoreceptors which initiate drinking in response to increased plasma osmolality are located in the lateral preoptic area. These are separate from the osmoreceptors involved in ADH release.

- The neurons that induce thirst in response to decrease ECFV are more diffusely spread in lateral hypothalamus.

### Role in control of water loss

The excretion of water is regulated by the kidneys via ADH. The hypothalamic nuclei that form the main source of ADH are the supraoptic nuclei which are called magnocellular neurosecretory neurons.

### Neurotransmitters and thirst

- A system of cholinergic neurons that subserve drinking converge on the lateral hypothalamus
- The renin angiotensin system is concerned with drinking caused by β-adrenergic stimulation.

## TEMPERATURE REGULATING MECHANISMS　　　2.5

Body temperature is always kept close to a normal range by maintaining a balance between heat production and heat loss:

### Heat Production (Thermogenesis)

- **Metabolic activities of the body:** Skeletal muscle, liver and heart
- Specific dynamic action of food
- Heat gained from the surrounding hot environment: Direct and reflected heating

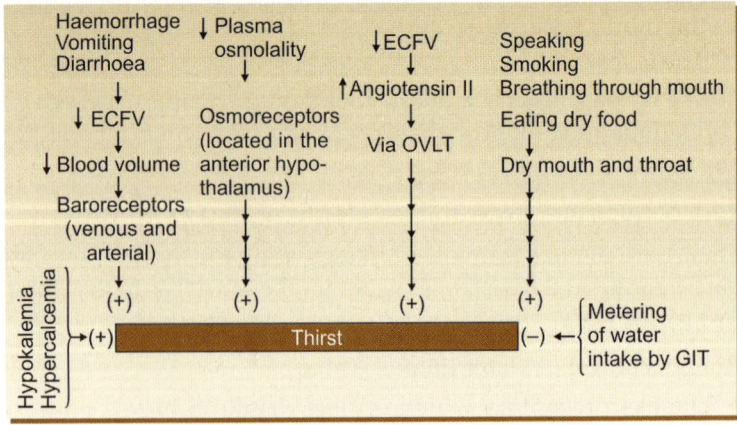

**Fig 10.10:** Inputs reflexly controlling thirst

- **Endocrine mechanisms:** Epinephrine, norepinephrine and $T_4$
- **Brown fat:** Especially in infants
- Exercise and increased voluntary activity
- Shivering
- Increased food intake

## Heat Loss

- To the surrounding: Radiation, conduction and convection
- **Evaporation:** Sweating, insensible water loss and respiration
- **Excretion:** Urine and faeces
- Cutaneous vasodilation
- Sweating
- Increased respiration
- Anorexia
- Apathy and inertia

## PATHOPHYSIOLOGY OF FEVER                    3 (2003)-IPU

- Bacterial endotoxins act on monocyte, macrophages and Kupffer cells to produce cytokines that act as endogenous pyrogens.
- IL- 1β, IL-6, β-IFN, γ-IFN and TNF-α can act independently to produce fever. These cytokines act on OVLT, a circumventricular organ, located outside the blood-brain barrier.
- These in turn activate the preoptic area of the hypothalamus. Cytokines are also produced by cells in the CNS when these are stimulated by infection and these may act directly on the thermoregulatory centre.
- The fever produced by cytokines is probably due to the release of prostaglandins in the hypothalamus ($PGE_2$).

Endotoxin inflammation and other pyrogenic stimuli
↓
Monocytes, macrophages and Kupffer cells
↓ Cytokines
Preoptic area of hypothalamus
↓ Prostaglandins
Raise temperature set point
↓
Fever

## CEREBRAL HEMISPHERES

### PREFRONTAL LOBE                              3 (1985)

Prefrontal lobe of cerebral cortex is the part of the cortex that lies anterior to Brodmann areas 4, 6 and 8 extending onto the medial aspect of the hemisphere including the cingulate gyrus.

It has extensive afferent connection with the following:

- Thalamus—dorsomedial, anterior and intralaminar nuclei.
- Hypothalamus—through thalamus.
- Other areas of the cerebral cortex—visual cortex.

It sends efferent fibres to:

- Temporal lobe
- Caudate nucleus
- Pontine nuclei going to cerebellum
- Midbrain tegmentum reticular formation
- Thalamic nuclei
- Hypothalamus
- Limbic cortex—hippocampus and amygdala

An interconnected nervous complex constituted by prefrontal cortex-thalamus-hypothalamus functions to perform higher intellectual activities like:

1. Personality
2. Emotional exteriorization
3. Appropriate social behaviour
4. Memory
5. Learning

### HIGHER FUNCTIONS OF THE CEREBRAL CORTEX

In human there is immense growth of the cerebral hemispheres.

Cerebral cortex is a six-layered neocortex. Cerebral hemisphere in addition to primary motor and sensory areas (in frontal, parietal, temporal and occipital lobes) also contain three association areas.

**Association areas are**

1. **Frontal**—anterior to premotor cortex.

2. **Parietotemporal-occipital area**—between general sensory and visual cortex extending up to posterior part of the temporal lobes.

**3. Temporal**—From lower part of temporal lobe to limbic cortex. Higher functions of the cerebral cortex are:

- Learning
- Memory
- Language
- Intellect, judgement and personality.

Language function and intellect is only present in humans by virtue of the immense growth of association areas of cortex.

In humans one of the hemispheres is involved more in categorisation and symbolisation functions like language and is called the **categorical hemisphere** (previously called the dominant hemisphere).

In 96% of right-handed individuals left is the categorical hemisphere and in 70% of left-handed individuals again left is the categorical hemisphere.

The other hemisphere which is more involved is spatiotemporal relations and concerned with stereognosis, recognition of faces and recognition of musical notes is called **the representational hemisphere.**

## LIMBIC SYSTEM

### SHAM RAGE                                      2.5 (1987)

Rage is violent behaviour of man or even animals in response to a major irritating stimulus.

Rage reaction has two components:

i.  Exteriorisation of rage is the physical component, e.g. in cat it is associated with hissing, spitting, piloerection, pupillary dilatation, cowering, clawing and biting.

ii. **Affect or the feeling of anger:** Somatic effects are mediated by hypothalamus and 'feeling' is the function of the limbic cortex. In experiments on cats when neocortex and limbic system was destroyed such an animal shows all the physical manifestations of rage. Previously it was thought that animals had no feelings and it was named as sham rage. Now it is known that animals also feel.

## KLÜVER-BUCY SYNDROME                     3 (2004)-IPU

Bilateral temporal lobe removal in monkeys produces Klüver-Bucy syndrome. This was first described by Klüver and Bucy and such animals are called Klüver-Bucy animals. The characteristic features are due to destruction of limbic system, especially amygdaloid nucleus and has the following features:

- Animals are obedient, hyperphagic and the males are hypersexual
- They become omniphagic—it starts taking diet like meat which it was not taking previously
- **Visual agnosia**—inability to identify objects in spite of good vision
- Marked increase in oral activity: Monkeys pick all movable objects in their environment. They manipulate each object in a compulsive way, mouth, lick and bite them and then unless it is edible, discard it. However, discarded objects are again picked up in a few minutes as if the animal has never seen them before and subjected to the same oral manipulation and exploration. This may be due to:
  - Inability to identify objects.
  - Manifestation of memory loss due to removal of hippocampus.
- The attention of the animal can be easily diverted.
- They have an inability to ignore peripheral stimuli called **hypermetamorphosis**.

### Clinical Significance

In humans with temporal lobe disease or lesions various above-mentioned symptoms are present. However, impairment of recent memory may also be due to bilateral damage to the hippocampus and hypersexuality may also be due to damage to amygdaloid nuclei and piriform cortex.

### PAPEZ CIRCUIT IN EMOTIONS                     (2000)

The Papez circuit was described by Papez JW (Fig. 10.11) where the prefrontal lobe forms a close circuit connection with the thalamus. This circuit is responsible for resting EEG and plays an important role in the control and genesis of emotions.

Fibres from the anterior nucleus of the thalamus project onto the precallosal part of the cingulate gyrus.

As the anterior nucleus of the thalamus receives afferents from the mammillary bodies of the hypothalamus which in turn receives afferents from the hippocampus via the fornix. The hippocampus is thus ultimately projected to the inhibitory area 24.

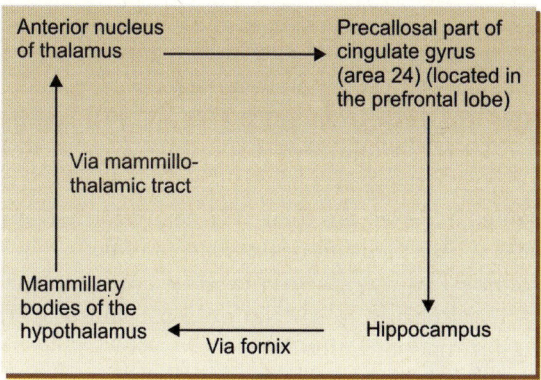

**Fig 10.11:** Papez circuit

## HIGHER FUNCTIONS OF NERVOUS SYSTEM

### CONDITIONED REFLEX                                      2.5 (2004)

A conditioned reflex is a reflex response to a stimulus that previously elicited little or no response acquired by repeatedly pairing the stimulus to another stimulus that normally does produce the response. It depends on the appearance of new functional connections in the CNS. They are primarily built up on the basis of inborn reflexes.

Example: **Pavlov's classical dog experiments**

- The introduction of food (unconditioned stimulus) into the mouth sets up reflex salivation in a dog. This is called the unconditioned reflex.

- Ringing of a bell just before the unconditioned stimulus produces salivation. After this procedure is repeated several times the ringing of the bell only produces salivation called the conditioned reflex. Therefore, the initial neutral stimulus finally develops new connections in the CNS and can now by itself produce salivation.

**The factors which influence condition reflexes to develop**

- The animal must be alert and in good health.
- For conditioning to occur the conditioned stimulus (CS) must begin to operate before the unconditioned stimulus (US) is applied. If the CS follows the US, no conditioned response develops.
- The CS must be allowed to continue to act so as to overlap the US. Almost any stimulus can become a CS.
- **Necessity for reinforcement:** For a CS to retain its new properties, it is essential that it should always be followed by US.
- Conditioned reflexes are relatively easily formed if the US is associated with a pleasant or unpleasant effect.
- The biochemical events involved in conditioned reflexes include: Habituation, sensitisation, post-tetanic potentiation and long-term potentiation.

## Physiological Basis of Conditioned Reflex

One of the essential features is the formation of new functional connections within the CNS, for example in Pavlov's experiments salivation in response to a bell-ringing indicates that a functional connection has developed between auditory pathway and the autonomic centres controlling salivation. The new functional connections develop at two levels: Intracortical (mainly) and subcortical level.

## Clinical Significance

A large number of somatic, visceral and other neural phenomena can be conditioned known as **biofeedback**. The changes that can be produced include alteration in bowel movements, heart rate and blood pressure. Conditioned decrease in BP has been used to lower BP in hypertensive individuals.

## LANGUAGE AND APHASIAS

Language is an elaborate form of communication present only in human species, through speech, reading and writing. In its classical form it is defined as the ability to understand the spoken and written words and to express ideas in speech and writing. It is considered as the most important trait that has made man more successful than other species.

The function is confined to parieto-occipitotemporal association area and a part of frontal association area in categorical hemisphere.

Various anatomical regions involved are:

- Secondary visual area
- Angular gyrus in occipital lobe
- Wernicke's area: An area behind the auditory cortex in posterior part of superior temporal lobe
- Secondary auditory cortex
- Broca's area of speech in the frontal cortex.

One speaks in response to a visual or an auditory stimulus.

## Mechanism of Speech

- Visual stimuli perceived in visual cortex are further processed in secondary visual area to understand their meaning.
- After processing impulses are conveyed to angular gyrus for their interpretation.
- From angular gyrus impulses are sent to Wernicke's area for comprehension.
- Auditory stimuli are also conveyed to the Wernicke's area after processing in secondary auditory cortex and comprehended there.
- Wernicke's area projects to the Broca's area of speech via arcuate fasciculus.
- Planning and programming of motor activity for vocalisation, i.e. to initiate appropriate movements of lips, tongue, larynx take place in the Broca's area of speech and conveyed to appropriate area of face in primary motor cortex.

For exteriorisation of speech, the excitomotor areas of brain, their descending motor pathways, related lower motor neurons and association motor structures, i.e. cerebellum and basal ganglion should also be intact.

## APHASIA                                           2.5 (2003)
## SENSORY APHASIA                              2.5 (2011)

Aphasia is the term used to describe the disorders of expression in speech, writing and sign language and disability in comprehension of spoken, written and sign language. Lesions causing aphasias are in association areas in categorical hemisphere, commonly due to thrombosis or embolism of cerebral vessels. It is divided into two types:

a. Non-fluent aphasia
b. Fluent aphasia

Non-fluent aphasia occurs when there is a lesion in the Broca's speech area. Interpretation and comprehension of language is there but the person is not able to say whatever he/she wants. Speech is not fluent and is slow, and words are hard to come out.

If the damage is extensive, speech is limited to 2–3 words to express a wide range of ideas and emotions, it is also called motor aphasia.

### Fluent Aphasias

No difficulty in speech but there is a defect in understanding and comprehension. It can occur in different forms. It is also called sensory aphasia.

a. **Lesion in angular gyrus:** If Wernicke's and Broca's areas are intact, there is no difficulty in comprehension of auditory information. There is a problem in understanding written words and pictures, as visual information is not processed completely and not transmitted to the Wernicke's area. It is also called *anomic aphasia*.

b. **Lesion in Wernicke's cortex:** Speech is fluent and at times person talks excessively but there is no comprehension and thoughts are incoherent. Speech is full of jargon and neologism, that makes little sense.

c. **Lesion of arcuate fasciculus:** Speech is good and auditory comprehension is there, but the person cannot put parts of words together or conjure up words. It is also known as **conduction aphasia** (Fig. 10.12).

**Dysarthria:** It is a defect in articulation of speech due to loss of performance of muscles of articulation. There is a lesion in motor system, e.g. cerebellar lesion.

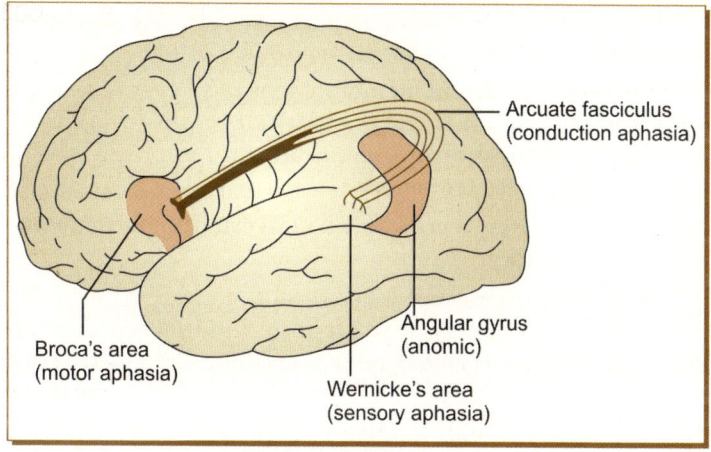

**Fig. 10.12:** Language pathway

## EXPLAIN WHY LESION IN WERNICKE'S AREA LEADS TO FLUENT APHASIA
**1 (2003)-IPU**

Lesion in the Wernicke's area leads to fluent or sensory aphasia. Speech is not disturbed but sometimes the patient talks excessively which makes little sense. He fails to understand spoken or written words, so other aspects of the use of a language are also compromised. This happens because the Wernicke's area is concerned with comprehension of auditory and visual information, whereas the motor functions are not compromised.

## MEMORY

### SHORT-TERM MEMORY
**3 (2004)-IPU**

Memory is one of the higher functions of brain. It is of two types:

a. **Reflexive or non-declarative:** It includes learning skills, classical conditioning and habits. It involves almost no conscious efforts. It involves activation and alteration in a number of central synapses.

b. **Declarative or explicit memory:** Declarative memory involves conscious recall of facts and events. In humans it is divided into three types.

1. **Working memory:** Temporary storage of bits of information for very short time. It needs lots of attention to be focussed,

e.g. memorising a telephone number before dialling. It involves activation of large areas of neocortex.

2. **Short-term or Recent memory:** Memory of events occurring few minutes, hours, days before. It requires the hippocampus and adjoining areas in the temporal lobe for encoding of recent memory.

It is vulnerable to erasure till converted to permanent or remote memory.

In lesions of temporal lobes recent memory is lost called retrograde amnesia. In such an individual working and remote memory is intact but no new long-term memory can be formed and stored.

3. **Long-term or Remote memory:** It is recall of past events which one never forgets. Once established it can be recalled by a large number of different associations. Encoding of permanent memory involves many areas of the brain.

**Encoding of long-term memory:** It involves hippocampus and its connections with other areas of the brain.

Hippocampus projects to mammillary bodies through fornix which in turn project to anterior thalamic nuclei via mammillothalamic tract (MTT).

Thalamus is connected to prefrontal cortex which sends diffuse cholinergic projections to neocortex by way of basal forebrain bundle thus forming permanent memories.

Hippocampus $\xrightarrow{\text{FORNIX}}$ Mammillary bodies $\xrightarrow{\text{MTT}}$

Anterior thalamic nuclei $\longrightarrow$ Prefrontal cortex

$\xrightarrow[\text{(Cholinergic)}]{\text{Basal forebrain bundle}}$ All areas of neocortex.

Degeneration of cholinergic neurons in basal forebrain bundle occurs in Alzheimer disease with progressive loss of short-term memory and loss of awareness of surroundings.

## WHAT WILL HAPPEN AND WHY TO CSF PRESSURE IN COMMUNICATING HYDROCEPHALUS  1 (2010)

There is an increase in CSF pressure in communicating hydrocephalus which is defined as a pathological accumulation of CSF within brain spaces.

Communicating hydrocephalus is produced due to excessive accumulation of fluid in the subarachnoid spaces. It may be produced due to the following two causes:

- When rate of CSF formation is more than its rate of absorption, for example, due to over development of choroid plexus.
- Decreased absorptive capacity of arachnoid villi due to thrombosis of venous sinuses or inflammatory changes in the meninges which causes accumulation of CSF.

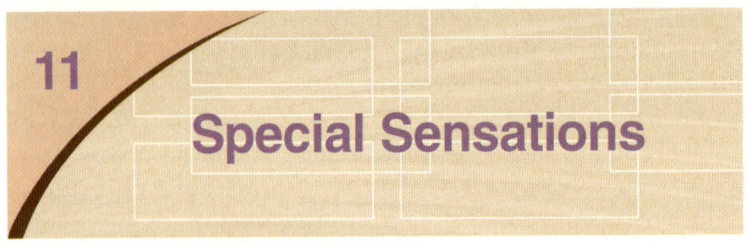

11

# Special Sensations

## EXPLAIN WHY LIGHT REFLEX IS LOST BUT ACCOMMODATION REFLEX IS PRESENT IN NEUROSYPHILIS (2006)

### ARGYLL ROBERTSON PUPIL 3 (1989)

The pathway for the pupillary light reflex is separate and dorsal to the pathway for the accommodation reflex. In neurosyphilis, a selective lesion in the midbrain (pretectal region and superior colliculi) occurs which damages the pathway of light reflex but the pathway for the accommodation reflex is spared. Consequently the light reflex is lost while the response to accommodation remains intact. This is called **Argyll Robertson** pupil and is typically seen in neurosyphilis but may also be produced in other diseases producing selective lesions in the midbrain.

## WHAT WILL HAPPEN AND WHY IF THERE IS BILATERAL DESTRUCTION OF THE VISUAL CORTEX 1 (2010)

In case of bilateral destruction of the visual cortex, patients will not be able to identify the object being shown to him or may not be able to tell about any details of the object other than colour or shape. This indicates that the visual centre of the brain is unable to interpret input from the eyes after its bilateral destruction.

## EXPLAIN WHY VISUAL ACUITY IS MAXIMUM AT THE FOVEA CENTRALIS 1 (2007)

The fovea centralis is a thinned out rod free portion of the retina that is present in humans and other primates. Over this area cones are densely packed and each synapses with a single bipolar cell which in turn synapses with a single ganglion cell providing a direct pathway to the brain. There are few overlying cells and no blood vessels in this region also. Consequently this is the site with maximum visual acuity. When attention is fixed on an object, the eyes are normally moved in such a way that light rays coming from the object fall on the fovea.

## EFFECT OF LESION OF OPTIC CHIASMA     2.5 (1992)

Optic chiasma is the site where the fibres from nasal halves of two retinae cross over to the opposite side. It carries visual impulses from nasal side of the two retinae. Any lesion involving optic chiasma produces loss of vision in temporal halves of both eyes known as bitemporal hemianopia. Optic chiasma lies in close relation with the pituitary gland hence a tumour of the pituitary gland can press upon the optic chiasma producing bitemporal hemianopia.

## EXPLAIN WHY RADIOLOGISTS AND AIRCRAFT PILOTS WEAR RED GLASSES IN BRIGHT LIGHT BEFORE GOING INTO DIM LIGHT     1 (2009)

Radiologists and aircraft pilots who need maximum visual sensitivity in dim light can avoid having to wait for 20 minutes in the dark to become dark adapted if they wear red goggles when in bright light. Light wavelengths in the red end of the spectrum stimulate the rods only to a slight degree while permitting the cones to function reasonably well. Therefore, a person wearing red glasses before entering a dark area can see in the dark during the time it takes for the rods to become dark-adapted.

## COMPARE MONOCULAR AND BINOCULAR VISION     2 (2003)

The visual field of a single eye is called **monocular vision**. The visual field seen with both eyes is the binocular field. The central parts of the visual field of the two eyes coincide therefore anything in this portion of the field is seen with both eyes called **binocular vision**. The difference between the two is the ability to judge distances or have depth perception. In binocular vision, two eyes work together to focus on a single point. The brain then processes that information to determine depth or distance to that point. Monocular vision exists in animals with eyes on opposite sides of the head, which prevents the two eyes from ever having a common focal point. It also exists in animals who may have formerly had binocular vision, but have lost vision in one eye.

## COMPARE PHOTOPIC VISION AND SCOTOPIC VISION (2001)

**Photopic vision:** It is the daylight or bright light vision which is the function of cones. It operates at higher intensity of illumination. The cones have a much higher threshold but a much greater acuity thus responsible for vision in bright light. They are also required for colour vision. The maximum sensitivity of photopic vision is for 560 nm, i.e. for greenish yellow light.

**Scotopic vision:** This is the vision in dim light and is the function of rods. It is the vision below 0.001 mA intensity of brightness since rods have much lower threshold and are extremely sensitive to light. The maximum sensitivity of scotopic vision is for 500 nm, i.e. for bluish green light.

## DARK ADAPTATION 3 (1993)

After a person stays in bright light for a considerable length of time and then enters a dimly lit environment, the person has initial difficulty in visualising objects, but gradually becomes adapted to darkness and can see again. This phenomenon is called **dark adaptation**.

Visual perception increases quickly at first followed by more gradual increase, reaching a maximum in 20–30 minutes. This is basically due to a fall in threshold of stimulation of photoreceptor. The first drop is due to dark adaptation of cones and later it is due to that of rods. In a completely dark adapted eye sensitivity to light is increased 10,000 fold.

**Mechanism of dark adaptation:** It is believed that in light photopigment rhodopsin is hydrolysed and in dark it is resynthesized. Regeneration of rhodopsin is essential for vision in dark. At the same time now it is believed that other unknown complex mechanisms are also involved in the phenomenon of dark adaptation.

### Applied

Deficiency of vitamin A is associated with poor dark adaptation and night blindness, as vitamin A is important for synthesis of rhodopsin.

## FUNCTIONS OF RODS AND CONES OF THE EYE    3 (1990)

Rods and cones are sensory receptors present in the retina of the eye. These receptors are stimulated by light falling on the eye and are hence called photoreceptors. Though both are photoreceptors, each has distinct functions.

### Functions of Rods

1. Rods are for dim light or night vision as their threshold is low, called **scotopic vision**.
2. These are responsible for vision in the peripheral part of field of vision as these are present mainly in peripheral retina.

### Functions of Cones

1. Responsible for vision in bright light or daytime called photopic vision as their threshold is higher than rods.
2. Essential for colour vision as they contain special colour pigments.
3. Provide greater visual acuity to appreciate minute details of the object.
4. Provide vision in the central part of visual field as they are mainly concentrated in the central part, i.e. fovea centralis in the retina.

## ACCOMMODATION REFLEX    2.5 (1988, 1991)

Accommodation reflex is a three part response when an individual looks at a near object, therefore, also called near response. It consists of contraction of ciliary muscles, constriction of pupils and convergence of visual axis by the contraction of medial rectus muscle.

Lens with its elastic capsule is suspended by means of zonule which in turn is attached to the ciliary muscle.

At rest anterior surface of lens is comparatively flattened as the zonule is kept under tension because the ciliary muscle is relaxed.

Normally, in an emmetropic eye when the ciliary muscle is relaxed, parallel light rays from an object at 6 metres are focussed on the retina.

If an object is brought nearer and relaxation of ciliary muscle is still maintained, the image will be formed behind the retina and object will appear blurred.

To overcome this problem there is an increase in the curvature of the anterior surface of the lens, its power is increased and rays from the object are focused on the retina and a clear image is formed.

An increase in curvature of anterior surface of lens occurs due to reflex contraction of ciliary muscles, in turn relaxing the zonule and thus allowing the lens to bulge more.

In addition there occurs:

a. Constriction of pupil due to contraction of constrictor pupillae.

b. Medial convergence of eyeball due to contraction of medial rectus (Fig. 11.1).

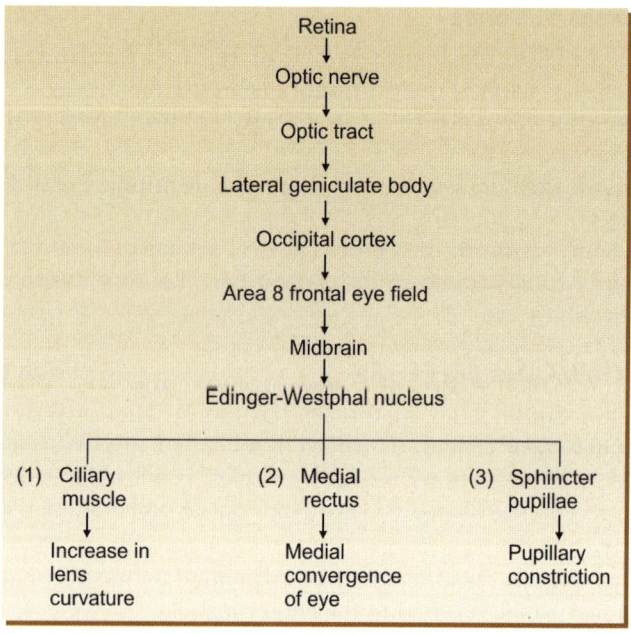

**Fig. 11.1:** Pathway for accommodation reflex

## LIGHT REFLEX                                    2.5 (1985, 1988, 1991)

Shining of light in one eye leads to constriction of pupil in the same eye called direct light reflex, in addition it leads to constriction of pupil in the other eye called indirect light reflex. As the pupil constricts light rays fall only on central foveal region stimulating the cones and thus ensure better acuity of vision and colour vision. It is a good clinical test while examining neurological patients. Absence of light reflex indicates brain oedema or damage to brain tissue (Fig. 11.2).

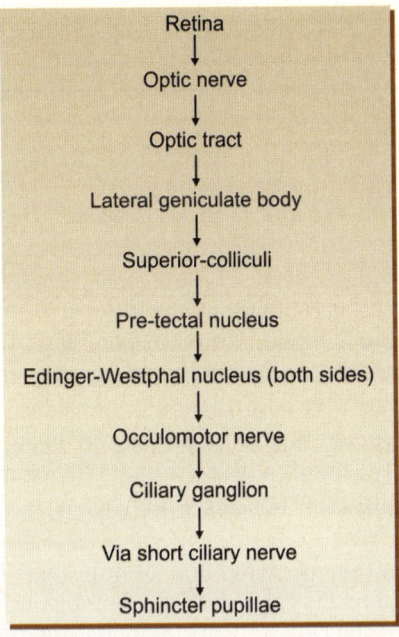

**Fig. 11.2:** Pathway for light reflex

## COLOUR BLINDNESS                                    3 (1992)

It is a clinical condition where a person is unable to distinguish some colours from each other. This happens due to the absence of a single type of cone. Normally, one can distinguish colour due to red and green cones. If any of them is missing, one will be colour blind and cannot distinguish red from green and said to be having red-green colour blindness.

Person with absence of red cones are called **protanope** and person who lacks green cones are called **deuteranope**. Some people have colour weakness for red called **protanomaly** or for green colour called **deuteranomaly**. Commonest type of colour blindness is **deuteranopia**.

Rarely blue colour cones may be absent and the condition is known as **tritanopia**.

Colour blindness is a genetic disorder due to defect in the gene in one of the X-chromosomes, coding for a respective colour cone. The other X-chromosome is almost always normal. Hence the disease is passed from females to males inheriting the defective X-chromosome. So, the sufferer is the male and female is the carrier of the defect. Colour blindness can be clinically detected by:

a. Yarn matching test or Holmgren's skeins of coloured wool test

b. Ishihara charts.

Detection of colour blindness is important for persons working as drivers or in textile and paint industries.

## MYOPIA                                             2.5 (1990)

Myopia is one of the common errors of refraction of the eye.

In a normal persons having emmetropic vision the parallel rays of light from infinity, i.e. more than 6 metres, are brought to a focus on the retina (Fig. 11.3).

In a myopic person rays from infinity are brought to a focus in front of the retina, hence a blurred image is formed. The person cannot see distant objects clearly and hence is said to be short sighted.

Commonest cause is elongation of anterioposterior diametre of the eye. The defect is corrected by using biconcave lens, which diverges the parallel rays appropriately before they enter the eye so that they are now focused on the retina and a clear image is formed (Fig.11.3).

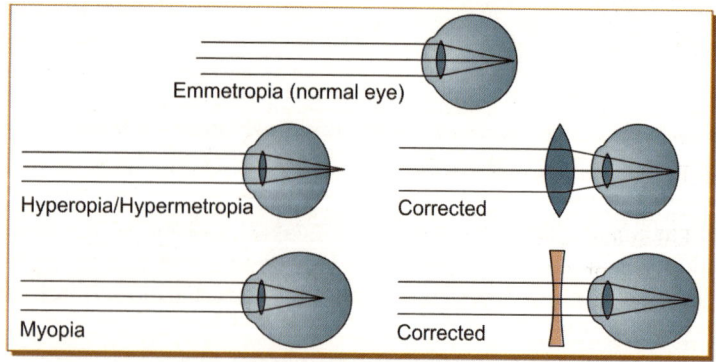

**Fig. 11.3:** Common defects of the optical system of the eye

## HYPERMETROPIA
**2.5 (1988, 1989)**

This is one of the common errors of refraction of the eye. In this clinical condition parallel rays from infinity are brought to focus behind the retina and hence a blurred image is formed. To focus rays on the retina the person uses power of accommodation to see distant objects but cannot focus near objects, as limit of accommodation is already reached. Continuous use of accommodation gives a headache.

The usual cause of defect is shortening of the anteroposterior diametre of the eyeball.

The defect is corrected by giving biconvex lenses to the person suffering from the defect. The lens converges the rays of light before their entry into eye and are hence focussed on the retina and a clear image is formed (Fig. 11.3).

## PRESBYOPIA
**2.5 (1988, 1989, 1990), 2 (2006)**

Presbyopia is a condition occurring at about the age of 45 years, when a person is unable to see near objects clearly. It is due to loss of power of accommodation for near objects.

It is a physiological aging process. The lens capsule becomes rigid and does not change its curvature in spite of ciliary muscle contraction. The major problem is in reading printed material held at the usual reading distance of 25 cm. Person may be able to read when the print is held further away from eye. Such a person is helped by giving convex lens of appropriate diaoptric strength, also called 'reading glasses' as they are required only during near work and while reading.

## DIFFERENCES BETWEEN HYPERMETROPIA AND PRESBYOPIA
**2.5 (1989), 2000, 2 (2004)**

| Hypermetropia | Presbyopia |
|---|---|
| 1. This occurs in young people | 1. This happens after 45 years of age generally |
| 2. Either length of the eyeball is too short (axial hypermetropic eye) or refractive power of the lens decreases (refractive hypermetropic eye) | 2. Anteroposterior diametre of the eyeball is not shortened |

*Contd.*

*Contd.*

| Hypermetropia | Presbyopia |
|---|---|
| 3. There is no change in the lens material, hence it can change its curvature | 3. There is increased sclerosis (hardening) of the lens substance. The loss of elasticity of the lens is due to the denaturation of proteins due to UV rays which are being absorbed by the lens. As a result of this irradiation proteins agglutinate and coagulate in the presence of calcium. Eventually the lens become swollen, hard and opaque |

## VISUAL FIELD/FIELD OF VISION                                      3, 4

It is the area seen by an eye at a given instant when the subject looks with one eye towards a central spot directly in front of the eye. Visual field of one eye is monocular field. Abnormalities in the fields of vision arise out of lesions in visual pathway. For example:

1. **Destruction of one optic nerve:** Blindness of affected eye.
2. **Lesion in central region of optic chiasma: Bitemporal hemianopia.**
3. **Lesion of the right optic tract:** Loss of vision of left half of both the eyes (homonymous hemianopia).
4. **Lesion of the left optic tract:** Loss of right half of both eyes.
5. **Lesion of occipital cortex:** Homonymous hemianopia with sparing of central vision (macular sparing). Representation of macula in visual area is separate and large.

Peripheral field is mapped with a perimetre and central field with a tangent screen.

## CRITICAL FUSION FREQUENCY                                        2, 3

It is the rate at which stimuli can be presented to the eye and still be perceived as discrete stimuli. Stimuli presented at a rate more than critical fusion frequency (CFF) are perceived as continuous stimuli.

CFF is 15–20/sec. In motion pictures various frames are presented at a rate more than CFF and hence motion is created. Movies start flickering when the speed of projector slows down to less than CFF.

## COLOUR VISION/PERCEPTION 5

Humans are capable of perceiving hundreds of different shades of colours and their intensity and saturation. There are three primary colours, viz. red, green and blue. Spectral as well as a large number of extraspectral colours can be created by mixing the primary colours in different proportions. For any colour there is a complementary colour which when mixed with it properly produces a sensation of white. The colour perceived is also affected by the colour of the background and the intensity of light illuminating the object.

Colour vision is the function of retinal cones. As proposed in **Young-Helmholtz** theory, there are 3 types of cones each having a different type of pigment and being maximally sensitive to one of three primary colours:

a. Blue sensitive or short wave pigment—absorbs light maximally in blue-violet part of spectrum (440 nm).

b. Green sensitive or middle wave pigment—absorbs light maximally in green part (535 nm).

c. Red sensitive or long wave pigment—absorbs maximally in red part (560 nm).

There is a considerable overlap in each spectra. Hence most stimuli influence the activity of at least two types of cones. The colour perceived depends on the ratio of excitation of the three types of cones. Hundreds of different patterns of excitation are possible and hence a large number of colours can be distinguished. Some distinction is possible at the level of ganglion cells, which are single opponent cells showing either red-green or blue-yellow sensitivity. Colour sensitive ganglion cells are also sensitive to brightness. This ambiguity is taken care of by double opponent cells in visual cortex.

### Encoding of Cone Pigments

Genes for red and green cone pigment are present on X-chromosome and for blue cone on autosome 7.

A normal person having all the three cone pigments is a trichromat. Dichromats are individuals with a two cone system and suffer from colour blindness of some type. Monochromats have only one cone system.

## DIFFERENCE BETWEEN PERIPHERAL AND CENTRAL RETINAE

| Peripheral | Central |
|---|---|
| 1. Photoreceptors are mainly rods and light passes through bipolar cells and ganglion cells before reaching these receptors | 1. Cones are the main photoreceptors. No rods, bipolar and ganglion cells are present |
| 2. Marked degree of convergence on neurons resulting in large receptive fields for bipolar and ganglion cells | 2. Convergence is less resulting in small receptive fields |
| 3. Sensitivity to light is high | 3. Sensitivity to light is low |
| 4. Visual acuity is low | 4. Visual acuity is high and colour vision is present |

## EAR

### WHAT WILL HAPPEN AND WHY TO HEARING IN OTITIS MEDIA 1 (2007)

Otitis media is a middle ear inflammatory disorder which damages the tympanic membrane or the ear ossicles. It may lead to temporary hearing problems of the conductive type.

### EXPLAIN WHY IRRIGATION OF THE EAR CANAL CAUSES VERTIGO IN SOME PATIENTS 1 (2003)

The semicircular canals can be stimulated by instilling water that is hotter or colder than the body temperature into the external auditory meatus. This temperature difference sets up convection currents in the endolymph with consequent motion of the cupula. This technique called caloric stimulation produces nystagmus, vertigo and nausea by stimulating semicircular canals. To avoid this while irrigating ear canal for treating ear infection, the water used should be at the body temperature.

## EXPLAIN WHY IN WEBER'S TEST AFFECTED EAR HEARS BETTER IN CONDUCTIVE DEAFNESS          1 (2002)

In Weber's test base of the vibrating tuning fork of 256 Hz or 512 Hz is placed on the vertex of the skull in the midline or over the mandible. Sound is better heard in the affected ear because masking effect of environmental noise is absent on the affected side.

## WHAT WILL HAPPEN AND WHY IF THE MEMBRANOUS LABYRINTH IS OVERDISTENDED          1 (2005)

Overdistension of the membranous labyrinth probably due to oversecretion (endolymphatic hydrops) leads to **Meniere's disease**. This disease originates in the labyrinth and is characterized by a triad of the following features:

* Fluctuating deafness of the sensorineural type
* Tinnitus
* Episodic attacks of rotatory vertigo.

Episodes of vertigo occur because the input from the two ears is not balanced, either because only one ear is affected or the process begins in one ear sooner than the other.

## COMPARE COCHLEAR MICROPHONIC POTENTIAL AND ACTION POTENTIAL          (2001)

Cochlear microphonic potential is a potential fluctuation that can be recorded by placing an active electrode on or near the cochlea and an indifferent electrode placed on the body. These are called **cochlear microphonic potentials** because they are amplified through a loudspeaker. It records pure tone up to frequencies of 20,000 Hz.

These potentials are considered similar to the generator potentials because:

* They show no latency or refractory period
* They do not obey all-or-none law
* They are resistant to anaesthesia and ischaemia

**(Please refer to difference between generator potential and action potential in nerve muscle physiology).**

## COMPARE ENDOCOCHLEAR POTENTIAL AND COCHLEAR MICROPHONICS 2 (2010)

## ELECTRIC RESPONSE OF HAIR CELLS IN THE ORGANS OF CORTI 2 (2004)

### Endolymphatic/Endocochlear Potential

### Definition

It is the potential difference recorded between two electrode, one inserted into the scala media containing endolymph and the other into the scala vestibuli containing perilymph.

**The value of this potential difference:** +50 to +100 mV

### Genesis

This potential difference is similar to potential generated due to the ionic difference between the ICF and the ECF separated by the plasma membrane. The endolymph is formed by stria vascularis having electrolyte composition similar to ICF, whereas perilymph is formed by the plasma and has a composition similar to ECF.

### Factors affecting endolymphatic potential

- The movements of the basilar membrane affect the endolymphatic potential by altering the forces acting on the hair cells which are embedded on the tectorial membrane. It can be increased by a downward movement of the basilar membrane and conversely an upward displacement of the basilar membrane reduces it.

- Injection of ringer solution (having the same composition as ECF) into the scala media (composition similar to ICF) abolishes the endolymphatic potential but it has no effect when injected into the scala tympani (which contains perilymph similar to the ECF).

- The injection of potassium rich, sodium poor solution into the scala media does not alter the endolymphatic potential but abolishes it if the injection is made into the scala tympani or vestibuli.

## Cochlear Microphonic Potential

### Definition

Cochlear microphonic potential is a potential fluctuation that can be recorded by placing an active electrode placed on or near the cochlea and an indifferent electrode placed on the body. These are called cochlear microphonic potentials because they are amplified through a loudspeaker, it records pure tone fed into the ears as sound waves up to frequencies of 20,000 Hz.

These potentials are considered similar to the generator potentials because:

- They show no latency or refractory period
- They do not obey all-or-none law
- They are resistant to anaesthesia and ischaemia.

### Genesis

1. The cochlear microphonic potentials are produced by transformation of mechanical energy (distortion affecting the outer hair cells) into electrical energy (generator potential).
2. These potentials are recorded by placing one electrode in the scala media and one in the scala tympani. Thus these potentials are developed as a modification of the endolymphatic potential.

### Factors affecting

Like the endolymphatic potentials, these potentials are also altered by movements of the basilar membrane and show linear relationship to the magnitude of the basilar membrane displacement.

## IMPEDANCE MATCHING                              2.5 (2006)

The middle ear contains air, whereas the inner ear contains fluid, hence sound is conducted from air to fluid during its transmission. As fluid has got inertia the sound is not so easily transmitted through the inner ear, hence this is made possible by increasing the pressure in the middle ear called **impedance matching**.

### Mechanism to increase sound pressure

1. **Lever action of ossicles:** The ossicles are connected to each other and move as a single unit which increases its force of movement by 1.3 times.

2. **Hydraulic action of tympanic membrane:** The effective surface area of the tympanic membrane is 50 mm$^2$ and that of the oval window is 3 mm$^2$, thus the reduction in surface area is 17 times during the transmission of sound at the oval window. This leads to a corresponding increase in pressure at the oval window.

Both the above factors increase the pressure within the middle ear by 22 times which is referred to as **impedance matching**. Thus when the stapes is pressed into the oval window, the pressure is transferred to the perilymph in the scala vestibuli (inner ear).

## ORGAN OF CORTI                    2.5 (1988), 2 (2006)

1. It is sense organ of hearing which is located on the basilar membrane extending from the apex to the base of the cochlea. On the membrane stand two rods called the rods of Corti which project into the scala media. In between the rods is the tunnel of Corti which is filled with perilymph.
2. Internal to the inner rod are the inner hair cells (3500 in number) and external to the outer rod are the outer hair cells (20,000 in number). The inner hair cells are supported by the phalangeal cells, while the outer hair cells are supported by the Deiter's cells.
3. From the upper surface of the hair cells project cilia that are called stereocilia which pass through a thin dense granular reticular lamina and get embedded in the tectorial membrane.

### Innervation

**Afferent innervations:** The hair cells are innervated by nerve fibres of the cochlear divison of the VIIIth nerve. Although the inner hair cells are less in number but they have greater density of innervations.

**Efferent innervations:** Efferent innervation arises from the ipsilateral and contralateral superior olivary nucleus via the olivocochlear bundle. These fibres descend to join the VIIIth nerve and end around the bases of outer hair cells of the organ of Corti. Activity in the efferent fibres inhibits the activity in the afferent fibres. Efferent fibres play an important role in auditory discrimination.

## Functions of Hair Cells

- The inner hair cells are the primary sensory cells that generate action potentials in the auditory nerve that are stimulated by fluid between the tectorial membrane and hair cells. These are responsible for fine auditory discrimination.
- Outer hair cells are responsible for detecting the presence of sound and they improve hearing by influencing the vibration patterns of the basilar membrane.

## ROLE OF INNER EAR IN HEARING          2.5 (2009)

1. **Vibration of the basilar membrane:** The movement of the foot plate of the stapes into the oval window sets up a pressure in the perilymph in the scala vestibuli. The basilar membrane is readily depressed into the scala tympani because of the pressure. Finally, the pressure is transmitted to the round window causing secondary tympanic membrane to bulge outwards into the middle ear. Conversely, an outward movement of the stapes and oval window causes an upward movement of the basilar membrane. Secondary tympanic membrane thus plays an important role in the proper vibration of the basilar membrane.

   As the stapes rocks to and fro in the oval window, it sets up wave motion in the membranous labyrinth. This stimulates movement of fluid within causing basilar membrane to vibrate. The site of the membrane at which the vibrations are maximal will be determined by the frequency of the sound waves.

2. **Stimulation of the hair cells:** When the basilar membrane moves, there is a sharp motion between two stiff structures—the tectorial membrane and the reticular lamina. This bends the processes of the hair cells and results in generation of action potentials in the VIIIth nerve.

3. **Mechanism of pitch discrimination**
   **Place theory or Beksey travelling wave theory**
   The basic pattern of movement of basilar membrane is that of a travelling wave. The apex of the cochlea is affected by only low frequency tones while the base of the cochlea though responding to low frequencies is mainly affected by high frequency.

## Volley Principle

The apex of the cochlea contains units that respond to lower octaves. Thus pure tones up to 2000 Hz produce clear synchronous volleys of action potential in the VIIIth nerve. This is called volley principle of frequency discrimination.

The place theory of coding of sensory information is responsible for discrimination of sound frequencies above 2000 Hz and the volley principle for coding of sound frequencies up to 2000 Hz. Together this is called **duplex theory of pitch discrimination.**

Factors affecting pitch discrimination:

- Frequency of the sound waves
- **Frequency affects loudness:** Low tones sound lower and high tones sound higher as their loudness increases
- The pitch of a sound cannot be perceived unless it lasts for more than 0.01 sec. With duration between 0.01 sec and 0.1 sec, pitch rises as duration increases.

## TESTS TO DIFFERENTIATE BETWEEN CONDUCTION DEAFNESS AND NERVE DEAFNESS      5, 2.5 (1985, 1987, 1989)

Clinically tuning fork tests are performed to differentiate between conduction and nerve deafness, once it is established that the person is deaf.

### Conduction Deafness

The fault is that sound waves are not conducted to internal ear, i.e. cochlea satisfactorily. It may be due to:

a. Accumulation of wax in external earcanal

b. Perforation of ear drum

c. Fixation of foot plate of stapes to oval window due to disease.

### Nerve Deafness

Due to damage in internal ear either to the organ of Corti or the cochlear nerve.

(The two conditions can be differentiated by the tuning fork tests)

| Test | Method | Normal | Conductive deafness | Sensorineural deafness |
|------|--------|--------|---------------------|------------------------|
| **1. Rinne test** | Base of the vibrating tuning fork is placed on the mastoid process until he no longer hears it **(bone conduction)** then it is held in air **(air conduction)** | Air conduction is better than bone conduction (Rinne test positive) | Bone conduction is better than air conduction (Rinne test– negative) | In partial deafness Rinne test is positive. In complete nerve deafness both air and bone conducted sounds are not heard |
| **2. Weber test** | Base of the vibrating tuning fork is placed on the vertex of the skull in the midline or over the mandible | Both the ears hear the sounds equally well | Sound is better heard in the affected ear | Sound is better heard and perceived by the normal ear, i.e. lateralised to the healthy ear |
| **3. Shwabach test** | Bone conduction of the patient is compared with the examiner, assuming the later to be normal | Both the subject and the examiner hear the sound equally well | Subject's bone conduction is better than the examiner | Subject's bone conduction is worse than the examiner |

## ROLE OF MIDDLE EAR IN HEARING    4 (1988), 5 (1992)

Middle ear is an air-filled cavity containing three small bones called the ossicles, namely malleus, incus and stapes. Its function is to transmit the sound waves from external to inner ear.

As the sound waves strike the tympanic membrane, it vibrates. Vibrations of tympanic membrane are transmitted to malleus as it is attached to the tympanic membrane through its handle.

Vibrations are in turn transmitted to the incus and then to the foot plate of stapes, which overlies the oval window of the cochlea. Foot plate of stapes develops rocking movements like a door hinge at the posterior end of oval window. The auditory ossicles of middle ear thus work as a lever system that converts resonant vibrations of tympanic membrane into movements of stapes against the perilymph filled sac of cochlea and sound is thus transmitted to the inner ear. This system increases the sound pressure as it arrives at the oval window (Fig. 11.4).

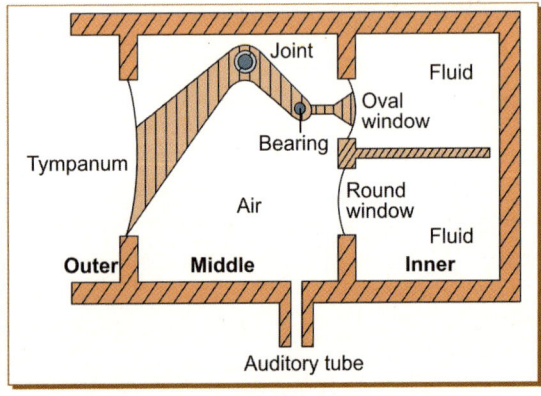

**Fig. 11.4:** Role of middle ear in hearing

## HEARING

- Audible frequency range—20–20,000 Hz
- Most sensitive range—1000–3000 Hz
- Frequency range of most common sounds—200–4500 Hz
- Pitch of male voice—120 Hz
- Pitch of female voice—250 Hz
- Intensity of common sounds
  a. Whisper—40 dB
  b. Conversation—70 dB
  c. Heavy traffic—80 dB
  d. Shouting—90 dB
  e. Rock-band—110 dB
  f. Discomfort—120 dB
  g. Pain—140 dB

## AUDIOMETRY

Audiometry is the determination of hearing threshold for pure tones in the range of 125–8000 Hz. The sounds of varying frequencies are presented to each ear separately through air conduction and bone conduction routes and plotted graphically. The normal threshold is depicted as zero dB in the graph and the hearing loss for each frequency is plotted.

## HEARING-AID (BASIC DESIGN)

These aids amplify the sounds so they are helpful in patients specially with conductive deafness and to some extent in sensorineural deafness.

**These have three basic components**

1. **Microphone**—a transducer to convert sound signals to electrical signals.
2. **Amplifier**—amplifies electrical signals of microphone.
3. **Earphone**—also a transducer to convert amplified electrical signals to sound signals.

Hence the sound delivered to the ear is louder than the original sound.

## FUNCTIONS OF VESTIBULAR APPARATUS 5 (1990), 3 (2003)-IPU

Vestibular apparatus is a sense organ present in the inner ear, containing specialized receptors and functions to maintain body equilibrium, by appreciating:

1. Position of the head in space
2. Movement of head in relation to the body
3. Rotational movement of the head
4. Linear acceleration of the head

Vastibular apparatus consists of two functionally distinct parts:

I. Sac-like structures—saccule and utricle
II. Semicircular canals—three in number and placed at right angle to each other, namely anterior, horizontal and posterior.

Saccule and utricle contains endolymph and have a projecting ridge the macula. Hair cells lie over the macula and their cilia are embedded in gelatinous material which contains dense particles made of chalky material called **otoliths** or **otoconia**.

## Semicircular Canals

Each canal has a dilatation at one end called ampulla, containing a ridge-like structure the crista ampullaris.

Crista ampullaris has hair cells with their cilia embedded in gelatinous cupula forming a partition in the ampulla and closes it. Hair cells are receptor cells having a row of small stercocilia and a large kinocillium at one end of the hair cells.

Base and sides of hair cells have synaptic connection with afferents of vestibular division of the vestibulocochlear nerve.

Hair cells are oriented in different direction so that different groups are activated in various positions of the head.

Activity of hair cell increases when stercocilia bend towards the kinocilium and decreases when they bend in the opposite direction.

I. **Functions of saccule and utricle**

   1. In maculae of saccule and utricle different hair cells are oriented in different direction. At a particular position of the head, pattern of stimulation of different hair cells apprises the nervous system of head position via the afferents from the vestibular nuclei, as a result appropriate muscles reflexly contract and the body equilibrium is maintained.

   2. **Detection of linear acceleration**

      When the body accelerates, the otolith organs which have greater inertia than surrounding fluid fall back and stimulate the hair cells. Information is relayed to higher centres and one feels that one is falling backwards, so one leans forward to correct the equilibrium. When one stops, the opposite happens. Impulses are also relayed to the cortex and are responsible for conscious perception of motion and orientation in space.

II. **Functions of semicircular canals:** These function to detect head rotation. As the head rotates, the canals move along with it, whereas endolymph in them remains stationary due to inertia. This causes motion of endolymph and subsequent movement of cupula in the ampulla. As an example, when head is rotated to right both canals are rotated to the right, but endolymph in them remains on the left side. Hence in the right canal endolymph moves toward the ampulla and in the left out of the ampulla. The two ampullae are stimulated in a different pattern and this information is fed into higher centres and movement of head is appreciated. After a short time if the rotation is continued, endolymph also starts moving with the canals at the same rate and no information is relayed from ampullae on both sides to the brain. When the person suddenly stops moving, the opposite happens. Endolymph moves in the opposite direction and information is again relayed to higher centre and one feels movement in opposite direction for a moment though one has stopped moving.

III. **Control of eye movements during head rotation:** During rotational movements of head, eyes, move in opposite direction, so that gaze is fixed at an object and vision is stabilized, called **vestibulo-ocular reflex**. This reflex occurs because of connections of vestibular nuclei with cranial nerve nuclei through medial longitudinal bundle.

## TESTS FOR VESTIBULAR FUNCTION ASSESSMENT      3 (1993)

Vestibular function can be assessed by stimulating semicircular canals and observing the response.

I. **Caloric test:** The head of the subject is thrown backward at 60 degree and one looks towards the opposite side. The ear, for example, the right ear is syringed with cold air or water at a temperature lower than body temperature. Convention currents are set up which cause movement of endolymph and stimulation of canals. As a result the subject complains of the following:
   1. Giddiness
   2. Nausea
   3. Vomiting
   4. Tends to fall towards right if allowed to stand.
   5. **Nystagmus:** A sharp jerk to opposite side, i.e. left and slow jerk to the right side.
   6. Past pointing of upper arm of the same side. Above signs and symptom occur if the vestibular apparatus is normal.

II. **Barany's test:** Person is made to sit in special Barany's chair which is rotated at a controlled speed. If semicircular canals are normal, nystagmus is seen.

## TASTE AND SMELL

### OLFACTORY PATHWAY                    2 (2003)-IPU

The axons from the olfactory receptor cells are fine unmyelinated fibres which pierce the cribriform plate of ethmoid bone and enter the olfactory bulb.

Within the olfactory bulb axons of the olfactory nerve enter the glomeruli and synapse with dendrites from the mitral and tufted cells which form second order neurons in the olfactory pathway. The glomeruli also contain periglomerular short axon cells which are inhibitory neurons connecting one glomerulus to another and mediating lateral inhibition.

The axons of the mitral cells (Fig. 11.5) form lateral olfactory stria and run to the olfactory cortex on the same side which lies between the anterior perforated substance and the uncus. The olfactory cortex contains parts of the limbic system, viz. anterior olfactory nucleus, piriform cortex, olfactory tubercle, amygdala and entorhinal cortex.

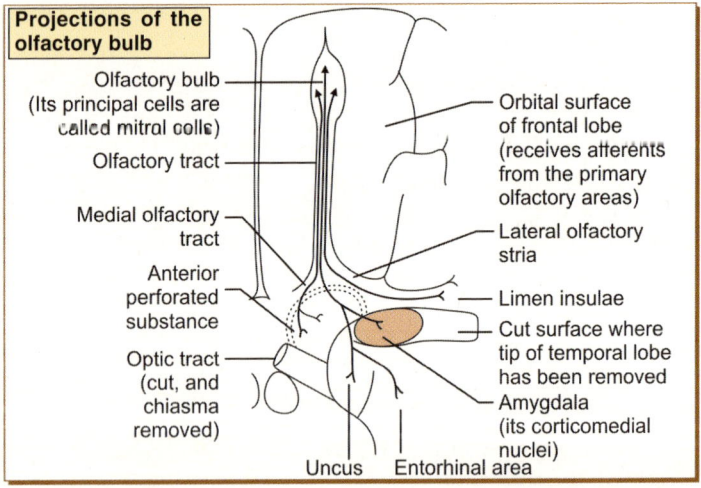

Central olfactory pathways projected onto the ventral surface of the left cerebral hemisphere. The tip of the temporal lobe has been cut off. (The ridge named "medial olfactory stria" does not contain fibres from the olfactory bulb.)

**Fig. 11.5:** Olfactory pathway

Other fibres run via the intermediate olfactory stria to connect with olfactory tubercle and hence with the limbic system.

The axons of the tufted cells run in the medial olfactory stria and cross the midline in the anterior commissure to form synapses with the granule cells in the opposite olfactory cortex.

There is point to point representation of the olfactory mucous membrane in the olfactory bulb. The upper part of the olfactory epithelium is represented in the anterior part of the bulb while lower part is represented posteriorly.

There are efferent fibres in the olfactory striae and stimulation of these fibres depresses the electrical activity in the olfactory bulb. These effects are mediated by the granule cells by releasing GABA that makes reciprocal synaptic connections with dendrites of the mitral cells.